Sleep Medicine

Sleep Medicine

Edited by
HAROLD R. SMITH
CYNTHIA L. COMELLA and
BIRGIT HÖGL

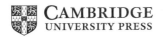
CAMBRIDGE
UNIVERSITY PRESS

CAMBRIDGE UNIVERSITY PRESS

Cambridge, New York, Melbourne, Madrid, Cape Town, Singapore, São Paulo, Delhi

Cambridge University Press
The Edinburgh Building, Cambridge CB2 8RU, UK

Published in the United States of America by Cambridge University Press, New York

www.cambridge.org
Information on this title: www.cambridge.org/9780521699570

First published 2008

Printed in the United Kingdom at the University Press, Cambridge

A catalog record for this publication is available from the British Library

Library of Congress Cataloging in Publication data

Sleep medicine / edited by Harold R. Smith, Cynthia L. Comella, and Birgit Högl.
    p. cm.
    Includes bibliographical references and index.
    ISBN 978-0-521-69957-0 (pbk.)
1. Sleep disorders. 2. Sleep–Physiological aspects. I. Smith, Harold R. II. Comella, Cynthia L.
III. Högl, Birgit.
    [DNLM: 1. Sleep Disorders. 2. Sleep–physiology. WM 188 S63239 2008]

    RC547.S5472   2008
    616.8'498–dc22

                            2007048759

ISBN 978-0-521-69957-0 paperback

This work is dedicated to the many who suffer from the maladies of sleep, and to those who research and care for those with sleep disorders.

For some must watch, while some must sleep

William Shakespeare, *Hamlet*, Act iii, Scene ii

Contents

Contributors

Irene Aricò
Sleep Medicine Center, Department of Neurosciences, Psychiatric and Anesthesiological Sciences, University of Messina, Messina, Italy

Alon Avidan
Neurology Clinic and Sleep Disorders Center, University of California Los Angeles Department of Neurology, Los Angeles, California, USA

Charles Bae
Sleep Disorders Center, Cleveland Clinic Neurological Institute, Cleveland, Ohio, USA

Paul Christian Baier
Department of Clinical Neurophysiology, Georg-August University Göttingen, Göttingen, Germany

Michel Billiard
Department of Neurology, University of Montpellier, Montpellier, France

Michel A. Cramer Bornemann
Minnesota Regional Sleep Disorders Center, University of Minnesota Medical School, Minneapolis, Minnesota, USA

M. Isabel Crisostomo
Sleep Disorders Service and Research Center, Department of Behavioral Sciences, Rush University Medical Center, Chicago, Illinois, USA

Antonio Culebras
Upstate Medical University, State University of New York, New York, USA

Ilonka Eisensehr
Department of Neurology, Ludwig Maximilian University, Munich, Germany

Christopher D. Fahey
Department of Neurology, Northwestern University Feinberg School of Medicine, Chicago, Illinois, USA

Stephany Fulda
Max Planck Institute of Psychiatry, Munich, Germany

Christian Guilleminault
Stanford University Sleep Medicine Program, Stanford, California, USA

Marcel Hungs
Center for Sleep Medicine, University of California Irvine Department of Neurology, Orange, California, USA

Andrea Iaboni
Sleep Disorders Clinic of the Centre for Sleep & Chronobiology, University of Toronto, Toronto, Canada

Roberta M. Leu
Department of Pediatrics, Case University School of Medicine, Rainbow Babies & Children's Hospital, Cleveland, Ohio, USA

Mark W. Mahowald
Minnesota Regional Sleep Disorders Center, University of Minnesota Medical School, Minneapolis, Minnesota, USA

Geert Mayer
Sleep Disorder Unit, Hephata Klinik, Schwalmstadt-Treysa, Germany

Harvey Moldofsky
Sleep Disorders Clinic of the Centre for Sleep & Chronobiology, University of Toronto, Toronto, Canada

Kannan Ramar
Stanford University Sleep Medicine Program, Stanford, California, USA

Carol L. Rosen
Department of Pediatrics, Case University School of Medicine, Rainbow Babies & Children's Hospital, Cleveland, Ohio, USA

Carlos H. Schenck
Minnesota Regional Sleep Disorders Center, University of Minnesota Medical School, Minneapolis, Minnesota, USA

Rosalia Silvestri
Sleep Medicine Center, Department of Neurosciences, Psychiatric and Anesthesiological Sciences, University of Messina, Messina, Italy

Harold R. Smith
Center for Sleep Medicine, University of California Irvine School of Medicine, Irvine, California, USA

Claudia Trenkwalder
Paracelsus-Elena-Klinik, Kassel, Germany

Thomas C. Wetter
Max Planck Institute of Psychiatry, Munich, Germany

James K. Wyatt
Sleep Disorders Service and Research Center, Department of Behavioral Sciences, Rush University Medical Center, Chicago, Illinois, USA

Phyllis C. Zee
Department of Neurology, Northwestern University Feinberg School of Medicine, Chicago, Illinois, USA

Elisabeth Zils
Max Planck Institute of Psychiatry, Munich, Germany

Foreword

Sleep in medicine has been important since the days of Hippocrates, when he wrote in Aphorism LXXI: SOMNUS, VIGILIA, UTRAQUE MODUM EXCEDENTIA, MORBUS – *Disease exists, if either sleep or watchfulness be excessive.* Sleep and its disorders were treated by poets, visionaries, medicine men, healers, psychiatrists – and by a few family physicians who since time immemorial had observed the influence of sleep in physical, mental, and emotional health. And yet, sleep was not established as a scientifically based medical discipline until the middle of the twentieth century, barely fifty years ago. It was the probing of the brain with recently developed EEG techniques that opened the window to the magnificent world of sleep. Searching for the source of dreams, like searching for the fountain of youth in centuries past, led to the discovery of a myriad of disorders that had been unimaginable only a few decades before. Today these conditions are placed in the forefront of medicine. Sleep apnea, restless legs syndrome, the insomnias, the hypersomnias, REM sleep behavior disorder, and so many others have become everyday diagnoses in clinical practice. The disorders of sleep have grown exponentially in complexity. The new *International Classification of Sleep Disorders* (ICSD-2) incorporates more than 80 recognized sleep diagnoses. To understand and be familiar with so many alterations of human physiology one has to delve into psychology, psychiatry, neurology, pulmonary medicine, cardiology, pediatrics, dentistry, and otorhinolaryngology. Nonetheless, sleep remains a function of the brain, a concept that should not be forgotten when attempting to research the pathophysiology of most sleep maladies.

Complex sleep alterations should be evaluated in the sleep center, because a precise diagnosis will lead to accurate management. And what a difference it makes! How many times have we heard, the morning after titration of a CPAP machine, "Doctor, I have not felt this good in years!"? Or, after the first interview, have alleviated the anxiety of a teenager with delayed sleep phase disorder who was about to be expelled from school? Or have soothed the fears of parents terrified by chilling screams in the middle of the night, proffered by their son with night terrors? And yet the disorders of sleep are not a subject just for the specialist. General practitioners should be well acquainted with the problems of sleep in the same way that they are knowledgeable about classical disorders of daily practice like anemias, heart dysrhythmias, and fainting spells.

It is with this vision of the whole that Dr. Harold Smith, accompanied by Dr. Cynthia Comella and Dr. Birgit Högl, has embarked upon the creation of a book on disorders of sleep, directed to all who care about human disease. Knowing Dr. Smith's and his coeditors' tenacity, efficiency, and attention to detail, it goes without saying that I expect to see the birth of a milestone book in the landscape of treatises devoted to the subject of sleep.

Antonio Culebras

Section 1 – Normal sleep

Introduction: the basic neurology of sleep

Harold R. Smith

Overview

Sleep is not an inactive state.

Dating back to early modern classifications of sleep based on electrophysiological measurements, the inherent activities of various neural substrates in sleep have been readily recognized.

Normal sleep has been classified as having two characteristic divisions: non-rapid eye movement (NREM) and rapid eye movement (REM) sleep. These sleep states are defined by neurophysiological parameters of electroencephalogram (EEG), electrooculogram (EOG), and surface electromyogram (EMG), as detailed by Dr. Billiard in the following chapter. These characteristics clearly distinguish the NREM and REM sleep states from the wakefulness state.

Behaviorally, sleep is a reversible state characterized by perceptual disengagement and apparent unresponsiveness to the environment with closed eyes, reduced movements, and recumbency. Early behaviorally based studies revealed that even in those with unequivocal electrophysiologic correlates of being asleep, arousal to one's own name and responsiveness to other auditory stimuli persist.

Additionally, the understanding that continues to evolve of the neurophysiology and neurochemistry of normal sleep suggests that many of the neurologic substrates involved are by no means passive, but rather very active in sleep. An example is the increase in cerebral blood flow that occurs in normal sleep. Both animal and human studies have shown that cerebral blood flow in NREM sleep may increase up to 25% greater than in wakefulness, and up to 80% greater in REM sleep. These changes in cerebral blood flow, at least in part, correlate with concomitant increased brain oxygen metabolism in sleep.

Wakefulness

In the late nineteenth century and early twentieth century, it was posited that a sleep/wake center existed in the midbrain and caudal diencephalon, based on clinical correlates of nervous system lesions. The ascending reticular activating system was defined as a center point in maintenance of wakefulness in a series of sophisticated

Sleep Medicine, ed. Harold R. Smith, Cynthia L. Comella, and Birgit Högl. Published by Cambridge University Press. © Cambridge University Press 2008.

animal studies. Electrical stimulation of the reticular formation in the brainstem of anesthetized cats resulted in cortical activation and EEG low-voltage fast activity. Lesions of the brainstem reticular formations, especially in midbrain tegmentum and oral pontine nuclei, resulted in EEG changes similar to sleep. Further studies revealed that the reticular formation receives collateral input from visceral, somatic, and special sensory systems, and projects ascending pathways to the forebrain by way of a dorsal path to the thalamus and a ventral projection through the hypothalamus, subthalamus, and ventral thalamus to the basal forebrain. An important role of the hypothalamus was suggested in *cerveau isolé* studies, and further clarified in subsequent animal studies with localization to the posterior hypothalamus.

Catecholamines are central to wakefulness. Levodopa may stimulate cortical activation and prolonged arousal but has also been reported to induce sleep in specific instances, and a biphasic effect of dopamine agonists on sleep and wakefulness has been described in animals. Amphetamines, which release dopamine and norepinephrine, also produce arousal and prolonged vigilance. Dopaminergic neurons are present in the substantia nigra, the midbrain ventral tegmentum, the posterior hypothalamus, and the subthalamus. Norepinephrine-containing neurons are most concentrated in the dorsolateral pontine tegmentum locus ceruleus and in the pontine and medullary reticular formation, projecting to the entire forebrain and all areas of the cortex.

Cholinergic contributions to cortical activation and wakefulness have been described. Both muscarinic and nicotinic cholinergic agonists can activate wakefulness. Cholinergic neurons in the caudal mesencephalic and oral pontine reticular formation project to the basal forebrain, thalamus, lateral hypothalamus, and frontal cortex, with cholinergic neurons also concentrated in the basal forebrain. Cortical activation and wakefulness have been associated with acetylcholine release in the cortex.

Histamine may have an effect on arousal, as may glutamate. Substance P and other peptides may be contributors to wakefulness. The understanding of the importance of the hypocretinergic hypothalamic system in wakefulness and in sleep/wake state control mechanisms continues to evolve.

NREM sleep

With the knowledge of the activating systems involved in wakefulness, there was a supposition early last century that sleep may be a result of inactivity of the wake-promoting pathways, that is, sleep as a passive state. Animal studies involving brainstem transsection at the oral pontine tegmentum, however, resulted in complete insomnia, connoting that sleep is an active state generated by structures in the lower brainstem. The concept of active sleep-generating structures was further supported in cat studies in which insomnia resulted from lesions of the raphe system from the medulla to the pontomesencephalic border, and from electrical stimulation of the solitary tract nucleus and dorsal reticular formation producing EEG cortical synchronization suggestive of NREM sleep. Indirect evidence of similar structures in humans is seen in reports of reduction or abatement of NREM sleep in raphe nucleus infarction and in other brainstem lesions.

Thalamic nucleus reticularis, to which projections arise from the midbrain reticular system, has been elegantly demonstrated to be the generator of NREM sleep spindle activity in the thalamic nuclei and in cortical projections.

Hypothalamic sleep synchrony centers, as well as wake centers, were implied in the *cerveau isolé* studies of Bremer in the 1930s. Anterior hypothalamic localization in humans as a sleep facilitatory center, in contradistinction to posterior hypothalamic wake centers, was proposed by Von Economo. Electrical stimulation studies in the cat of the preoptic area and basal forebrain resulted in synchronized NREM sleep. Thus the anterior hypothalamus, preoptic area, and basal forebrain, in conjunction with brainstem reticular formation, appear to be central to generation of NREM sleep. Additionally, recent work has shown that the amygdala may also, in part, be related to NREM sleep.

Serotonin appears to have a role in the induction of NREM sleep, as demonstrated in reserpine studies nearly 50 years ago. Blocking of serotonin either pharmacologically or by lesions of raphe serotonin nuclei leads to severe insomnia in animal studies, which is reversible by reinstituting serotonin. Similar restoration of NREM sleep in humans by administration of the serotonin precursor 5-hydroxytryptamine in a severe case of insomnia has been reported. Single unit recordings have shown that raphe neurons reduce firing with NREM sleep and cease firing in REM sleep. This has led to the conclusion that serotonergic neurons facilitate NREM sleep onset, but are not singularly essential for the occurrence of NREM sleep.

Adenosine may contribute to NREM sleep in that caffeine, which blocks adenosine receptors, can block NREM sleep. Adenosine release in the basal forebrain in NREM sleep has been demonstrated. A model of adenosine contributing to sleep/wake homeostatic regulation has been proposed. There is an evolving understanding of the importance of the interactions of adenosine, basal forebrain cholinergic cell groups, and numerous central nervous system sites in sleep homeostasis. Gamma-aminobutyric acid (GABA) may also play a role in NREM sleep synchrony.

REM sleep

Rapid eye movement (REM) sleep is characterized by desynchronized low-voltage EEG patterns, in contradistinction to the synchronized EEG of NREM sleep. In addition, REM sleep also is characterized by skeletal muscle atonia.

Episodic bursts of rapid eye movements, which are at times concurrent with transitory muscle activity and cardiorespiratory changes, are an additional hallmark of REM sleep. Interestingly, though the REM sleep cortical EEG is desynchronized, depth electrode studies in the cat reveal highly synchronized theta rhythm in the hippocampus, and also subcortically the presence of ponto-geniculo-occipital (PGO) phasic spikes.

In investigating where REM sleep is generated, transection between the midbrain and pons in the cat resulted in absence of REM sleep characteristics rostrally but maintenance of REM sleep caudally, indicating that the neural structures important to REM sleep generation must be located caudal to this transection.

In humans, high cervical lesions interrupting continuity between the medulla and spinal cord have been shown to disrupt spinal innervated REM atonia, but to preserve other characteristics of REM sleep, thus further localizing the neural structures generating REM sleep to rostral to the spinal cord, but caudal to the midbrain.

When transection studies were completed in cats between the medulla and pons, caudal medullary cycles of activated and quiescent states, respectively similar to wakefulness and NREM sleep, were seen. Rostral to the transection three states were seen, similar to wakefulness, NREM sleep, and REM sleep. Thus the pons is central in generating the characteristics of REM sleep. Additional investigations localized REM sleep-generating phenomena to the lateral region of the reticularis pontis oralis lateral to the locus ceruleus. Further, atonia can be elicited in the medial medulla at the nucleus reticularis magnocellularis. Recordings of cellular unit firing in the lateral pontine reticular formation and medial medulla have revealed very high discharges in REM sleep and minimal to no firing in NREM sleep or wakefulness. These cells have been described as REM "sleep-on" cells and are present in the lateral pons, with projections to the medial medulla. The amygdala may also be modulatory or contributory to REM sleep.

Acetylcholine appears to be important in REM sleep components. Acetylcholine depletion reduces EEG desynchronization and REM sleep. Acetylcholinesterase inhibitors increased some REM sleep characteristics. The lateral pontine REM "sleep-on" cells are cholinoceptive. Injection of cholinomimetics into the pontine tegmentum in cats resulted in atonia, rapid eye movements, and PGO spikes. Though acetylcholine may not be the exclusive neurochemical component of REM sleep, it does appear to contribute to EEG desynchrony, muscle atonia, and PGO spikes.

Serotonergic cells of the midline raphe system and noradrenergic cells of the locus ceruleus may have a role in gating, inhibiting, or disinhibiting some aspects of REM sleep. This raises the possibility of a reciprocal interaction of REM "sleep-off" cells in these systems, though the relation is not absolute. A recent study using microinjection into pedunculopontine tegmentum of norepinephrine, serotonin, and adenosine in the rat did not suppress REM sleep, which will further prompt revisiting of the reciprocal interaction model.

Conclusion

Though there clearly appears to be a biological requirement for sleep, the physiological role of sleep remains unclear. Ongoing investigations and sleep research continue to move forward, and we await exciting developments that will help solve the many questions yet to be answered.

ACKNOWLEDGMENT

Excerpts of this Introduction were previously published in *The Interface of Sleep and Neurological Disorders*, © American Academy of Neurology 2007. Used with permission.

FURTHER READING

Adey WR, Bors E, Porter RW. EEG sleep patterns after high cervical lesions in man. *Arch Neurol* 1968; **19**: 377–83.

Basheer R, Strecker RF, Thakkar MM, McCarley RW. Adenosine and sleep–wake regulation. *Prog Neurobiol* 2004; **73**: 379–96.

Batini C, Moruzzi G, Palestini M, Rossi GF, Zanchetti A. Effects of complete pontine transections of the sleep–wakefulness rhythm: the midpontine pretrigeminal preparation. *Arch Ital Biol* 1959; **97**: 1–12.

Belsky G, Henriksen S, McGarr K. Effects of anticholinesterase (DFP) on the sleep–wakefulness cycle of the cat. *Psychophysiology* 1968; **5**: 243.

Blanco-Centurion C, Xu M, Murillo-Rodriguez E, *et al.* Adenosine and sleep homeostasis in the basal forebrain. *J Neurosci* 2006; **26**: 8092–100.

Bremer F. Cerveau "isolé" et physiologie du sommeil. *C R Soc Biol (Paris)* 1935; **118**: 1235–41.

Carlsson A, Lindqvist M, Magnusson T. 3,4-Dihydroxyphenylalanine and 5-hydroxytryptophan as reserpine antagonists. *Nature* 1957; **180**: 1200.

Carskadon MA, Dement WC. Normal human sleep: an overview. In: Kryger MH, Roth T, Dement WC, eds. *Principles and Practice of Sleep Medicine*, 2nd edn. Philadelphia, PA: Saunders, 1994: 16–25.

Celesia GG, Jasper HH. Acetylcholine released from the cerebral cortex in relation to state of activation. *Neurology* 1966; **16**: 1053–63.

Datta S, Mavanji V, Patterson EH, Ulloor J. Regulation of rapid eye movement sleep in the freely moving rat: local microinjection of serotonin, norepinephrine, and adenosine into the brainstem. *Sleep* 2003; **26**: 513–20.

Dement W, Kleitman N. Cyclic variations in EEG during sleep and their relation to eye movements, body motility, and dreaming. *Electroencephalogr Clin Neurophysiol* 1957; **9**: 673–90.

Dinner DS. Physiology of sleep. In: Levin KH, Lüders HO, eds. *Comprehensive Clinical Neurophysiology*. Philadelphia, PA: Saunders, 2000: 589–96.

Domino EF, Yamamoto K, Dren AT. Role of cholinergic mechanisms in states of wakefulness and sleep. *Prog Brain Res* 1968; **28**: 113–33.

Drucker-Colin R, Pedraza JGB. Kainic acid lesions of gigantocellular tegmental field (FTG) neurons do not abolish REM sleep. *Brain Res* 1983; **272**: 387–91.

Fischer-Perroudon C, Mouret J, Jouvet M. Sur un cas d'agrypnie (4 mois sans sommeil) au cours d'une maladie de Morvan: effet favorable du 5-hydroxytryptophane. *Electroencephalogr Clin Neurophysiol* 1974; **36**: 1–18.

Freemon FR, Salinas-Garcia RF, Ward JW. Sleep patterns in a patient with a brain stem infarction involving the raphe nucleus. *Electroencephalogr Clin Neurophysiol* 1974; **36**: 657–60.

Friedman L, Jones BE. Computer graphics analysis of sleep–wakefulness state changes after pontine lesions. *Brain Res Bull* 1984; **13**: 53–68.

Heller, HC. A global rather than local role for adenosine in sleep homeostasis. *Sleep* 2006; **29**: 1382–3.

Hobson JA, Alexander J, Frederickson CJ. The effect of lateral geniculate lesions on phasic electrical activity of the cortex during desynchronized sleep in the cat. *Brain Res* 1969; **14**: 607–21.

Jones BE. The respective involvement of noradrenaline and its delaminated metabolites in waking and paradoxical sleep: a neuropharmacological model. *Brain Res* 1972; **39**: 121–36.

Jones, BE. Basic mechanisms of sleep–wake states. In: Kryger MH, Roth T, Dement WC, eds. *Principles and Practice of Sleep Medicine*, 2nd edn. Philadelphia, PA: Saunders, 1994: 145–62.

Jones BE, Beaudet A. Distribution of acetylcholine and catecholamine neurons in the cat brainstem: a choline acetyltransferase and tylosine hydroxylase immunohistochemical study. *J Comp Neurol* 1987; **261**: 15–32.

Jones BE, Cuello AC. Afferents to the basal forebrain cholinergic cell area from pontomesencephalic catecholamine, serotonin, and acetylcholine neurons. *Neuroscience* 1989; **31**: 37–61.

Jones BE, Yang TZ. The efferent projections from the reticular formation and the locus coeruleus studied by anterograde and retrograde axonal transport in the rat. *J Comp Neurol* 1985; **242**: 56–92.

Jouvet M. The role of monoamines and acetylcholine-containing neurons in the regulation of the sleep–waking cycle. *Ergeb Physiol* 1972; **64**: 166–307.

Jouvet M, Renault J. Insomnie persistante après lesions des moyaux du raphe chez le chat. *C R Soc Biol (Paris)* 1966; **160**: 1461–5.

Lindsley D, Bourden J, Bagoun H. Effects upon the EEG of acute injury to the brain stem activating system. *Electroencephalogr Clin Neurophysiol* 1949; **1**: 475–86.

Madsen PL, Schmidt JF, Wildschiodtz G, *et al.* Cerebral O_2 metabolism and cerebral blood flow in humans during sleep and rapid-eye movement sleep. *J Appl Physiol* 1991; **70**: 2597–601.

Magnes J, Moruzzi G, Pompeiano O. Synchronization of the EEG produced by low frequency electrical stimulation of the region of the solitary tract. *Arch Ital Biol* 1961; **99**: 33–67.

Mangold R, Sokoloff K, Conner E, *et al.* The effects of sleep and lack of sleep on the cerebral circulation and metabolism of normal young men. *J Clinical Invest* 1955; **34**: 1092–100.

Markand ON, Dyken ML. Sleep abnormalities in patients with brain stem lesions. *Neurology* 1976; **26**: 769–76.

Mauthner L. Zur pathologie und physiologie des schlafes nebst bermerkungen ueber die "Nona." *Wein Klin Wochenschr* 1890; **40**: 961.

McGinty D. Somnolence, recovery and hyposomnia following ventro-medial diencephalic lesions in the rat. *Electroencephalogr Clin Neurophysiol* 1969; **26**: 70–9.

McGinty D, Harper RM. Dorsal raphe neurons: depression of firing during sleep in cats. *Brain Res* 1976; **101**: 569–75.

Mendelson WB. GABA-benzodiazepine receptor-chloride ionophore complex: implications for the pharmacology of sleep. In: Wauquier A, Monti JM, Gaillard JM, Radulovacki M, eds. *Sleep: Neurotransmitters and Neuromodulators*. New York, NY: Raven Press, 1985: 229 ff.

Mignot E. A year in review: basic science, narcolepsy, and sleep in neurologic diseases. *Sleep* 2004; **27**: 1209–12.

Monnier M, Sauer R, Hatt AM. The activating effect of histamine on the central nervous system. *Int Rev Neurobiol* 1970; **12**: 265–305.

Moruzzi G. The sleep–waking cycle. *Ergeb Physiol* 1972; **64**: 1–165.

Moruzzi G, Mogoun H. Brainstem reticular formation and activation in the EEG. *Electroencephalogr Clin Neurophysiol* 1949; **1**: 455–73.

Nauta W. Hypothalamic regulation of sleep in rats: experimental study. *J Neurophysiol* 1946; **9**: 285–316.

Noor Alam MD, Szymusiak R, McGinty D. Adenosinergic regulation of sleep: multiple sites of action in the brain. *Sleep* 2006; **29**: 1384–5.

Oswald I, Taylor AM, Treisman M. Discriminative responses to stimulation during human sleep. *Brain* 1960; **83**: 440–53.

Porkka-Heiskanen T, Strecker RE, Thakkar M, *et al.* Adenosine: a mediator of the sleep-inducing effects of prolonged wakefulness. *Science* 1997; **276**: 1265–8.

Radulovacki M, Virus RM. Purine, 1-methylisoguanosine and pyrimidine compounds and sleep in rats. In: Wauquier A, Monti JM, Gaillard JM, Radulovacki M, eds. *Sleep: Neurotransmitters and Neuromodulators*. New York, NY: Raven Press, 1985: 221 ff.

Rechtschaffen A, Kales A. *A Manual of Standardized Terminology, Techniques and Scoring System for Sleep Stages of Human Subjects*. Los Angeles, CA: UCLA Brain Information Service/Brain Research Institute, 1968.

Reivich M, Issacs G, Evarts E, Kety S. The effect of slow wave sleep and REM sleep on regional cerebral blood flow in cats. *J Neurochem* 1968; **15**: 301–6.

Riou F, Cespuglio R, Jouvet M. Endogenous peptides and sleep in the rat. I: Peptides decreasing paradoxical sleep. *Neuropeptides* 1982; **2**: 243–54.

Sakai K. Some anatomical and physiological properties of pontomesencephalic tegmental neurons with special reference to the PGO waves and postural atonia during paradoxical sleep in the cat. In: Hobson JA, Brazier MA, eds. *The Reticular Formation Revisited*. New York, NY: Raven Press, 1980: 427–47.

Santiago TV, Guerra E, Neubauer JA, Edelman NH. Correlation between ventilation and brain blood flow during sleep. *J Clin Invest* 1984; **73**: 497–506.

Sastre J, Sakai K, Jouvet M. Persistence of paradoxical sleep after destruction of the pontine gigantocellular tegmental field with kainic acid in the cat. *C R Acad Sci (Paris)* 1979; **289**: 959–64.

Siegel JM. Brainstem mechanisms generating REM sleep. In: Kryger MH, Roth T, Dement WC, eds. *Principles and Practice of Sleep Medicine*, 2nd edn. Philadelphia, PA: Saunders, 1994: 125–44.

Siegel JM, Tomaszewski KS, Nienhuis R. Behavioral organization of reticular formation: studies in the unrestrained cat, II. Cells related to facial movements. *J Neurophysiol* 1983; **50**: 717–23.

Siegel JM, Nienhuis R, Tomaszewski KS. REM sleep signs rostral to chronic transections at the pontomedullary junction. *Neurosci Lett* 1984; **45**: 241–6.

Simon-Arceo K, Ramirez-Salado I, Calvo JM. Long-lasting enhancement of rapid eye movement sleep and pontogeniculooccipital waves by vasoactive intestinal peptide microinjection into the amygdala temporal lobe. *Sleep* 2003; **26**: 259–64.

Smith HR. Stimulant-dependent sleep disorder. In: Gilman S, ed. *MedLink Neurology [online]*. www.medlink.com. Accessed December, 2007.

Steriade M. Brain electrical activity and sensory processing during waking and sleep states. In: Kryger MH, Roth T, Dement WC, eds. *Principles and Practice of Sleep Medicine*, 2nd edn. Philadelphia, PA: Saunders, 1994: 105–24.

Steriade M, Hobson JA. Neuronal activity during the sleep–waking cycle. *Prog Neurobiol* 1976; **6**: 155–376.

Sterman MB, Clemente CD. Forebrain inhibitory mechanisms: cortical synchronization induced by basal forebrain stimulation. *Exp Neurol* 1962; **6**: 91–102.

Sterman MB, Clemente CD. Forebrain inhibitory mechanisms: sleep patterns induced by basal forebrain stimulation in the behaving cat. *Exp Neurol* 1962; **6**: 103–17.

Townsend RE, Prinz PN, Obrist WD. Human cerebral blood flow during sleep and waking. *J Appl Physiol* 1973; **35**: 620–5.

Villablanca J. The electrocorticogram in the chronic cerveau isolé cat. *Electroencephalogr Clin Neurophysiol* 1965; **19**: 576–86.

Von Economo C. *Encephalitis Lethargica: Its Sequelae and Treatment*. London: Oxford University Press, 1931.

Williams HL, Hammack JT, Daly RL, Dement WC, Lubin A. Responses to auditory stimulation, sleep loss and the EEG stages of sleep. *Electroencephalogr Clin Neurophysiol* 1964; **16**: 269–79.

Zepelin H, Rechtschaffen A. Mammalian sleep, longevity and energy metabolism. *Brain Behav Evol* 1974; **10**: 425–70.

OTHER SOURCES OF INFORMATION RELATED TO SLEEP

National Institutes of Health. *MedlinePlus: Sleep Disorders.* www.nlm.nih.gov/medlineplus/sleepdisorders.html.

American Academy of Sleep Medicine. www.aasmnet.org.

1 Normal sleep

Michel Billiard

Introduction

The state of wakefulness regularly alternates with the states of sleep. Our initial knowledge of the states of sleep was based on observations of individual subjects while asleep. The beginning of the scientific era of research in normal humans dates back to the sleep deprivation studies conducted by Kleitman in the 1920s. In the following decade, the first classification of sleep stages was published by Loomis *et al.* in 1937, and Kleitman's comprehensive landmark monograph *Sleep and Wakefulness* was published in 1939. Loomis's classification was based on electroencephalographic (EEG) criteria alone and distinguished five different sleep states, from wakefulness (A) to deep sleep (E). In 1953, Aserinsky and Kleitman described a special type of sleep with rapid eye movements, and sleep was subsequently classified based on EEG and electrooculographic (EOG) parameters. This classification system distinguished four stages of sleep without rapid eye movements (NREM sleep) and a state of sleep with rapid eye movements (REM sleep). Following the discovery of muscle atonia accompanying REM sleep by Jouvet in 1962, a revised classification of sleep was developed using the three parameters of EEG, EOG, and electromyography (EMG). In 1968 this staging system was published in the *Manual of Standardized Terminology, Techniques, and Scoring System for Sleep Stages of Human Subjects*, under the leadership of Rechtschaffen and Kales, and is still used worldwide.

Polysomnography

Polysomnography (PSG) is the recording of several electrophysiologic signals during sleep. Polysomnography uses the 10–20 international electrode placement system for EEG recording (Fig. 1.1). The minimum monitoring requires one EEG lead with electrode positions at either C3–A2 or C4–A1. It is standard practice to add a frontal electrode, most commonly F2. To record eye movements, electrodes are placed on the skin at the outer canthus of both eyes. The electrodes are placed so that eye movements result in signals going in the opposite direction, and head movements or EEG artifacts are recorded as signals going in the same directions. The electromyogram of the chin muscles is monitored with two electrodes placed under the chin. In order to obtain reliable identification of sleep stages, three EEG, two EOG, and one EMG channels are necessary. An electrocardiographic channel is mandatory, with

Sleep Medicine, ed. Harold R. Smith, Cynthia L. Comella, and Birgit Högl. Published by Cambridge University Press. © Cambridge University Press 2008.

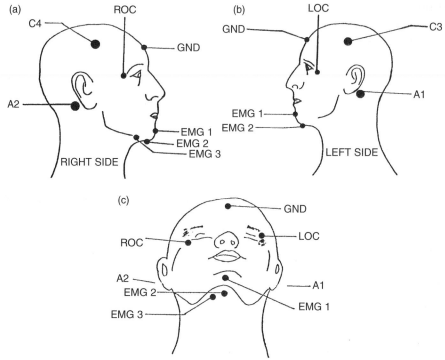

Fig. 1.1. Diagrammatic representation of electrode placements for recording the electrophysiologic phenomena of sleep. GND, ground electrode.

electrodes usually placed on the right shoulder and left leg. In a standard montage, leg muscles and respiration are monitored. The electrode placement for leg EMG is on the skin above right and left anterior tibialis muscles. Respiration is monitored by different methods. The most common montage comprises a nasal cannula/ pressure transducer system, a mouth thermistor, a neck microphone, a thoracic and an abdominal band, and a pulse oximeter. Depending on the reason for the test, other variables may be added. The most common additions are esophageal pressure measurement, pulse transit time, body temperature, and additional EEG leads.

The signals obtained from these sensors are amplified and recorded on special systems. A minimum of 16 channels is recommended. The recording of sleep must be accompanied by a video recording of the sleeping subject, which can be synchronized with the polysomnographic recording. The frequency of sampling is important. The normal frequency is 128 cycles/second (Hz), although frequencies up to 500 Hz are used when doing a spectral analysis. Of note, most of the variables collected during sleep are qualitative or semi-quantitative at best.

Conventional analysis of wakefulness and sleep
Sleep macrostructure
Sleep is generally scored in 20- or 30-second segments or epochs. The scoring is performed using two international scoring systems. The Rechtschaffen and Kales

Manual gives specific instructions on the scoring of sleep states and stages, based on a 20- or 30-second epoch. However, this scoring system was developed to score the sleep of normal subjects and not for disordered sleep. The American Sleep Disorders Association Atlas Task Force has developed a scoring system to complement the international *Manual* and to provide specific rules for evaluating sleep pathology. It examines smaller epochs (3 seconds and longer) and abnormal events. Both atlases are used simultaneously to study sleep disorders.

There are three states of sleep and wakefulness: NREM sleep, REM sleep, and wakefulness (Fig. 1.2). Wakefulness includes calm and active wakefulness. Calm wakefulness is recorded at rest with eyes closed, and is characterized by alpha rhythm (8–12 Hz) on EEG, the presence of muscle tone, and the lack of eye movements. In contrast, active wakefulness is associated with fast low-voltage activity, eye and eyelid movements, and the presence of muscle tone.

Sleep is divided into NREM and REM sleep. NREM sleep is subdivided into four sleep stages. Stage 1 occurs at sleep onset and is defined by low-voltage mixed-frequency (2–7 Hz) waves, slow eye movements with a frequency less than 1 Hz, and preserved muscle tone. Stage 2 is scored when sleep spindles and/or K complexes are present against a background activity of relatively low-voltage mixed EEG frequency. Sleep spindles have a frequency of 12–14 Hz and should be at least 0.5 s duration. K complexes are EEG wave forms having a well-delineated negative sharp wave which is immediately followed by a positive component, of more than 0.5 s duration. During stage 2 sleep, muscle tone is present and eye movements are absent. Stage 3 is scored when a moderate amount (20–50%) of high-amplitude (75 µV or greater) slow-wave (0.5–2 Hz) activity is seen, and stage 4 when the high-amplitude slow-wave activity predominates (greater than 50%). In stages 3 and 4 muscle tone tends to decrease and eye movements are absent.

REM sleep is defined by the concomitant appearance of relatively low-voltage, mixed-frequency EEG activity, episodic rapid eye movements, and low tonic EMG activity. The EEG pattern resembles stage 1, but distinctive "saw-tooth" waves may often appear in vertex and frontal regions, and trains of alpha activity may be seen. Rapid eye movements occur, isolated or in bursts. The tonic mental–submental EMG activity reaches its lowest levels during REM sleep. There are frequent occasions when the EMG tracing may show bursts of phasic activity or twitches for several seconds. REM sleep is not divided into stages. One can distinguish two types of activity, however, referred to as phasic events (bursts of eye movements, saw-tooth waves, and twitches) occurring on a background of tonic muscle inhibition, called tonic REM sleep.

Polysomnography recordings are also scored for movement time. Movement time is assigned to epochs which immediately precede or follow sleep stages, but in which the EEG and EOG tracings are obscured for more than half the epoch by muscle tension and/or amplifier blocking artifacts associated with movement of the subject.

Nocturnal sleep is associated with a pattern of regular reoccurrence of "sleep cycles" (Fig. 1.3). Individuals first enter NREM sleep, with stage 1 NREM sleep lasting a few minutes. This stage may be interrupted by wakefulness. Stage 2 NREM sleep

Awake – low voltage – random, fast

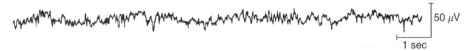

50 μV

1 sec

Drowsy – 8 to 12 cps – alpha waves

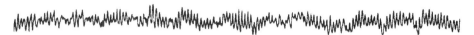

Stage 1 – 3 to 7 cps – theta waves

Theta Waves

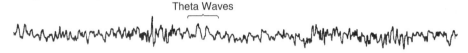

Stage 2 – 12 to 14 cps – sleep spindles and K complexes

Sleep Spindle   K Complex –

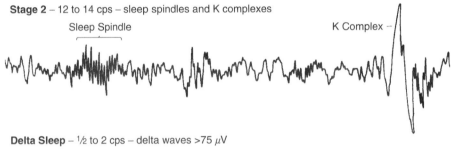

Delta Sleep – ½ to 2 cps – delta waves >75 μV

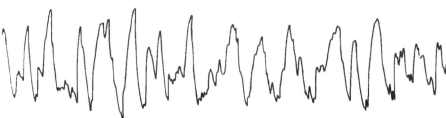

REM Sleep – low voltage – random, fast with sawtooth waves

Sawtooth Waves   Sawtooth Waves

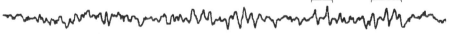

Fig. 1.2. EEG patterns of human sleep states and stages.

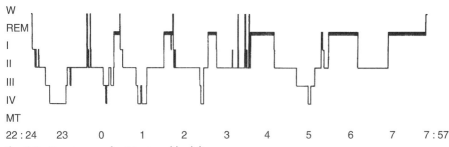

Fig. 1.3. Hypnogram of a 24-year-old adult.

follows and continues for 10–25 minutes. The gradual appearance of high-voltage slow waves signals the onset of stage 3 followed by stage 4 NREM sleep, lasting between 20 and 40 minutes. A fleeting switch to stage 2 may precede the occurrence of REM sleep. The first REM period is of short duration, between 4 and 8 minutes. REM sleep often ends with a brief body movement, and a new sleep cycle begins. NREM and REM sleep continue to alternate throughout the night in a cyclical fashion. The average length of the first sleep cycle is approximately 90 minutes, and the average length of the following cycles 100–120 minutes. Stages 3 and 4 are abundant in the first two cycles, and rare or nonexistent in the following ones. In contrast, REM sleep is of longer duration during the last cycles. In the young adult NREM sleep comprises 75–85% of total sleep and REM sleep 15–25%. Stage 1 occupies 5% of total sleep, stage 2, 50%, and stages 3 and 4, 20–25%.

Sleep microstructure

In addition to the states and stages of sleep as defined above, there is another view of sleep, first developed by Terzano *et al.* in 1985, that integrates the more dynamic features of sleep, referred to as CAP (cyclic alternating pattern). This applies to the transient EEG phenomena, lasting less than the scoring epoch, that occur within the sleep recordings (phasic events). The measurement of these allows identification of the microstructure of sleep.

The concept of CAP is based on the observation of repetitive stereotyped EEG patterns lasting less than 60 seconds, separated by time-equivalent intervals of background activity (Fig. 1.4). CAP translates a sustained oscillatory condition between a greater arousal level referred to as phase A and phase B. Phase A is identified by the presence of EEG arousal-related phasic events, and phase B is a lesser arousal level (intervals between the successive clusters of EEG transients). In NREM sleep, the A phases are formed by the EEG arousal-related phasic events peculiar to the single stages (Table 1.1) and the B phases by the intervals of background theta–delta activity.

The absence of CAP within the sleep EEG coincides with a condition of sustained arousal stability, which is defined as non-CAP. CAP time is the temporal sum of all CAP sequences. CAP time can be calculated throughout total NREM sleep and within the single NREM stage. The percentage ratio of CAP time to sleep time is referred to as the CAP rate. CAP rate can be measured in NREM sleep (ratio of total CAP time to total

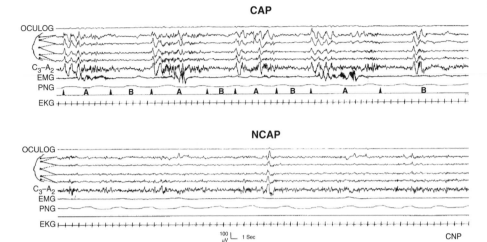

Fig. 1.4. CAP time and non-CAP time in stage 2 NREM sleep. CAP time: alternance of arousal-related phasic events (A) and of the background EEG activities (B) EMG, electromyogram; PNG, pneumogram; EKG, electrocardiogram; CNP, Clinica Neurologica Parma. From Terzano and Parrino, *Sleep* 1992; **15**: 64–70.

Table 1.1. *Phase A phasic events peculiar to the single NREM sleep stages (from Terzano MG, Parrino L. Sleep Med Rev 2000; 4: 101–23).*

Stage 1	Intermittent alpha rhythms (EEG synchronization) and sequences of vertex sharp waves (EEG synchronization)
Stage 2	Sequences of two or more K complexes alone (EEG synchronization) or followed by alpha-like components (EEG desynchronization)
Stages 3 and 4	Delta bursts (EEG synchronization) which exceed by at least a third the amplitude of the background activity
All stages	Transient activation phases (EEG desynchronization) and EEG arousals (EEG desynchronization).

NREM sleep time) and in the single NREM sleep stage (ratio of CAP time in a given stage to the total duration of that stage throughout sleep). In human sleep, the CAP rate is an index of arousal instability that shows a U-shaped evolution during the life span (teenagers, mean 43.4%; young adults, 31.9%; middle-aged, 37.5%; elderly, 55.3%). A CAP atlas has been recently published (Terzano *et al.* 2001) to facilitate scoring sleep with this approach.

Automatic analysis of sleep

The Rechtschaffen and Kales *Manual* has greatly advanced sleep medicine by providing a common language for clinicians and scientists to communicate about sleep. Today it remains the gold standard for interpretation of sleep studies across sleep centers internationally. However, there are some limitations to this scoring method. Scoring by epochs of 20 or 30 seconds is a compromise between accuracy and laboriousness, with the consequence that short state changes are ignored and the microstructure of sleep is not taken into account. The stepwise transitions of sleep stages are probably far from physiological changes, and quantitative determination of EEG components in the low frequency range, 0.5–4.75 Hz (slow-wave activity), an indicator of "sleep intensity", is left out. Moreover, pathological sleep is not adequately analyzed in most cases.

Hence the interest in computer-based sleep recordings and analysis, a comprehensive account of which can be found in Penzel and Conradt (2000). Automatic sleep analysis consists of two main steps: first, signal preprocessing and, second, combining the extracted features and waveforms into a limited number of sleep stages.

Signal preprocessing

The aim of preprocessing is to reduce the enormous amount of raw data to an amount which can be managed by statistical tools. Typically the resolution of 100 Hz for raw data is reduced to a resolution of 1 Hz as the result of preprocessing. The preprocessing yields a number of features: the amplitude or power of regular waves, such as beta, alpha, theta, or delta waves, and the specific patterns such as K complexes, sleep spindles, and vertex sharp waves. In EOG the specific patterns are rapid eye movements and slow eye movements, which have to be distinguished from each other. Signal preprocessing may use two methods, spectral analysis and period analysis.

Spectral analysis is easily performed with the help of fast Fourier transform algorithms (FFT). The technique relies on two basic hypotheses: (1) the normality of signal amplitude distribution; (2) the stationarity of the signal, as the Fourier transform can only be applied to static signals. Therefore the choice of the length of epoch to which FFT is applied will determine the frequency resolution of the spectrum corresponding to the inverse duration of the epoch. Thus for a 2-second epoch, resolution will be 0.5 Hz, and for a 4-second epoch it will be 0.25 Hz. The latter resolution is usually chosen for sleep EEG spectral analysis. The majority of studies with spectral analysis use two bands of frequency, the 0.5–4.75 Hz band or slow-wave activity and the 13–16 Hz band or sigma activity. The derivations used are C3–A2 and C4–A1 with a low-pass 40 Hz filter and a high-pass 0.5 Hz filter. The elimination of epochs with artifacts (eye movements, body movements, electrodermal reactions, etc.) is indispensable. Slow wave activity provides a marker of sleep intensity. It predominates during the first part of sleep and then decreases in an exponential manner throughout the night. The analysis of sigma activity by FFT cannot identify sleep spindles and their density. It assesses the power density in this frequency band. However, the power density of the sigma band is tightly correlated with the variations of sleep spindle density. In contrast to slow wave activity, the sigma band power progressively increases with the successive cycles of sleep. There is an inverse relationship between slow wave activity and sigma activity. Sleep deprivation leads to an increase of slow-wave activity and a decrease of sigma activity. Spectral analysis may also be performed through autoregressive filtering, the latter allowing continuous calculation of spectral power. Using this approach, spectral analysis is no longer bound to consecutive segments of fixed duration and values can be updated every second.

Period analysis is a method that more closely approximates the visual analysis performed by human sleep scorers. It is a time domain analysis implemented either as zero crossing or as peak detection of the EEG waveform. A systematic comparison of period amplitude analysis and spectral analysis by Geering and colleagues showed that the two methods are equivalent for low delta frequencies, while spectral analysis is superior for higher frequencies.

Finally, another EEG quantification technique has been used recently, based on *transformation into wavelets.* This technique enables quantification of short-life graphoelements (1 or 2 seconds) which are difficult to detect using standard spectral analysis. These include spindles and transient arousals.

Combination of features

The second step in automatic sleep analysis is the combination of features, either into a limited number of sleep stages in accordance with the customary criteria or into newly developed variables that may be a better reflection of the sleep process and avoid the limitations of the *Manual.*

The first approach uses logic rules either set for once or adapted, taking into account newly recorded data and subject to continuous improvement (neural network). Assessment of human–machine agreement in this context has generally produced figures in the range 70–90%. A recent report by Anderer and others, adhering to the decision rules for visual scoring as closely as possible and including a structured quality control procedure, sets performance standards for the automatic sleep stager that are almost indistinguishable from a human expert. Nonetheless, there is still dissatisfaction concerning Rechtschaffen and Kales sleep staging, owing to:

- a low temporal resolution of 20–30 seconds
- neglect of the microstructure of sleep
- too much room for subjective interpretation because it is rule-based
- the standards being designed for young normal subjects
- the standards being based on a single electroencephalogram (EEG) channel neglecting spatial EEG information.

Hence the second approach, based on different techniques such as adaptive segmentation and fuzzy subsets, quantitative analysis of EEG waves, continuous parameters. Within the last technique several probabilistic continuous models have been developed by the SIESTA group, but they have yet to prove their usefulness in large clinical trials.

Factors modifying sleep stage distribution

Age

Infants, children, and adolescents show different stages of maturation of sleep, in terms of polysomnographic patterns, architecture, and duration of sleep. Aging is characterized by modifications of the morphology, architecture, and duration of sleep as well as of the situation of sleep within the 24-hour cycle.

Full-term newborn

Active wakefulness is characterized by a continuous EEG theta activity associated with eye movements and muscular artifacts. Active sleep is marked by rapid eye movements, phasic activity of the limbs, face, and body, muscular atonia interrupted by sudden movements, irregular respiration, and unstable heart rate. EEG shows continuous theta activity of moderate amplitude. Quiet sleep is characterized by regular respirations, regular heart rate that is lower than in wakefulness, tonic muscular activity, and an EEG showing slow bursts that are predominantly anterior, interspersed with theta elements and separated by phases of irregular activity of weak amplitude and variable duration, referred to as *tracé alternant*. Transitional sleep precedes, follows, or replaces active sleep. It corresponds to a stage in which the characteristics of the two stages previously referred to are incomplete. The transition from wakefulness to sleep is often accomplished through active sleep. The cyclical alternation of active and quiet sleep is present from birth, but with a period of approximately 50–60 minutes in the newborn compared with approximately 90 minutes in the adult. Total sleep duration is approximately 16 hours with 40–50% active sleep, 30–40% quiet sleep and 10–15% transitional sleep. Periods of sleep and wakefulness are equally distributed during day and night, during the first 3 weeks of life.

From birth to 1 year of age, polysomnographic features rapidly evolve. The *tracé alternant* disappears around the age of 6 weeks, to slow, irregular, and continuous delta rhythms which clearly predominate in the anterior regions. The first bursts of spindles appear at the age of 6 weeks. At 5–6 months of age a basic rhythm of wakefulness of 5–6 Hz is clearly differentiated in the occipital regions. REM sleep is clearly identified with all its EEG, EOG, and EMG features. Between 6 months and 1 year, NREM sleep is distinguishable, with deep sleep stages 3 and 4. During the same period the duration of daytime sleep decreases. Quiet sleep increases and REM sleep decreases from 35% at 6 months of age to 25% between 8 and 20 months. Transitional sleep is replaced by REM sleep. At the age of 1 year the child sleeps 12–14 hours per day with 10–11 hours of night sleep, and daytime sleep is split into two episodes, one at the end of the morning (11:00) and the other one at the beginning of the afternoon (14:00).

Children aged 1 to 3 years

The basic theta rhythm of wakefulness is increasingly associated with frequencies of 7–8 Hz, well localized in the occipital region. NREM sleep can be distinguished in stages 2, 3, and 4. K complexes only appear clearly around the age of 3 years. At around the age of 2 years, children transition from two naps a day to a single postprandial nap.

Children aged 3 to 12 years

Children in this age range have a reduction in total sleep time. At 6 years, total sleep time is about 11 hours; by the age of 10, total sleep time is about 9 hours. The afternoon nap disappears between 4 and 6 years.

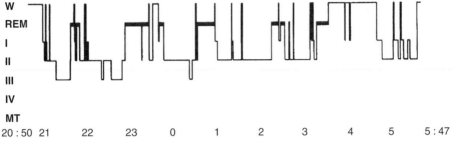

Fig. 1.5. Hypnogram of a 76-year-old male. Note the almost complete absence of NREM sleep stages 3 and 4.

Adolescence

The quantitative change in stages 3 and 4 may be seen across adolescence, when these stages decrease by nearly 40% even if length of nocturnal sleep remains constant.

Normal aging

The modifications of the morphology, duration, architecture, slow-wave activity, and situation of sleep within the 24 hours are a hallmark of the normal aging process (Fig. 1.5). The morphologic modifications consist mainly of a decrease in amplitude of delta waves and a decrease in frequency and amplitude of sleep spindles. Total sleep duration is reduced in comparison with young adults. Extended periods of wakefulness and brief arousals both increase with aging. Stage 3 and 4 NREM sleep is reduced in duration and percentage with aging. The effects of aging on REM sleep are more controversial. Slow-wave activity diminishes with aging. In contrast, spectral power increases in beta frequencies. Elderly subjects retire and get up earlier than young subjects. These changes of the sleep schedule may be linked to an age-dependent modification of the phase of the internal circadian pacemaker. One of the most pronounced findings regarding sleep in the elderly is the profound increase in inter-individual variability, which precludes generalization.

Duration of sleep

The duration of nocturnal sleep depends on several factors. Voluntary control of the sleep time is among the most significant in human beings. Young adults report sleeping approximately 7.5 hours a night on weekday nights and 8.5 hours on weekend nights.

However, sleep length may also be determined by genetics, with several family members reporting similar sleep durations. People sleeping less than 6–6.5 hours per night are called "natural short sleepers" and those sleeping more than 9.5 hours per night are called "natural long sleepers." Comparisons of sleep architecture between short and long sleepers show that the normal final 2 hours of sleep made up of REM sleep and stage 2 NREM sleep disappears in the short sleeper, rather than a compression of all cycles into the shortened sleep time.

In addition, short sleepers have little wake time after sleep onset and stage 1 sleep, suggesting that their sleep is more efficient. Conversely, long sleepers seem to have an additional sleep cycle compared with normal 7.5-hour sleepers, hence the additional stage 2 and REM sleep for the long sleepers. One of the most interesting findings is that stages 3 and 4 are remarkably similar in short and long sleepers, in both cases being equivalent to normal sleepers (Fig. 1.6).

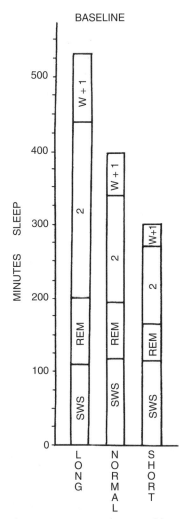

Fig. 1.6. Sleep stage amounts for natural long, normal, and short sleepers. There are similar amounts of NREM sleep stages 3 and 4 for the three groups. The differences lie with the other stages, particularly NREM sleep stage 2. From Benoit *et al.*, *Electroencephalogr Clin Neurophysiol* 1980; **50**: 477–85.

Timing of sleep

The timing of sleep has obvious repercussions both on the duration and on the architecture of sleep. Akerstedt and Gillberg carried out a study 25 years ago in which sleep was displaced to seven different times of day (one displacement per week) in six male volunteers. The baseline bedtime was scheduled at 23:00 after 16 hours of wakefulness. Then sleep was progressively postponed by 4 hours, with bedtimes scheduled at 03:00, 07:00, 11:00, 15:00, 19:00, and 23:00. The longest delay was preceded by 40 hours of continuous wakefulness. They found that the longest sleep (8–10 hours) occurred after evening bedtimes (at 19:00 and 23:00), coinciding with the beginning of the falling arm of the temperature cycle. The shortest (4–5 hours) sleep periods occurred with the morning bedtimes (at 07:00 and 11:00), coinciding with the beginning of the rising arm of the circadian body temperature (Fig. 1.7).

Sleep loss and differential sleep deprivation

Sleep loss on one or more nights is followed by a sleep pattern that favors stages 3 and 4 during recovery. Following sleep deprivation, REM sleep tends to rebound on the second or subsequent recovery nights. Therefore, with total sleep loss, stages 3 and 4 are preferentially recovered before REM sleep.

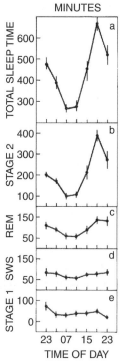

Fig. 1.7. Total sleep time and the amounts of various sleep stages for each experimental sleep condition. From Akerstedt and Gillberg, *Sleep* 1981; **4**: 159–69.

When an individual is selectively deprived of REM sleep or stages 3 and 4 sleep, either by being awakened each time the sleep pattern occurs or by the use of pharmacologic agents, there is a preferential rebound of that stage of sleep when natural sleep is resumed.

Sleep in extreme environments
Sleep in polar regions
Subjects living in temporal isolation, in a completely natural environment with constant light, in the Arctic, develop a free-running sleep/wake cycle longer than 24 hours, with a high degree of inter-subject variability in circadian patterns. However, most subjects participating in polar expeditions are not in temporal isolation and their sleep varies with the degree of comfort or discomfort of their environment, with the altitude of the station, with the light level, and with the possibility of no outdoor exposure. In an uncomfortable situation sleep latency increases, and NREM sleep stages 3 and 4 and REM sleep are reduced.

Sleep in the tropics
Night sleep in sedentary African subjects living in the Sahel region lasts 7–8 hours. While nocturnal sleep is frequently interrupted by awakenings, it contains high amounts of NREM sleep stages 3 and 4 and REM sleep. Interestingly, NREM sleep stages 3 and 4 are at their highest and stage 2 at its lowest in March, when the climatic heat load increases most rapidly. Similar results have been observed in European expatriates living in the same tropical climate.

Sleep at altitude
Sleep may deteriorate at an altitude of around 2000 meters, depending on the subject and the adaptation to fatigue, exposure to cold or heat, and poor conditions of sleep in mountain cabins. Sleep is fragmented by frequent awakenings. NREM sleep stages 3 and 4 decrease markedly and REM sleep is variably affected. At higher altitudes of 4000 meters or more, periodic breathing occurs in almost all subjects, likely in association with the hyperventilation induced by the hypoxia encountered at high altitudes. It is characterized by recurrent central apneas (more than 5 per hour) primarily during NREM sleep, with the consequences of severe sleep fragmentation, reduced stages 3 and 4 NREM sleep, and a variable reduction of REM sleep. Remarkably, Tibetans seem better adapted to life and work at high altitude as compared to other populations. They maintain higher arterial oxygen saturation at rest and during exercise, and they have greater hypoxic and hypercapnic ventilatory responsiveness. This superior adaptation to high altitude may be inborn.

Sleep in space
Field data demonstrate that sleep times and performance of crew members can be compromised by extended duty days, irregular work schedules, high workload, and highly variable light/dark cycles on the flight deck. By developing special strategies,

such as artificial bright lights to reset the physiologic circadian pacemaker, it has been shown that astronauts can at least partially remedy the problem of circadian adaptation in space.

Conclusion

Sleep is a complex behavior. It may be altered by many different factors including age, genetics, volitional control, timing, previous time awake, and environment. Over the course of the last 40 years, major advances have included the recognition of different sleep stages and the development of a uniform sleep scoring system that allows communication between sleep researchers and clinicians. However, the limitations of this system have been recognized and new methodologies have been created to better understand sleep. Nonetheless, there is still a need for sleep researchers and clinicians to find new approaches to sleep analysis that will lead to further improvement in our understanding of normal sleep.

FURTHER READING

Akerstedt T, Gillberg M. The circadian variation of experimentally displaced sleep. *Sleep* 1981; **4**: 1159–69.

American Academy of Sleep Medicine. *The International Classification of Sleep Disorders: Diagnostic and Coding Manual*, 2nd edn (ICSD-2). Westchester, IL: American Academy of Sleep Medicine, 2005.

Anderer P, Gruber G, Parapatics S, *et al.* An E-health solution for automatic sleep classification according to Rechtschaffen and Kales: validation study of the Somnolyzer 24 × 7 utilizing the Siesta database. *Neuropsychobiology* 2005; **53**: 360–63.

Aserinsky E, Kleitman N. Regularly occurring periods of eye motility and concomitant phenomena during sleep. *Science* 1953; **118**: 273–4.

Atlas Task Force. EEG arousals: scoring rules and examples. A preliminary report from the Sleep Disorders Atlas Task Force of the American Sleep Disorders Association. *Sleep* 1992; **15**: 173–84.

Benoit O, Foret J, Bouard G, *et al.* Habitual sleep length and patterns of recovery sleep after 24 hour and 36 hour sleep deprivation. *Electroencephalogr Clin Neurophysiol* 1980; **50**: 477–85.

Bliwise DL. Normal aging. In: Kryger MH, Roth T, Dement WC, eds. *Principles and Practice of Sleep Medicine*, 4th edn. Philadelphia, PA: Saunders, 2005: 24–38.

Carskadon MA, Brown ED, Dement WC. Sleep fragmentation in the elderly: relationship to daytime sleep tendency. *Neurobiol Aging* 1982; **3**: 321–7.

Davis KF, Parker KP, Montgomery GL. Sleep in infants and young children. Part one: normal sleep. *J Pediatr Health Care* 2004; **18**: 65–71.

Dement WC, Kleitman N. The relation of eye movements during sleep to dream activity: an objective method for the study of dreaming. *J Exp Psychol* 1957; **53**: 339–46.

Dijk DJ, Neri DF, Wyatt JK, *et al.* Sleep, performance, circadian rhythms, and light–dark cycles during two space shuttle flights. *Am J Physiol Regul Integr Comp Physiol* 2001; **281**: R1647–64.

Dorffner G. Toward a new standard of modeling sleep based on polysomnograms: the SIESTA project. *Electroencephalogr Clin Neurophysiol* 1998; **106** (suppl. 1001): 28.

Flexer A, Gruber G, Dorffner G. A reliable probabilistic sleep stager based on a single EEG signal. *Appl Artif Intell* 2004; **33**: 209–22.

Gati R, Pétieu R, Wamba B, Buguet A. Human sleep in dry tropical Africa. In: Horne J, ed. *Sleep 90*. Bochum: Pontenagel Press, 1994: 39–41.

Geering BA, Achermann P, Eggimann F, Borbely AA. Period-amplitude analysis and power spectral analysis: a comparison based on all-night sleep EEG recordings. *J Sleep Res* 1993; **2**: 121–9.

Grigg-Damberger M, Gozal D, Marcus CL, *et al.* The visual scoring of sleep and arousal in infants and children. *J Clin Sleep Med* 2007; **3**: 201–40.

Hjorth B. EEG analysis based on time domain properties. *Electroencephalogr Clin Neurophysiol* 1970; **29**: 306–10.

Jouvet M. Récherches sur les structures nerveuses et les mécanismes responsables des différentes phases du sommeil physiologique. *Arch Ital Biol* 1962; **1090**: 125–206.

Kahn A, Dan B, Groswasser J, Franco P, Sottiaux M. Normal sleep architecture in infants and children. *J Clin Neurophysiol* 1996; **13**: 184–97.

Karacan I, Moore CA. Genetics and human sleep. *Psychiatr Ann* 1979; **9**: 11–23.

Kleitman N. *Sleep and Wakefulness*. Chicago, IL: University of Chicago Press, 1939.

Kubicki S, Höller L, Berg I, Pastelack-Price C, Dorow R. Sleep EEG evaluation: a comparison of results obtained by visual scoring and automatic analysis with the Oxford sleep stager. *Sleep* 1989; **12**: 140–9.

Loomis AL, Harvey EN, Hobart GA. Cerebral states during sleep, as studied by human brain potentials. *J Exp Psychol* 1937; **21**: 127–44.

Louis RP, Lee J, Stephenson R. Design and validation of a computer-based sleep-scoring algorithm. *J Neurosci Methods* 2004; **133**: 71–80.

Mallis MM, De Roshia CW. Circadian rhythms, sleep, and performance in space. *Aviat Space Environ Med* 2005; **76** (6 suppl): B94–107.

Montmayeur A, Buguet A. Sleep problems in Melanoids and Caucasians living in the tropics. *J Sleep Res* 1994; **3** (suppl 1): 171.

Natani K, Shurley JT, Pierce CM, Brooks RE. Long-term changes in sleep patterns in men on the south polar plateau. *Arch Intern Med* 1970; **125**: 655–9.

Pardey J, Roberts S, Tarassenko L. A new approach to the analysis of the human sleep/wakefulness continuum. *J Sleep Res* 1996; **5**: 201–10.

Penzel T, Conradt R. Computer-based sleep recording and analysis. *Sleep Med Rev* 2000; **4**: 131–48.

Rechtschaffen A, Kales A. *A Manual of Standardized Terminology, Techniques and Scoring System for Sleep Stages of Human Subjects*. Los Angeles, CA: UCLA Brain Information Service/Brain Research Institute, 1968.

Robert C, Guilpin C, Limoge A. Review of neural network application in sleep research. *J Neurosci Meth* 1998; **79**: 187–93.

Steel GD, Callaway M, Suedfeld P, Palinkas L. Human sleep–wake cycles in the high Arctic: effects of unusual photoperiodicity in a natural setting. *Biol Rhythm Res* 1995; **26**: 582–92.

Terzano MG, Parrino L. Evaluation of EEG cyclic alternating pattern during sleep in insomniacs and controls under placebo and acute treatment with zolpidem. *Sleep* 1992; **15**: 64–70.

Terzano MG, Parrino L. Origin and significance of the cyclic alternating pattern (CAP). *Sleep Med Rev* 2000; **4**: 101–23.

Terzano MG, Mancia D, Salati MR, *et al.* The cyclic alternating pattern as a physiologic component of normal NREM sleep. *Sleep* 1985; **8**: 137–45.

Terzano MG, Parrino L, Mennuni GF, eds. *Phasic Events and Microstructure of Sleep*. Consensus conference, Italian Association of Sleep Medicine (AIMS). Lecce: Martano Editore, 1997.

Terzano MG, Parrino L, Smerieri A, *et al*. Atlas, rules, and recording techniques for the scoring of cyclic alternating pattern (CAP) in human sleep. *Sleep Med* 2001; **2**: 537–53.

Webb WB, Agnew HW. Sleep stage characteristics of long and short sleepers. *Science* 1970; **168**: 146–7.

Wu T, Kayser B. High altitude adaptation in Tibetans. *High Alt Med Biol* 2006; **7**: 193–208.

2 Evaluation and testing of the sleepy patient

Charles Bae and Alon Avidan

Introduction

Sleep disturbances can affect people throughout their life span, and the frequency of sleep disturbances increases as we age. Currently, there are more than 80 sleep disorders that are described in the second edition of the International Classification of Sleep Disorders (ICSD-2). There is mounting evidence showing that sleep disorders are closely related to comorbid medical and neurological diseases. Sleep deprivation has been shown to be a possible risk factor for obesity. Untreated obstructive sleep apnea (OSA) is associated with an increased risk of having elevated blood pressure and insulin resistance. Untreated OSA may also be associated with an increased risk of heart attack or stroke. Specific epilepsies occur exclusively during sleep, and sleep deprivation may provoke seizures. Individuals with REM sleep behavior disorder (RBD) are at a higher risk for developing a neurodegenerative disorder such as Parkinson's disease or dementia.

It is the responsibility of healthcare providers to inquire about sleep quality and any possible sleep disruptions in their patients. People with sleep disturbances may complain of difficulty falling asleep or maintaining sleep, abnormal behaviors during the night, daytime sleepiness or fatigue. Multiple sleep disorders can be present in one individual, causing a decreased quality of life. A systematic approach is therefore crucial in facilitating the evaluation, diagnosis, and treatment of sleep disorders.

When evaluating someone for sleep disorders, a comprehensive and detailed sleep history is often the most important part of the evaluation. Many of the sleep disorders in the ICSD-2 can be diagnosed by history alone without the need for sleep tests. It is a common occurrence to see someone present to the sleep clinic only when sleep is so severely interrupted as to produce daytime sleepiness and cognitive difficulties. Many times, the visit to the sleep clinic occurs at the urging of a bed partner whose sleep is disrupted as well. Patients can provide important historical facts and details about their sleep patterns and nocturnal arousals; often the best source of information is a bed partner, since the affected person is asleep and is not fully aware of what occurs during the night. This is especially true when inquiring about snoring, apneic episodes, periodic leg movements, and parasomnias such as RBD or sleepwalking.

Sleep Medicine, ed. Harold R. Smith, Cynthia L. Comella, and Birgit Högl. Published by Cambridge University Press. © Cambridge University Press 2008.

Table 2.1 shows a list of questions that can help screen for sleep problems. As is illustrated in the table, a detailed sleep history consists of information regarding bedtime habits and rituals that precede the typical sleep period and wake time, along with daytime function. Some individuals may be affected by daytime sleepiness severe enough to cause motor vehicle accidents, while others may only complain of daytime fatigue which is relatively manageable. Symptoms that are associated with mood disorders (poor concentration or memory, irritability, change in appetite) may be a prominent feature of unrefreshing sleep and an important cause of early morning awakenings. As a result, a comprehensive sleep history involves a thorough review of current medical and psychiatric problems, medications, social history, and family history.

A special consideration is sleep in women. During pregnancy, women experience an increased incidence of snoring, which may be associated with a higher incidence of sleep-disordered breathing. In addition, the prevalence of restless legs syndrome (RLS) is high in pregnancy, especially in the third trimester. Progesterone may provide a stimulatory effect on the upper airway musculature that is protective against obstructive sleep apnea (OSA) before menopause. A decrease in progesterone may increase the risk for sleep-disordered breathing

Table 2.1. *Sleep history template: questions that can help to screen for sleep problems.*

Do you have difficulties falling asleep or maintaining sleep?
Do you feel excessively sleepy, tired, or fatigued during the day?
What is your sleep schedule during the weekdays and on the weekends?
Are you a night owl or early bird?
How many hours do you sleep during the night?
How long does it take you to fall asleep once deciding to go to sleep?
How many times do you wake up during a typical night?
Do you take any daytime naps?
Do you feel refreshed when you wake up in the morning?
Do you have loud snoring and do you stop breathing at night?
Has your snoring intensity increased recently?
Is it associated with increased weight? Increased neck circumference? Is it positional
   (i.e., worse on your back)?
Do you ever experience loss of muscle tone triggered by a strong emotional stimulus
   (laughter/anger)?
Do you have any difficulties with feeling completely paralyzed upon awakening?
Do you have any vivid dream episodes upon falling asleep or upon awakening?
Do you have an urge to move your legs due to restlessness, crawling, or aching sensations
   when trying to fall asleep?
Do you repeatedly kick your legs during sleep?
Do you act out your dreams?
Do you grind your teeth?
Do you have any acid reflux symptoms at the beginning of the night?

in postmenopausal women. The apnea threshold has been shown to be higher in premenopausal women when compared to postmenopausal women, putting them at greater risk for sleep apnea.

People with a number of chronic comorbid diseases such as hypertension, diabetes mellitus, obesity, epilepsy, fibromyalgia, and depression may have sleep disturbances associated with these conditions. Many medications that are taken for chronic conditions can affect the quality of sleep or may contribute to daytime sleepiness and fatigue. Certain antidepressants, antipsychotics, antiepileptic agents, pain medications, and antihistamines can cause daytime sleepiness or fatigue. Beta-blockers have been associated with vivid dreams and nightmares. Selective serotonin reuptake inhibitors may increase periodic limb movements (PLMs) during sleep, in addition to exacerbating restless legs syndrome (RLS). Medications that can worsen OSA include long-acting benzodiazepines (muscle relaxation) and opioids (respiratory depression). Corticosteroids may cause difficulties with sleep onset.

The social history can provide a wealth of helpful information: stresses at home or at work may contribute to difficulties falling asleep. Illicit drug use may be contributing to sleep difficulties and daytime dysfunction, due to direct effects or from withdrawal symptoms. Other useful questions include an inventory of childhood sleep problems such as sleepwalking, sleeptalking, or enuresis. These behaviors may be a risk factor for similar activities in adulthood, especially with potential triggers such as sleep deprivation or alcohol use.

There may be a strong family history for some sleep disorders such as OSA, narcolepsy, circadian rhythm disorders, and RLS. Certain genes have been identified that may increase the risk for OSA. Narcolepsy with cataplexy has a strong association with the HLA DQB1*0602 allele, though a mode of inheritance has not been identified. Familial advanced sleep phase syndrome is an autosomal dominant circadian rhythm sleep disorder. An autosomal dominant inheritance pattern has also been described in families with early-onset RLS.

The physical examination is an important part of the evaluation of sleep disorders, especially for sleep-disordered breathing. The male gender and a large neck circumference (> 43cm [17 inches] in men and > 41cm [16 inches] in women) have been shown to be independent risk factors for OSA. Obesity and increased body mass index (BMI > 30 kg/m^2) is also associated with a higher risk for OSA. Other phenotypic features that can raise the suspicion of sleep-disordered breathing include a crowded posterior airspace and retrognathia of the mandible relative to the maxilla. A useful way to grade the posterior airspace is the Mallampati score, which assesses the relationship between the soft palate and the base of the tongue while the tongue is protruded (Fig. 2.1). The Mallampati classification was designed as a means of predicting the degree of difficulty in laryngeal exposure. More recently, it has been shown that a high Mallampati score and nasal obstruction are associated risk factors for obstructive sleep apnea. The Mallampati score can be used to predict the presence and severity of OSA. The Friedman palate position score is a modification of the Mallampati score in which the tongue is not protruded.

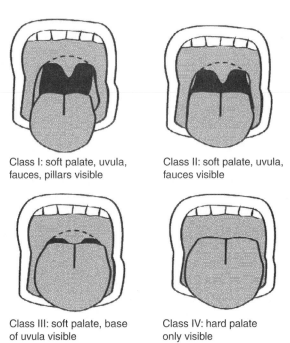

Class I: soft palate, uvula, fauces, pillars visible

Class II: soft palate, uvula, fauces visible

Class III: soft palate, base of uvula visible

Class IV: hard palate only visible

Fig. 2.1. The Mallampati classification is a relatively simple grading system for evaluating airway size, taking into account the relative size of the tonsillar pillars, soft palate, and base of uvula. It was designed as a means of predicting the degree of difficulty of laryngeal intubation but more recently has been demonstrated to correlate with the severity of obstructive sleep apnea. Image reproduced with permission from the *Canadian Journal of Anaesthesia* (Mallampati SR, Gatt SP, Gugino LD, *et al.* A clinical sign to predict difficult tracheal intubation: a prospective study. *Can Anaesth Soc J* 1985; **32**: 429–34).

An examination of the oral pharynx is useful in the treatment of snoring if the airway is small or crowded, or if there is inflammation present. However, a detailed examination by an otolaryngologist using fiberoptic nasendoscopy may be helpful in snorers presenting with these symptoms. Evidence of cardiovascular status (i.e., pulse rate, blood pressure) should be documented during the physical examination. In many individuals, the physical exam may be normal, so a normal physical exam cannot exclude sleep apnea.

In people with RLS or excessive movements during sleep, it is important to examine the lower extremities to see if a peripheral neuropathy is present. A sensory examination consisting of light touch, pinprick, vibration, and proprioception should be performed. If there is evidence of neuropathy, treatable causes should be evaluated utilizing HgbA1C, vitamin B12, TSH, two-hour fasting oral glucose tolerance test. Other potential neurologic causes for periodic leg movements may be detected by looking for asymmetric weakness or muscle stretch reflexes.

When RBD is suspected, a focal neurologic exam evaluating for Parkinsonism (masked facies, resting tremor, postural reflexes, cogwheel rigidity, decreased arm swing when walking), and other neurodegenerative conditions should be performed.

Subjective and objective assessment of sleep habits

Asking about typical bedtime rituals, sleep times and habits is a good place to start in the assessment of any sleep disorder. It is important to note typical bed and wake times during the week and on weekends, if schedules are different. The length of time it takes to fall asleep (sleep latency), and nighttime rituals before getting to bed (and while in bed) can trigger further discussion about patterns or conditions that could be contributing to insomnia. A person may be frustrated as he or she lies in bed for hours tossing and turning, while planning and worrying about the next day. Watching the time pass while trying to fall asleep may exacerbate the frustration experienced, further prolonging the process. A description of the general bedroom environment can be helpful to determine whether the environment is conducive for sleep. Excessive light or noise, uncomfortable temperature, and a ticking clock next to the bed can further delay sleep onset. The number and frequency of awakenings during the night should be elicited from the patient and from a bed partner if available. An obese individual who snores loudly and wakes up multiple times gasping for air may have OSA. If someone takes naps, one needs to describe the frequency, duration, and timing of naps in addition to how refreshing they may or may not be.

Sleep logs are completed by the person with a sleep problem, and are a subjective way to assess sleep habits. They can provide a wealth of information including the sleep and wake times, nap times, level of energy or fatigue in the morning, and any rituals such as caffeine ingestion or use of hypnotic agents. Sleep logs (Fig. 2.2) can be picture-based or word-based, and should be completed for several weeks at a time and brought in for the clinical sleep evaluation.

The person is instructed to record the following data:

- the time he/she wanted to fall asleep
- the time he/she thinks they fell asleep
- the number, time, and length of any nocturnal awakenings
- the time he/she woke up
- the time he/she got out of bed
- the time he/she had wanted to wake up
- a comment on how he/she felt during the day
- the start and end times of any daytime naps
- any medications used.

An accurate sleep log may help a person see his or her sleep problem from another perspective, looking at trends or patterns rather than focusing on the details of the sleep difficulty. Sleep logs are not only helpful with the evaluation and diagnosis of sleep disorders, but can also help people see that they are able to sleep better over time.

Actigraphy is an objective way to assess sleep habits. An actigraph is a small device worn by an individual to measure movement throughout a day, using an accelerometer. Lack of motion is assumed to represent sleep periods, and motion represents the awake state. This information, in combination with sleep-log data,

NAME _____

SLEEP DISORDERS CENTER

SLEEP CHART

1. MARK EACH TIME OF GETTING INTO BED WITH AN ARROW POINTING DOWNWARDS...............↓
2. MARK EACH TIME OF GETTING OUT OF BED WITH AN ARROW POINTING UPWARDS...............↑
3. MARK PERIODS OF SLEEP AS SHADED AREAS BETWEEN VERTICAL BARS.............................▨

(example of a period of waking)

DAY	DATE	MN 1AM 2AM 3AM 4AM 5AM 6AM 7AM 8AM 9AM 10AM 11AM NOON 1PM 2PM 3PM 4PM 5PM 6PM 7PM 8PM 9PM 10PM 11PM MN
MON	1/3	SLEEP ... ↑ ... ↓
TUES	1/4	SLEEP ... ↑ ... ↓ NAP ↑ ... ↓

Fig. 2.2. Sample sleep log. A sleep log is a record of an individual's sleeping and waking times, usually tabulated over a period of several weeks.

can provide a reasonable "snapshot" of activity during wake-to-sleep transition. A recent position paper from the American Academy of Sleep Medicine (AASM) suggests that actigraphy can be useful in the routine evaluation of insomnia, excessive daytime sleepiness, and circadian rhythm disorders.

Evaluation of excessive daytime sleepiness (EDS)

Daytime sleepiness can be caused by a variety of sleep disorders such as insufficient sleep time, acute and chronic sleep deprivation, OSA, insomnia, RLS, circadian rhythm sleep disorders, and narcolepsy. It may be difficult for some individuals to differentiate between daytime sleepiness and fatigue. Daytime sleepiness is typically characterized by a difficulty staying awake, while daytime fatigue is characterized by a lack of energy or motivation. The use of three objective self-assessment questionnaires can help differentiate between sleepiness and fatigue (Tables 2.2, 2.3, 2.4).

In the case of EDS, it is mandatory to investigate whether sleepiness affects driving (accidents or near-accidents) and whether sleepiness has any impact on safety in work environments using heavy machinery. The chronicity and emergence of clinically significant EDS may be helpful; this is especially true when severe EDS that has been present since childhood (despite an opportunity for adequate sleep) may be suggestive of narcolepsy. Figure 2.3 shows a possible algorithm for the workup of EDS/hypersomnia.

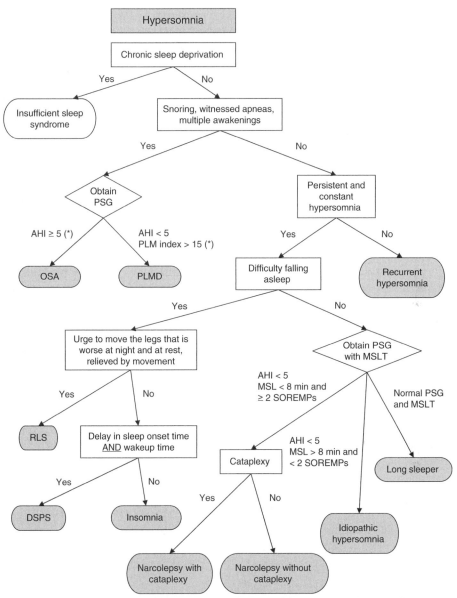

Fig. 2.3. EDS/hypersomnia algorithm: a general schematic of the workup of chronic and persistent EDS. AHI, apnea–hypopnea index; DSPS, delayed sleep phase syndrome; MSL, mean sleep latency; MSLT, multiple sleep latency test; OSA, obstructive sleep apnea; PLMD, periodic limb movement disorder; PSG, polysomnogram; RLS, restless legs syndrome; SOREMP, sleep onset REM period; (*), with consideration of the clinical symptoms.

The most common reason for both acute and chronic hypersomnia is sleep deprivation due to behaviorally induced insufficient sleep. Insufficient sleep syndrome occurs when an individual experiences less than optimal sleep periods, resulting in sleep deprivation.

If the chief complaint is loud snoring or witnessed apneas, OSA needs to be considered. People with OSA may experience frequent nocturnal awakenings, sometimes culminating in episodes of waking up gasping for air. Breathing during sleep may be adversely affected by recent weight gain and sleep in the supine position. Mouth breathing may contribute to a dry mouth in those who have difficulties breathing through the nose due to nasal congestion, nasal polyps, enlarged adenoids, or a deviated septum.

A diagnostic polysomnogram (PSG) may be suggested to evaluate for the presence of sleep apnea. If the PSG demonstrates evidence of an apnea–hypopnea index (AHI) greater than 5 with associated arousals or oxygen desaturations in the setting of daytime problems (sleepiness, tiredness, poor concentration), a diagnostic consideration of obstructive sleep apnea syndrome may be made. If the diagnostic PSG demonstrates an abnormally elevated periodic limb movements index, a consideration of periodic limb movement disorder of sleep is considered. If the hypersomnia is not persistent, but is rather episodic and severe, the possibility of a recurrent hypersomnia such as Kleine–Levin syndrome or menstruation-associated hypersomnia should be entertained. When the hypersomnia is pathologic and persistent, narcolepsy or idiopathic hypersomnia can be considered.

When the chief complaint is primarily that of severe EDS, it is important to screen for other symptoms that can be seen with narcolepsy such as cataplexy, hypnagogic hallucinations, disrupted nocturnal sleep, and sleep paralysis. Cataplexy with EDS is the symptom that defines the narcolepsy syndrome and is sometimes difficult to assess clinically. Cataplexy is often preceded by a strong emotional trigger such as laughter or anger, which precipitates a sudden loss of muscle tone that is brief in duration. As a rule, consciousness is preserved during episodes of cataplexy, which helps distinguish it from other spells such as atonic seizures. The loss of muscle tone does not have to be profound, is typically brief, and may only be noticeable by the affected person. Individuals with hypnagogic hallucinations typically describe sensory misperceptions that occur as they are falling asleep (hypnagogic) or waking up (hypnopompic). Sleep paralysis, which typically occurs on waking up, consists of a brief inability to move all skeletal muscles even when fully awake. An important question to ask individuals with sleep paralysis is how they felt during the episode, since true episodes of sleep paralysis are frequently associated with a sensation of overwhelming fear.

Restless legs syndrome (RLS) is a clinical diagnosis consisting of four essential criteria: (a) an urge to move the legs that may or may not be related to an uncomfortable sensation; (b) the urge to move begins or worsens with inactivity or rest; (c) the urge to move is worse in the evening or night; (d) the urge to move is partially or totally relieved with movement. A bed partner may provide additional information that the person is kicking during sleep, suggesting the presence of periodic leg movements, a condition that can be seen in up to 85% of people with RLS.

The Epworth Sleepiness Scale (ESS) is a widely used validated subjective self-assessment questionnaire to assess daytime sleepiness. A person is asked to rate the likelihood of dozing off or falling asleep in eight common situations that are sedentary

Table 2.2. *The Epworth Sleepiness Scale (ESS): a standardized self-administered eight-item questionnaire commonly used to assess sleepiness.*

The questionnaire asks you to rate the chances that you would doze off or fall asleep during different routine situations. Answers to the questions are rated from 0 to 3, with 0 meaning you would never doze or fall asleep in a given situation, and 3 meaning that there is a very high likelihood that you would doze or fall asleep in that situation. Use the following scale to choose the most appropriate number for each situation:

0 = would **never** doze
1 = **slight** chance of dozing
2 = **moderate** chance of dozing
3 = **high** chance of dozing

	Chance of dozing			
Situation	Never	Slight	Mod	High
Sitting and reading	0	1	2	3
Watching TV	0	1	2	3
Sitting inactive, in a public place (e.g. a theater or meeting)	0	1	2	3
As a passenger in a car for an hour without a break	0	1	2	3
Lying down to rest in the afternoon when circumstances permit	0	1	2	3
Sitting and talking to someone	0	1	2	3
Sitting quietly after a lunch without alcohol	0	1	2	3
In a car, while stopped for a few minutes in traffic	0	1	2	3

Total score of less than 10 suggests that you may not be suffering from excessive sleepiness. A total score of 10 or more suggests that you may need further evaluation by a physician to determine the cause of your excessive sleepiness and whether you have an underlying sleep disorder.

or involve little activity (Table 2.2). The maximum total score is 24, which implies the highest severity of sleepiness, and a score of greater than 10 has been shown to be correlated with significant EDS. The ESS has good test–retest reliability and good internal consistency. The ESS can be a useful tool to help assess the effectiveness of a particular treatment over time. However, the ESS should not be used as a substitute for the multiple sleep latency test (MSLT), which together with a nocturnal polysomnogram is the current gold standard for assessing and measuring sleepiness. A recent study showed that ESS scores correlated negatively, but not strongly, with MSLT scores. The ESS score correlated with the degree to which a person complained of sleepiness, and may be useful as an otherwise elusive link between those complaints and the objective findings on the MSLT.

The Stanford Sleepiness Scale (SSS) is another subjective self-rating scale to assess daytime sleepiness. A person is asked to select one out of seven statements that best describes his or her current level of sleepiness (Table 2.3). The SSS may be used during

Table 2.3. *The Stanford Sleepiness Scale (SSS): an introspective measure of sleepiness.*

The Stanford Sleepiness Scale is a quick way to assess how alert you are feeling. If it is
during the day when you go about your business, ideally you would want a rating of a
one. Take into account that most people have two peak times of alertness daily, at about
9 a.m. and 9 p.m. Alertness wanes to its lowest point at around 3 p.m.; after that it begins
to build again. Rate your alertness at different times during the day. If you go below a
three when you should be feeling alert, this is an indication that you have a serious sleep
debt and you need more sleep.

Degree of sleepiness	Scale rating
Feeling active, vital, alert, or wide awake	1
Functioning at high levels, but not at peak; able to concentrate	2
Awake, but relaxed; responsive but not fully alert	3
Somewhat foggy, let down	4
Foggy; losing interest in remaining awake; slowed down	5
Sleepy, woozy, fighting sleep; prefer to lie down	6
No longer fighting sleep, sleep onset soon; having dream-like thoughts	7
Asleep	X

the MSLT, before each nap trial, to assess whether the subjective assessment of
sleepiness correlates with an objective measure of sleepiness. The SSS has been
shown to be a reliable measure of the effects of partial sleep deprivation, although it
does not reliably measure performance after sleep deprivation.

Subjective fatigue scales such as the Fatigue Severity Scale (FSS) can be used. The
FSS is a self-assessment scale designed to determine the extent to which fatigue
affects the level of functioning in different areas of daily life. Individuals are asked
to rate nine statements that describe how fatigue may affect different aspects of
their lives (Table 2.4). The responses are averaged, and the score can range between
one and seven. Normal controls have a mean of 2.3, compared to a mean of 4.7 in
people with systemic lupus erythematosis and a mean of 4.8 in those with multiple
sclerosis. The FSS has a good test–retest reliability and can therefore be used in the
measurement of the effect size of treatments for fatigue.

A nocturnal polysomnogram (PSG) is indicated when primary sleep disorders
such as sleep apnea, periodic leg movements, and parasomnias are suspected.
A PSG is performed in the sleep laboratory under the watchful eye of a trained sleep
technologist. Recently, ambulatory sleep studies have been introduced to allow for
sleep recording at home. Currently, home monitoring is not considered to be an
acceptable alternative to an attended study. An attended PSG typically results in a
better-quality study since electrodes and respiratory monitors can be replaced as
needed during the study. A technologist also is able to provide a log of events during
the study that may help with interpretation of the study. All of these factors should
increase the diagnostic yield of a PSG and reduce the need to repeat a study, making
an attended PSG more cost-effective.

Table 2.4. *The Fatigue Severity Scale (FSS): a self-reported questionnaire used to measure a person's perceived level of fatigue in a variety of situations. The test was developed at the Multiple Sclerosis (MS) Comprehensive Care Center at State University of New York Stony Brook, to assist physicians in recognizing and diagnosing fatigue. It is also designed to differentiate fatigue from clinical depression, since both share some of the same symptoms.*

Choose a number from 1 to 7 that indicates the degree of agreement with each statement. 1 indicates strongly disagree, 7 indicates strongly agree.

	Disagree/ agree (1–7)
(1) My motivation is lower when I am fatigued	—
(2) Exercise brings on my fatigue	—
(3) I am easily fatigued	—
(4) Fatigue interferes with my physical conditioning	—
(5) Fatigue causes frequent problems for me	—
(6) My fatigue prevents sustained physical functioning	—
(7) Fatigue interferes with carrying out certain duties and responsibilities	—
(8) Fatigue is among my three most disabling symptoms	—
(9) Fatigue interferes with my work, family, or social life	—

The scoring is done by calculating the average response to the questions (adding up all the answers and dividing by nine).

A polysomnogram is not needed in the evaluation of RLS, unless comorbid OSA is a possibility. The PSG can be helpful for diagnosing periodic limb movement disorder (PLMD), which can only be diagnosed by PSG, although it can sometimes be suspected clinically. Periodic leg movement disorders of sleep consist of periodic contractions of the extremities recurring every 5–90 seconds with a burst duration of 0.5–5 seconds. The main indication for a multiple sleep latency test (MSLT) is to evaluate or document the severity of daytime sleepiness and when narcolepsy or idiopathic hypersomnia are diagnostic considerations. An overnight PSG is recommended the night prior to an MSLT to assess for other comorbid sleep disturbances and for objectively recording total sleep time.

Evaluation of insomnia

Many people who present with the classic symptom of "insomnia" may have more than one problem with sleep. A recent NIH State-of-the-Science Conference identified three types of problems associated with insomnia: difficulty falling asleep, difficulty maintaining sleep, and early morning awakenings. A fourth type consisting of nonrestorative sleep has been included in the definition of insomnia, but the underlying mechanism may be different than for the first three types.

Acute insomnia was defined as the aforementioned sleep disturbances occurring at any one time or another (in relation to a stressor), while the sleep disturbances for chronic insomnia had to be present for at least 30 days. A final distinction was made between primary and comorbid insomnias. The term primary insomnia is used when the sleep disturbance is not related to any other medical, psychiatric, or sleep disorder. Insomnia is currently thought to be comorbid with other medical, psychiatric, or sleep disorders; in the past, insomnia associated with other medical or psychiatric illnesses was referred to as secondary insomnia.

A classic model of insomnia takes into consideration three factors: predisposing, precipitating, and perpetuating factors. In this model, everyone has a certain propensity (insomnia threshold) to experience insomnia based on biologic, psychological, and social factors. When stressful events occur, a person may have trouble sleeping when the insomnia threshold is crossed. Acute insomnia can develop into chronic insomnia when perpetuating factors such as poor stress management or maladaptive sleep habits keep an individual above the insomnia threshold.

Time needs to be spent asking about sleep habits, starting with activities before entering the bedroom and activities while in bed. Maladaptive sleep habits that may interfere with falling asleep include watching television and reading in bed and checking the time regularly. A precipitating factor can often be identified in people who have transient or acute insomnia. This is in contrast to those who have chronic insomnia, who may have had a precipitating factor as well but over time have continued to have difficulty sleeping due to perpetuating behaviors and habits that have become established. It is important to review all chronic medical and psychiatric conditions and how they may be contributing to the insomnia.

The ESS and FSS can be used to assess how much daytime sleepiness or fatigue is present. A sleep log can be helpful to document sleep patterns and habits. A PSG is not indicated in the routine evaluation of insomnia unless OSA is suspected. An MSLT is not indicated when evaluating someone for insomnia.

Figure 2.4 demonstrates a possible algorithm for the evaluation of insomnia. This algorithm assumes that an individual presents with insomnia as a result of inadequate sleep habits (e.g., using caffeine, alcohol and tobacco, watching TV, reading in bed). Once inadequate sleep habits are found, the clinician typically recommends relaxation techniques before bedtime to help a person "turn off" his or her mind before going to bed, and staying out of bed until he or she feels sleepy and ready to fall asleep. These methods are a part of what is known as behavioral therapy. A common reason for patients to experience difficulties falling asleep is poor sleep hygiene. Sometimes an acute stressor prior to the onset of insomnia is the etiology. When the insomnia is more chronic, a triggering stressor may not be identified, and the difficulty falling asleep may be due to negative learned behaviors (i.e., conditioned insomnia). Insomnia may be comorbid with underlying illnesses such as restless legs syndrome (RLS), sleep apnea, depression, anxiety, or an underlying circadian rhythm sleep disorder such as delayed sleep phase syndrome, jet lag, or shift-work sleep disorder.

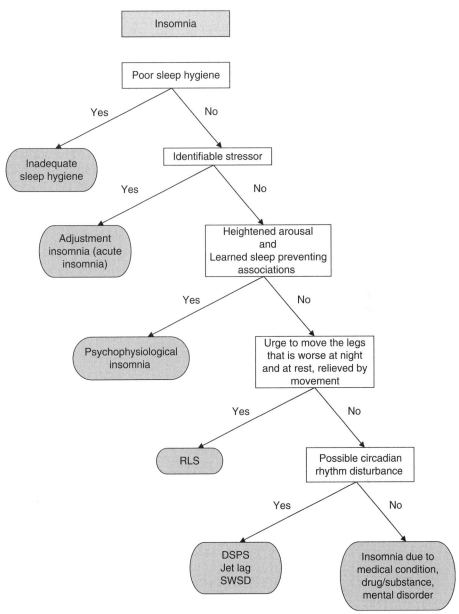

Fig. 2.4. Insomnia algorithm. DSPS, delayed sleep phase syndrome; RLS, restless legs syndrome; SWSD, shift work sleep disorder.

Evaluation of difficulties staying asleep

OSA is a one of the most common causes of difficulties maintaining sleep, and bed partners may complain of snoring, which may be loud and interrupted. Patients and their bed partners may complain about unusual or excessive movements during sleep. Non-REM or REM parasomnias such as confusional arousals, episodes of sleepwalking or talking, or REM sleep behavior disorder (RBD) may cause inappropriate awakenings during the night, resulting in poor and fragmented sleep. Besides parasomnias, other potential causes of abnormal behaviors during sleep include nocturnal seizures, which may be difficult to distinguish from parasomnias since many behaviors may appear similar in semiology and there may be a lack of information about the events, especially when no bed partner is present.

Useful questions in situations where parasomnias or nocturnal seizures are suspected include potential triggers, such as sleep deprivation, alcohol use at bedtime, recent emotional stressors, shift work, and changes in typical sleep/wake patterns. If a person acts out dreams, it is important to ask a bed partner about dream enactment behaviors, since RBD is often associated with violent dream content (typically fighting or being chased). Other sleep disorders may serve as a trigger for

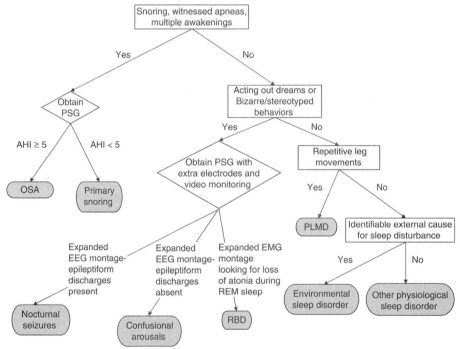

Fig. 2.5. Algorithm for difficulties maintaining sleep. This is complex but can be approached from the point of view that difficulties maintaining sleep arise due to underlying comorbid sleep disorders. Since sleep-disordered breathing is one of the most important and frequent causes of difficulties with sleep maintenance, it serves as the main fork in the decision tree analysis. This algorithm then takes into account the potential presence of underlying motor and neurological disorders of sleep (including parasomnias and seizures) and uses the diagnostic polysomnogram (PSG) to provide evidence for or against the possible diagnosis. AHI: apnea–hypopnea index; EEG, electroencephalogram; EMG, electromyogram; OSA, obstructive sleep apnea; PLMD, periodic limb movement disorder; RBD, REM sleep behavior disorder.

parasomnias. Frequent awakenings due to interruptions in breathing may trigger NREM parasomnias such as sleepwalking or talking. If the behavior in question is very unusual or stereotyped, a nocturnal seizure may be responsible. Figure 2.5 demonstrates an algorithm for the evaluation of difficulties maintaining sleep.

Polysomnography is indicated for the evaluation of abnormal or unusual movements during sleep. A full 10–20 EEG can be added to a PSG to determine if nocturnal behaviors are related to epileptiform discharges.

Interpretation of polysomnography (PSG)

Sleep disorders such as OSA, parasomnias, narcolepsy, and nocturnal seizures sometimes require formal evaluation in the sleep laboratory. The most commonly used techniques used in recording and evaluating sleep disorders include the polysomnogram (PSG), the multiple sleep latency test (MSLT), and under special circumstances, the maintenance of wakefulness test (MWT). The accurate interpretation of these studies requires a comprehensive sleep and medical history. Polysomnography is an electrographic recording of simultaneous physiologic parameters occurring during sleep and wakefulness. It describes the interaction of multiple organ systems (nervous system, respiratory, and sometimes genitourinary) during sleep and wakefulness. The PSG is used in the evaluation of abnormalities of sleep and sleep–wake transition, EDS, excessive nocturnal awakenings, abnormal behavioral events in sleep, and to assess the efficacy of treatments for various sleep disorders.

International standards require polysomnography to include four neurophysiologic channels at a minimum:

(1) one electroencephalography (EEG) channel (central with an ear reference provides the best amplitude) to monitor sleep staging
(2) two electrooculogram (EOG) channels to monitor both horizontal and vertical eye movements
(3) one electromyography (EMG) channel (usually chin or mentalis and/or submentalis) to record atonia of rapid eye movement (REM) sleep.

Based on the clinical indication, extended montages incorporating additional physiologic parameters are sometimes added. Examples include the following:

(1) additional EEG channels, particularly in individuals with sleep-related epilepsy
(2) additional EMG channels, particularly anterior tibialis, to detect periodic limb movements of sleep and parasomnias such as RBD
(3) airflow
(4) electrocardiography
(5) pulse oximetry
(6) abdominal and thoracic respiratory efforts
(7) snorogram: sound recordings to measure snoring
(8) position: monitored utilizing position sensors or direct observation by the technologist.

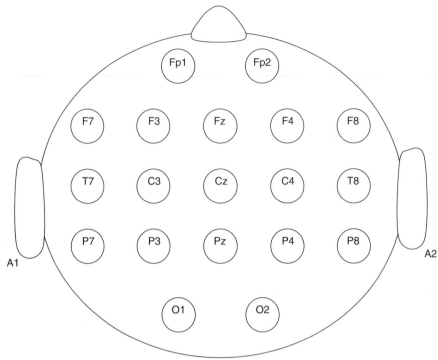

Fig. 2.6. The 10–20 system is an internationally standardized method to record the spontaneous EEG. It refers to the 10% and 20% inter-electrode distances. When recording a more detailed EEG with more electrodes, extra electrodes are added, utilizing the spaces in between the existing 10–20 system. F, frontal lobe; T, temporal lobe; C, central lobe; P, parietal lobe; O, occipital lobe; Fp, frontal polar. Even electrode numbers (2, 4, 6, 8) refer to the right hemisphere and odd electrode numbers (1, 3, 5, 7) refer to the left hemisphere. The smaller the number, the closer the position to the midline, and Z refers to an electrode placed on the midline.

Optional parameters include the following:
(1) Continuous video monitoring of unusual nocturnal events or seizures.
(2) Esophageal pressure (PES) monitoring, for the evaluation of upper airway resistance syndrome. Esophageal manometry is the measurement of esophageal pressure and provides a reflection of intrathoracic pressure fluctuations associated with breathing efforts.
(3) Nasal cannula-pressure transducer systems are useful in the detection of increased respiratory effort by its effects on the inspiratory airflow wave contour.
(4) Nocturnal penile tumescence, for the assessment of erectile dysfunction.
(5) Esophageal–gastric pH at various esophageal levels.
(6) Carbon dioxide (CO_2) monitoring may be indicated in the assessment of sleep-related hypoventilation and for the evaluation of sleep-disordered breathing in children.

Basic sleep architecture terms are defined as follows:
- Lights out: the beginning of sleep recording
- Lights on: the end of sleep recording
- Recorded time or total bedtime (TBT): time from lights out to lights on
- TST: total sleep time, the sum of all recorded sleep time in minutes
- Sleep efficiency: (TST/TBT) × 100
- WASO: wake after sleep onset
- Sleep latency: time from lights out to the first epoch of recorded sleep
- REM latency: time from the first epoch of sleep to the first epoch of REM sleep.

Figure 2.6 demonstrates the proper EEG electrode placement montage according to the 10–20 system. Figure 2.7 shows a typical recording from the nocturnal polysomnogram, demonstrating an obstructive respiratory event.

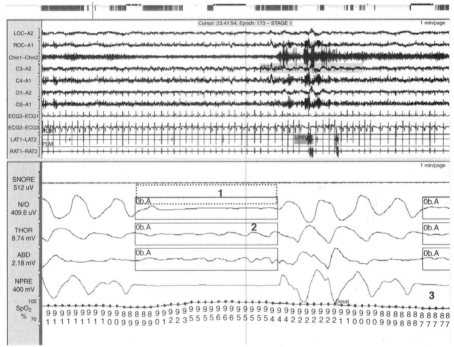

Fig. 2.7. A 60-second sleep epoch from a diagnostic polysomnogram (PSG) of a 71-year-old obese male who presented with a 7-year history of loud snoring and apneas witnessed by his wife. This figure illustrates obstructive sleep apnea characterized by nasal-oral (N/O) breathing cessation (dashed box 1) in the presence of persistent respiratory effort (2), and hypoxemia (3). Snoring was noted electrographically and heard by the monitoring technicians. Channels are as follows: electrooculogram (left, LOC–A2; right, ROC–A1), chin EMG (Chin1–Chin2), EEG (left central, C3–A2; right central, C4–A1; left occipital, O1–A2; right occipital, O2–A1), electrocardiogram (ECG), limb EMG (left leg, LAT; right leg, RAT), snoring (SNORE), nasal-oral airflow (N/O), respiratory effort (thoracic, THOR; abdominal, ABD), nasal pressure (NPRE), and oxygen saturation (SpO2).

Multiple sleep latency test (MSLT) and maintenance of wakefulness test (MWT)

It is suggested that the assessment of sleepiness or wakefulness should involve a comprehensive integration of findings from the clinical history, along with objective data from the MSLT or the MWT. Absence of sleepiness on these tests should not be taken to imply that a person does not have sleepiness.

Indications for use of the MSLT

(1) In a person with suspected narcolepsy, to confirm the diagnosis of narcolepsy.
(2) In a person with suspected idiopathic hypersomnia, to help differentiate idiopathic hypersomnia from narcolepsy.
(3) The MSLT is not typically needed in the diagnosis of obstructive sleep apnea or in the assessment of sleepiness in medical and neurological disorders (other than narcolepsy), insomnia, or circadian rhythm abnormalities.
(4) Repeat MSLT testing may be indicated in circumstances where an initial test might have been affected by extraneous factors or when appropriate study conditions were not present during initial testing, when ambiguous or uninterpretable findings were present, or when narcolepsy was suspected but earlier tests did not provide polygraphic confirmation.

Indications for use of the MWT

(1) The MWT may be used in the assessment of an individual's ability to remain awake when his or her inability to remain awake constitutes a public or personal safety issue.
(2) The MWT may be indicated in persons with excessive sleepiness to assess response to treatment.

Sleep hypnogram

Shown in Fig. 2.8 is a sample sleep hypnogram. On the vertical axis, the graph may depict the sleep stages (wake, stages 1–4, slow wave, REM, awakenings), respiratory data (number of obstructive, central, mixed apneas, hypopneas, and oxygen desaturations), position during the night, periodic leg movements, all against a horizontal axis depicting time (usually in 1-hour intervals).

Conclusion

Sleeping well is important for a good quality of life. There are many sleep disorders that can cause sleep disruption, resulting in daytime dysfunction. A significant overlap exists among sleep disorders, chronic medical and psychiatric conditions. Many people have problems with sleep due to chronic conditions and the associated

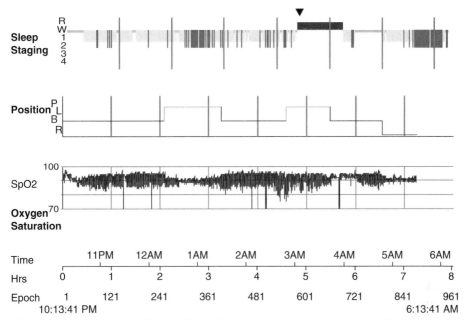

Fig. 2.8. A sleep hypnogram from a diagnostic polysomnogram of a 71-year-old obese male with a history of loud snoring and apneas witnessed by his wife. The sleep hypnograms summarize a recorded night of sleep. Sleep staging shows stage R (REM), W (wake), and stages 1, 2, 3, 4. Position of the patient during the study shows P (prone), L (left), B (back), R (right). In this study oxygen saturation is clearly worse during supine and REM sleep, and is as low as 75%. Time is indicated by increments of one hour beginning at 22:13 and ending at 06:13. Notable in this patient is the absence of slow-wave sleep (stages 1 and 2, SWS), sleep fragmentation caused by severe obstructive sleep apnea (as illustrated in Fig. 2.7), and delayed REM sleep latency noted by ▼.

treatment for each. A comprehensive sleep history and a focused physical examination can help identify potential sleep disorders and help determine the proper testing and treatment.

FURTHER READING

Agnew HW, Webb WB, Williams RL. The first-night effect: an EEG study of sleep. *Psychophysiology* 1966; **2**: 263–6.

Aldrich MS. Approach to the patient with disordered sleep. In: Kryger MH, Roth T, Dement WC, eds. *Principles and Practice of Sleep Medicine*, 3rd edn. Philadelphia, PA: Saunders, 2000: 521–5.

Allen RP, Earley CJ. Restless legs syndrome: a review of clinical and pathophysiologic features. *J Clin Neurophysiol* 2001; **18**: 128–47.

Allen RP, Picchietti D, Hening WA, Trenkwalder C, Walters AS, Montplaisi J. Restless legs syndrome: diagnostic criteria, special considerations, and epidemiology. A report from the restless legs syndrome diagnosis and epidemiology workshop at the National Institutes of Health. *Sleep Med* 2003; **4**: 101–19.

American Academy of Sleep Medicine. *The International Classification of Sleep Disorders*: *Diagnostic and Coding Manual*, 2nd edn (ICSD-2). Westchester, IL: American Academy of Sleep Medicine, 2005.

Arand D, Bonnet M, Hurwitz T, *et al.* The clinical use of the MSLT and MWT. *Sleep* 2005; **28**: 123–44.

Arzt M, Young T, Finn L, Skatrud JB, Bradley TD. Association of sleep-disordered breathing and the occurrence of stroke. *Am J Respir Crit Care Med* 2005; **172**: 1447–51.

Carskadon MA, Dement WC, Mitler MM, *et al.* Guidelines for the multiple sleep latency test (MSLT): a standard measure of sleepiness. *Sleep* 1986; **9**: 519–24.

Chervin RD, Aldrich MS, Pickett R, Guilleminault C. Comparison of the results of the Epworth Sleepiness Scale and the Multiple Sleep Latency Test. *J Psychosom Res* 1997; **42**: 145–55.

Chervin RD, Murman DL, Malow BA, Totten V. Cost-utility of three approaches to the diagnosis of sleep apnea: polysomnography, home testing and empirical therapy. *Ann Intern Med* 1999; **130**: 496–505.

Chesson AL Jr, Berry RB, Pack A. Practice parameters for the use of portable monitoring devices in the investigation of suspected obstructive sleep apnea in adults. *Sleep* 2003; **26**: 907–13.

Cizza G, Skarulis M, Mignot E. A link between short sleep and obesity: building the evidence for causation. *Sleep* 2005; **28**: 1217–20.

Dittner AJ, Wessely SC, Brown RG. The assessment of fatigue: a practical guide for clinicians and researchers. *Psychosom Res* 2004; **56**: 157–70.

Dixon JB, Schachter LM, O'Brien PE. Predicting sleep apnea and excessive daytime sleepiness in the severely obese: indicators for polysomnography. *Chest* 2003; **123**: 1134–41.

Doghramji K, Mitler MM, Sangal RB, *et al.* A normative study of the maintenance of wakefulness test (MWT). *Electroencephalogr Clin Neurophysiol* 1997; **103**: 554–62.

Driver HS, McLean H, Kumar DV, *et al.* The influence of the menstrual cycle on upper airway resistance and breathing during sleep. *Sleep* 2005; **28**: 449–56.

Foldvary-Schaefer N, Grigg-Damberger M. Sleep and epilepsy: what we know, don't know, and need to know. *J Clin Neurophysiol* 2006; **23**: 4–20.

Franklin KA, Holmgren PA, Jonsson F, *et al.* Snoring, pregnancy-induced hypertension, and growth retardation of the fetus. *Chest* 2000; **117**: 137–41.

Friedman M, Ibrahim H, Bass L. Clinical staging for sleep-disordered breathing. *Otolaryngol Head Neck Surg* 2002; **127**: 13–21.

Goldberg AN, Schwab RJ. Identifying the patient with sleep apnea: upper airway assessment and physical examination. *Otolaryngol Clin North Am* 1998; **31**: 919–30.

Hauri PJ, Olmstead EM. Reverse first night effect in insomnia. *Sleep* 1989; **12**: 97–105.

Hening W. The clinical neurophysiology of the restless legs syndrome and periodic limb movements. Part I: diagnosis, assessment, and characterization. *Clin Neurophysiol* 2004; **115**: 1965–74.

Herscovitch J, Broughton R. Sensitivity of the Stanford sleepiness scale to the effects of the cumulative partial sleep deprivation and recovery oversleeping. *Sleep* 1981; **4**: 83–91.

Hoddes E, Dement W, Zarcone V. The development and use of the Stanford Sleepiness Scale [abstract]. *Psychophysiology* 1972; **9**: 150.

Hoffstein V. Snoring. In: Kryger MH, Roth T, Dement WC, eds. *Principles and Practice of Sleep Medicine*, 3rd edn. Philadelphia, PA: Saunders, 2000: 813–26.

Ip MS, Lam B, Ng MM, *et al.* Obstructive sleep apnea is independently associated with insulin resistance. *Am J Respir Crit Care Med* 2002; **165**: 670–6.

Iranzo A, Molinuevo JL, Santamaria J, *et al.* Rapid-eye-movement sleep behaviour disorder as an early marker for a neurodegenerative disorder: a descriptive study. *Lancet Neurol* 2006; **5**: 572–7.

Jasper HH. The 10–20 electrode system of the International Federation. *Electroencephalogr Clin Neurophysiol* 1958; **10**: 370–5.

Johns M, Hocking B. Daytime sleepiness and sleep habits of Australian workers. *Sleep* 1997; **20**: 844–9.

Johns MW. A new method for measuring daytime sleepiness: The Epworth sleepiness scale. *Sleep* 1991; **14**: 540–5.

Johns MW. Reliability and factor analysis of the Epworth Sleepiness Scale. *Sleep* 1992; **15**: 376–81.

Krupp LB, LaRocca NG, Muir-Nash J, Steinberg AD. The fatigue severity scale: application to patients with multiple sclerosis and systemic lupus erythematosus. *Arch Neurol* 1989; **46**: 1121–3.

Kushida CA, Littner MR, Morgenthaler T, *et al.* Practice parameters for the indications for polysomnography and related procedures: an update for 2005. *Sleep* 2005; **28**: 499–521.

Le Bon O, Hoffmann G, Tecco J, *et al.* Mild to moderate sleep respiratory events: one negative night may not be enough. *Chest* 2000; **118**: 353–9.

Liistro G, Rombaux P, Belge C, *et al.* High Mallampati score and nasal obstruction are associated risk factors for obstructive sleep apnoea. *Eur Respir J* 2003; **21**: 248–52.

Littner M, Kushida CA, Anderson WM, *et al.* Practice parameters for the role of actigraphy in the study of sleep and circadian rhythms: an update for 2002. *Sleep* 2003; **26**: 337–41.

Mallampati SR, Gatt SP, Gugino LD, *et al.* A clinical sign to predict difficult tracheal intubation: a prospective study. *Can Anaesth Soc J* 1985; **32**: 429–34.

Manconi M, Govoni V, De Vito A, *et al.* Restless legs syndrome and pregnancy. *Neurology* 2004; **63**: 1065–9.

McConnell CF, Bretz KM, Dwyer WO. Falling asleep at the wheel: a close look at 1,269 fatal and serious injury-producing crashes. *Behav Sleep Med* 2003; **1**: 171–83.

Meyer TJ, Eveloff SE, Kline LR, Millman RP. One negative polysomnogram does not exclude obstructive sleep apnea. *Chest* 1993; **103**: 756–60.

National Institutes of Health State of the Science Conference statement on Manifestations and Management of Chronic Insomnia in Adults, June 13–15, 2005. *Sleep* 2005; **28**: 1049–57.

Nuckton TJ, Glidden DV, Browner WS, Claman DM. Physical examination: Mallampati score as an independent predictor of obstructive sleep apnea. *Sleep* 2006; **29**: 903–8.

Ohayon MM, Caulet M, Priest RG. Violent behavior during sleep. *J Clin Psychiatry* 1997; **58**: 369–76.

Parish JM, Somers VK. Obstructive sleep apnea and cardiovascular disease. *Mayo Clin Proc* 2004; **79**: 1036–46.

Pien GW, Fife D, Pack AI, Nkwuo JE, Schwab RJ. Changes in symptoms of sleep-disordered breathing during pregnancy. *Sleep* 2005; **28**: 1299–305.

Raizen DM, Mason TB, Pack AI. Genetic basis for sleep regulation and sleep disorders. *Semin Neurol* 2006; **26**: 467–83.

Rechtschaffen A, Kales A. *A Manual of Standardized Terminology, Techniques and Scoring System for Sleep Stages of Human Subjects.* Los Angeles, CA: UCLA Brain Information Service/Brain Research Institute, 1968.

Riedel BW, Winfield CF, Lichstein KL. First night effect and reverse first night effect in older adults with primary insomnia: does anxiety play a role? *Sleep Med* 2001; **2**: 125–33.

Rowley JA, Zhou XS, Diamond MP, Badr MS. The determinants of the apnea threshold during NREM sleep in normal subjects. *Sleep* 2006; **29**: 95–103.

Schweitzer PK. Drugs that disturb sleep and wakefulness. In: Kryger MH, Roth T, Dement WC, eds. *Principles and Practice of Sleep Medicine*, 4th edn. Philadelphia, PA: Elsevier Saunders; 2005: 499–518.

Sharma S, Kurian S, Malik V, *et al*. A stepped approach for prediction of obstructive sleep apnea in overtly asymptomatic obese subjects: a hospital based study. *Sleep Medicine* 2004; **5**: 351–7.

Spielman AJ, Caruso LS, Glovinsky PB. A behavioral perspective on insomnia treatment. *Psychiatr Clin North Am* 1987; **10**: 541–53.

Standards of Practice Committee of the American Academy of Sleep Medicine. Practice parameters for using polysomnography to evaluate insomnia: an update. *Sleep* 2003; **26**: 754–60.

Wolk R, Shamsuzzaman AS, Somers VK. Obesity, sleep apnea, and hypertension. *Hypertension* 2003; **42**: 1067–74.

Section 2 – Sleep disorders

3 Parasomnias

Rosalia Silvestri and Irene Aricò

Introduction

Parasomnias, as described in the recent second edition of the *International Classification of Sleep Disorders*, are "undesirable physical events or experiences" occurring during sleep transition, during arousal from sleep, or within the sleep period. They correspond to CNS patterns of activation expressed through either muscle/motoric or autonomic functions. Therefore they may range from abnormal sleep-related movements to emotions, perceptions, dreaming, or behaviors. In the most complex forms even "basic drive state" may emerge, resulting in complex abnormal behaviors such as sleep-related eating disorder (SRED) or abnormal sexual behaviors.

The pathophysiology of the parasomnias does not rely on an altered sleep structure, and physiological sleep processes are not involved. Rather the concept that sleep and wakefulness are not invariably mutually exclusive states is the main pathophysiology underlying parasomnias. Yet they are included among clinical disorders due to the resulting injuries, and adverse health and psychosocial effects, which may affect the bed partner as well as the patient. The word parasomnia derives from the Greek *para* combined with the Latin *somnus*: events accompanying sleep. Parasomnias often involve automatic behavior, i.e., seemingly goal-directed, complex purposeful behaviors enacted without the conscious awareness and volition of the individual, who cannot exercise conscious deliberate control over his or her behaviors and sleep-related experiences.

Parasomnias could be subdivided by taking into account the motoric versus autonomic/sensory activation (i.e., sleepwalking, REM sleep behavior disorder, sleep paralysis, versus sleep terrors, nightmares, enuresis) or, as most recently preferred, according to the type of sleep they are associated with (Table 3.1).

This chapter will deal with the most common disorders, covering the appropriate diagnostic and therapeutic strategies.

Sleep Medicine, ed. Harold R. Smith, Cynthia L. Comella, and Birgit Högl. Published by Cambridge University Press. © Cambridge University Press 2008.

Table 3.1. *Types of parasomnias.*

Disorders of arousal (from NREM sleep):
Confusional arousals
Sleepwalking
Sleep terrors
Parasomnias associated with REM sleep:
REM sleep behavior disorder (RBD)
Recurrent isolated sleep paralysis
Nightmare disorder
Other parasomnias:
Sleep enuresis
Catathrenia
Sleep-related eating disorder (SRED)
Sleep-related hallucination
Sleep-related dissociative disorders

Disorders of arousal

This term was first used by a Canadian neurologist, Robert Broughton, referring to the pathophysiology supporting those events characterized by incomplete dissociated arousal from sleep. They include sleepwalking or somnambulism, sleep terrors, and confusional arousals. Besides sharing a common pathogenic substrate (arousal from slow-wave sleep [SWS] with motor or sensory activation) they share other common features and often co-occur in the same predisposed individual.

Other sleep disorders may be comorbid and actually precipitate the arousal from SWS, such as obstructive sleep apnea (OSA), upper airway resistance syndrome (UARS), periodic limb movement of sleep (PLMS), restless legs syndrome (RLS). Disorders of arousal are often comorbid with other neurological conditions such as migraine, benign partial epilepsies of childhood, and attention-deficit/hyperactivity disorder (ADHD). They are most typical of developmental age and often interpreted as a dismaturative EEG/clinical pattern. However, they may persist or start later in life. In this case, or when lacking some of the most typical features depicted in Table 3.2, differential diagnosis is needed to distinguish from other disorders, especially epilepsy, dissociative disorders, and REM sleep behavior disorder (RBD). In this case, although not mandatory for simple diagnostic purposes, polygraphic recordings with extensive EEG and EMG leads could help the diagnosis.

Sleepwalking and confusional arousals

These disorders consist of a series of complex motor behaviors precipitated by arousal from SWS, often walking automatisms in a state of altered consciousness and impaired judgment. Episodes may be incomplete or abortive, stopping at the stage of confusional arousal with the person sitting up in bed, staring with a fixed gaze,

Table 3.2. *Typical features of disorders of arousal.*

First third of the night
Emerging from SWS
Typical childhood disorders disappearing post puberty
Strong familial trait
Usually benign (but be aware of potential risk of injury)
Sleep deprivation and sleep disruption are precipitating factors
Mostly non-stereotypical, non-aggressive behavior
Retrograde amnesia for event

C3–A2
O1–A2
ROC–A1
LOC–A1
EMG subm
O–N flow
Thor PNG
Abd PNG
EMGs tib R
EMGs tib L
EKG
Fp2–C4
C4–O2
O2–T4
T4–C4
Fp1–C3
C3–O1
O1–T3
T3–C3

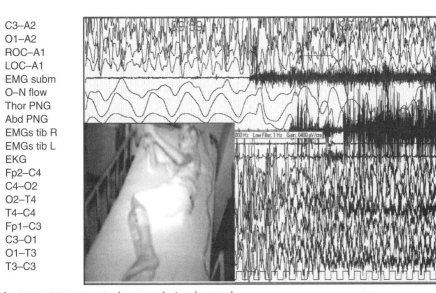

Fig. 3.1. NREM stage 4: abrupt confusional arousal.

performing bimanual automatisms or going as far as running out of a door or window, or driving for miles after getting up from bed. Subjects appear difficult to wake, often resistant and belligerent upon forced wakening. They may utter simple iterations or speak complex, often unintelligible conversations; they may entrain in complex routine behaviors such as eating (SRED); they may urinate or get involved in sexual intercourse, with different grades of amnesia following in the morning upon final awakening. Sleepwalking prevalence is high in childhood (17%) with no gender differences. Adult sleepwalkers (4% prevalence) are often males who persist in this behavior into adult life. The incidence of SW increases in proportion to the number of affected first-degree relatives, up to 60% with both parents sleepwalking. Concordance is highest for monozygotic twins. All-night video-polygraphic recordings show an intact sleep structure with an increased number of arousals and SWS instability as reflected by a higher CAP (cyclic alternating pattern) rate. The actual "arousal" response is more often described as a run of hypersynchronous delta waves intermixed with muscle and movement artifacts (Fig. 3.1). Type 3 arousal (low voltage, fast frequencies) are mostly typical of adult more complex and violent behaviors. Typically adult sleepwalking may also arise (22%) from NREM stage 2 instead of SWS. Precipitating aspects besides sleep deprivation include alcohol or cocaine abuse and, to a lesser extent, benzodiazepines, gamma hydroxybutyrate, psychotropic and anti-arrhythmic medications. Recently zolpidem has been reported as a specific trigger for SRED.

Treatment may not be necessary, especially during childhood for typical benign episodes. Generic precautionary measures to provide a safe environment for the subject are advisable, including avoiding high floors, unlocked doors and windows, and loose objects in the bedroom. It is also recommended that all sources of sleep fragmentation, and precipitating factors such as OSA, when co-diagnosed, should be treated by CPAP or other measures. Medications are used only when frequent long-lasting injurious episodes are reported: preferably benzodiazepines such as bedtime clonazepam 0.5 mg or diazepam (2–5 mg); alternatively trazodone and SSRIs have also been successfully employed, and most recently levetiracetam has been shown to be efficacious in suppressing disorders of arousal and normalizing sleep disruption in ADHD children. Hypnosis and psychotherapy alone or in combination has proved helpful in some cases, with cognitive behavioral treatment holding more promising results for children than for adults.

Sleep terrors

Sleep terrors represent the sensory/autonomic alter ego of sleepwalking, consisting of brisk SWS arousal accompanied by screaming or weeping with intense autonomic arousal and behavioral manifestations of fear. Dysautonomic features including increased heart and respiratory frequency, along with mydriasis, diaphoresis, and increased muscle tone, are prominent and immediately recognizable features. Episodes may be long-lasting and the child is typically inconsolable, with complete amnesia upon morning awakening. There is no gender preference and prevalence is lower than sleepwalking (1–6.5% in childhood, 2% in adults). Precipitating factors are as for other disorders of arousal, and a familial pattern of occurrence, although less definite than in sleepwalking, is observed. Psychopathology plays a role in the affected adult population, where a higher prevalence of anxiety disorders and bipolar depression has been reported. Diagnostic and therapeutic strategies overlap with those recognized for sleepwalking and confusional arousal.

Nightmares

Nightmares occur out of REM sleep in the form of terrifying dreams, usually in the middle or last part of the night. They are remembered by the individual, who usually wakes up suddenly with minor autonomic changes, in contrast to the distinctive and disturbing dream content. Nightmares usually start as early as age 3 and generally decrease in frequency and intensity over successive decades. Twin-based studies disclosed some genetic effects on the distribution for age and co-occurrence with other parasomnias. People with posttraumatic stress disorder (PTSD) show a high incidence of posttraumatic dreams spread out in NREM sleep across the night. PLMS is frequently recorded in both REM and NREM, and patients have a paradoxically higher than normal awakening threshold. PSG is not routinely performed, nor is it advisable unless a dissociative disorder problem arises. Differential diagnosis should consider night terrors, RBD (history of violent injurious acted-out behavior), nocturnal panic attacks (usually first part of the night), and sleep-related dissociative disorders including multiple personality disorder and dissociative fugues, during which, however, the subject is awake. Reassurance and cognitive behavioral therapy have proved useful in most cases. REM-suppressing antidepressants (SSRIs or tricyclics) may help, especially when a clinical depressive episode is comorbid.

REM sleep behavior disorder (RBD)

RBD is characterized by abnormal violent behavior emerging during REM sleep in the form of enacted dreams leading to sleep disruption and injury. The pathophysiology of RBD lies in a dysfunction of the brainstem structures modulating REM sleep. The disorder is in fact due to failure to suppress antigravitary muscle tone during sleep (REM physiologic muscle atonia) along with an excess of phasic EMG twitch activity during REM sleep. Enacted dreams are distinctively unpleasant, violent, and action-filled, while the enacting subject appears usually threatened or chased by confronting people or animals. The observed sleep behaviors are coherent with the dream content (isomorphism) and may include simple subclinical (groaning, laughing, screaming) or more complex (sitting, kicking, grabbing, punching, running) clinical behaviors. Walking is unusual, and vigorous violent episodes tend to progress in intensity and frequency to the point of injury to self and others. This is usually when medical attention is sought. Typical features of RBD are shown in Table 3.3.

The disorder exists in two forms: acute, from drug withdrawal (especially alcohol, delirium tremens syndrome) or intoxication, and chronic, either idiopathic ($> 40\%$), neurologic (48%), psychiatric, or endocrine. All medications potentially interfering with REM physiology are capable of inducing RBD reversible episodes. Among the most common are biperiden, caffeine, tricyclic antidepressants (especially clomipramine), SSRIs, venlafaxine, mirtazapine, monoamine oxidase inhibitors, selegiline, and cholinesterase inhibitors. RBD is often a sign or precursor of a neurodegenerative disease (Table 3.4), most frequently synucleinopathies, and may be a heralding sign of

Table 3.3. *Features of REM sleep behavior disorder (RBD).*

Typical presenting complaints	Demographics
Sleep injury 79%	Male 87.5%
Altered dreams 87.5%	Typical late onset (5th–6th decade)
Dream-enacting behavior 87.5%	Non-familial
Sleep disruption 20.8%	Often symptomatic of neurodegenerative disorders

Table 3.4. *RBD in neurodegenerative diseases.*

Disease	Percentage with RBD comorbidity	Reference
Multiple system atrophy	90–100%	Plazzi *et al.*, *Neurology* 1997
		Iranzo *et al.*, *Neurology* 2005
Dementia with Lewy bodies	72%	Boeve *et al.*, *Neurology* 2003
Machado–Joseph disease	55%	Iranzo *et al.*, *Mov Disord* 2003
Parkinson's disease	16–33%	Wetter *et al.*, *Wien Klin Wochenschr* 2001
		Gagnon *et al.*, *Neurology* 2002
Progressive supranuclear palsy	20%	Arnulf *et al.*, *Sleep* 2005

Parkinson's disease. Recently it has also been diagnosed in a large group of tau- and glutamine-related neurodegenerative disorders, as in the course of focal brainstem lesions such as stroke, tumors, demyelinating disorders, and in potassium-channel antibody-associated limbic encephalitis. RBD is also frequent in people with narcolepsy, even young women.

Many years before the clinical description of RBD by Carlos Schenck in 1986, Michel Jouvet described "REM sleep without atonia" in cats with bilateral perilocus ceruleus lesions, which could result in a spectrum of behaviors. Nowadays RBD is thought to result from impairment of the anatomic structures and pathways in the brainstem that modulate motor and affective components of REM sleep. The sub-ceruleus is still believed to be a crucial point in these connections but afferent and efferent pathways from the hypothalamus, amygdalae, PPN/LDT, periaqueductal gray, and medulla may represent equally important up- or downstream lesion sites.

RBD is the only parasomnia where video-PSG is mandatory for diagnostic purposes, to demonstrate REM origin of the episodes, sustained or intermittent loss of physiological atonia or excessive phasic muscle twitch activity of the submental or limb EMG during REM sleep, in association with sleep-related potentially injurious or disruptive behavior by history or abnormal REM behaviors documented during video-PSG monitoring (Fig. 3.2). Besides confirmation of these diagnostic criteria, PSG usually shows increased SWS, reduced autonomic activity during arousals, and increased percentage of PLMs during NREM sleep, infrequently associated with arousals.

RBD may be associated with different sleep disorders such as narcolepsy (both male and female subjects affected at a younger age, primitively or as a result of anticataplectic drug therapy), OSA (it can be an arousal-precipitating factor and suggest a misleading diagnosis), nocturnal ictal and interictal epileptic disorder, parasomnia overlap disorder (POD) when coexisting with disorders of arousal in adolescents or young adults, to the extreme of status dissociatus, where besides RBD occurrence the formal sleep markers are scanty and unevenly distributed so that definition of sleep stages and the demarcation between sleep and wakefulness

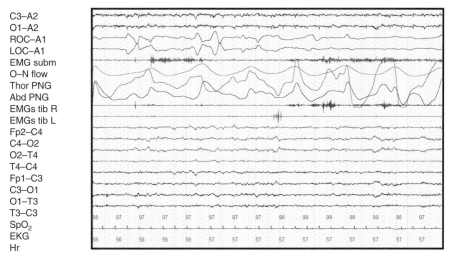

C3–A2
O1–A2
ROC–A1
LOC–A1
EMG subm
O–N flow
Thor PNG
Abd PNG
EMGs tib R
EMGs tib L
Fp2–C4
C4–O2
O2–T4
T4–C4
Fp1–C3
C3–O1
O1–T3
T3–C3
SpO$_2$
EKG
Hr

Fig. 3.2. An epoch of REM without atonia.

becomes impossible, as in fatal familial insomnia (FFI) with related prion disorders and delirium tremens. Current evidence argues against the existence of RBD as an idiopathic disorder. Recent studies have shown that in "idiopathic" RBD there are often subtle neurologic and neurodegenerative signs, including reduced olfactory function, praxic abilities, and visuospatial memory, and slowing of wake EEG frequencies. Furthermore, a presynaptic dopaminergic deficit resembling that seen in Parkinson's disease has been demonstrated consistently by PET and SPECT studies in "idiopathic" RBD.

Clonazepam is considered the standard treatment for RBD, although controlled trials are lacking. The dose of clonazepam is typically small, ranging from 0.5 to 1 mg. Melatonin in larger doses has also been reported to be of benefit. Other treatments that have been anecdotally reported include myorelaxant, administered at bedtime, or imipramine as a second choice. Levodopa and the dopamine agonists pramipexole and cabergoline have been employed with mixed results.

Sleep paralysis

Recurrent sleep paralysis refers to the inability to make voluntary movements upon falling asleep or awakening from sleep. The subject is typically awake or semiawake, and frightened by their vain efforts to move for seemingly endless seconds. While sleep paralysis is part of the classic narcoleptic tetrad, it may be seen in isolation and is equally common in men and women, often with a previous family history (20%). This is a common sporadic disorder, affecting up to 50% of normal people at least once during their lifetime. Episodes may be precipitated by sleep deprivation, emotional stress, and sleep/wake rhythm irregularities. Its pathophysiology relies on a state of REM sleep/wake dissociation likely due to a neurochemical dysfunction rather than a structural brain abnormality. Often, specifically in individuals with daytime somnolence, a full polysomnography plus multiple sleep latency test (MSLT) is recommended to rule out the diagnosis of narcolepsy. HLA typing can be additionally performed. When an episode is recorded by PSG, it shows wakeful EEG activity with muscle atonia and abundant muscle twitches and REMs. Treatment is directed toward improved sleep hygiene. If symptoms are frequent or severe, suppression of REM sleep by SSRIs or tricyclic antidepressants may be beneficial. If not responsive, treatment approaches used for cataplexy may be helpful.

Enuresis

This disorder consists of recurrent involuntary urination during sleep. It includes primary forms (up to 80% of all cases), where bladder control has never been achieved, and secondary variants occurring after a period of bladder control. Symptomatic enuresis due to kidney, bladder, and urinary tract abnormalities or infections or to neurological lesions is to be excluded from the parasomnia classification. The general prevalence is estimated at around 8% in healthy children aged 7–15 years, with a strong male preponderance. There is a strong familial trait for primary idiopathic enuresis, with 44% of those affected having one parent and 77% having both parents with enuresis. The disorder is more frequent among institutionalized children and often comorbid with sickle cell anemia, OSA, and ADHD. First-line diagnostic screening includes urinalysis and a comprehensive sleep and urinary history. Further workup may involve radiographic and cystoscopic examination, cystometric and sphincter EMG. All-night PSG is recommended only to evaluate the contributory role of OSA and disorders of arousal, and it should include a full seizure montage if epilepsy is suspected. Therapeutic strategies include behavioral techniques such as an enuresis alarm combined with positive reinforcement and retention control. Psychotherapy and hypnosis have shown highly variable results. Pharmaceutical options include antidepressants (imipramine 25 mg at bedtime), antidiuretics (desmopressine 200–600 mg), antispasmodics for children with detrusor instability (oxybutinin), and prostaglandin synthesis inhibitors.

Catathrenia

This disorder, also known as nocturnal groaning or expiratory vocalization during sleep, is a rare parasomnia occurring out of sleep stage 2 or REM in subjects with normal ventilatory effort and nocturnal SpO_2. It consists of the emission of an unusual expiratory noise occurring in bursts without associated motor phenomena. Affected individuals are often unaware but bed partners are disturbed by the unusual sound and report the episodes. Symptoms occur capriciously, are often long lasting and may have a familial trait. Differential diagnosis includes OSA, stridor, and nocturnal seizures, all of which may be excluded by video-PSG. Other than reassurance for the bed partner, there is no need for specific therapy.

Conclusion

Marked by the undesirable physical or experiential phenomena occurring exclusively during the sleep period or exacerbated by sleep, parasomnias represent fascinating experiments in the nature of state dissociation. They involve an admixture or rapid oscillation of the three primary states of being (REM sleep, NREM sleep, or wakefulness). Their study underscores the importance of close collaboration between clinicians and researchers to better characterize the already identified parasomnias and to be vigilant in the identification of new disorders that may still be awaiting description and explanation.

FURTHER READING

American Academy of Sleep Medicine. *The International Classification of Sleep Disorders: Diagnostic and Coding Manual*, 2nd edn (ICSD-2). Westchester, IL: American Academy of Sleep Medicine, 2005.

Arnulf I, Merino-Andreu M, Bloch F, *et al.* REM sleep behavior disorder and REM sleep without atonia in patients with progressive supranuclear palsy. *Sleep* 2005; **28**: 349–54.

Boeve BF, Silber MH, Parisi JE, *et al.* Synucleinopathy pathology and REM sleep behavior disorder plus dementia or Parkinsonism. *Neurology* 2003; **61**: 40–5.

Broughton RJ. Sleep disorders: disorders of arousal? *Science* 1968; **159**: 1070–8.

Gagnon JF, Bedard MA, Fantini ML, *et al.* REM sleep behavior disorder and REM sleep without atonia in Parkinson's disease. *Neurology* 2002; **59**: 585–9.

Hobson JA. A new model of brain mind state: activation level, input source, and mode of processing (AIM). In: Antrobus J, Bertini M, eds. *The Neuropsychology of Sleep and Dreaming*. Rahway, NJ: Lawrence Erlbaum, 1992.

Iranzo A, Munoz E, Santamaria J, *et al.* REM sleep behavior disorder and vocal cord paralysis in Machado–Joseph disease. *Mov Disord* 2003; **18**: 1179–83.

Iranzo A, Santamaria J, Rye DB, *et al.* Characteristics of idiopathic REM sleep behavior disorder and that associated with MSA and PD. *Neurology* 2005; **65**: 247–52.

Mahowald MW, Schenck CH. Evolving concepts of human state dissociation. *Arch Ital Biol* 2001; **139**: 269–300.

Mazza M, Faia V, Paciello N, Della Marca G, Mazza S. Sleep disorders in childhood: a review. *Clin Ter* 2002; **153**: 189–93.

Nielsen T, Zadra A. Dreaming disorders. In: Kryger MH, Roth T, Dement WC, eds. *Principles and Practice of Sleep Medicine*, 3rd edn. Philadelphia: Saunders, 2000: 753–72.

Ohayon M, Zulley J, Guilleminault C, Smirne S. Prevalence and pathologic associations of sleep paralysis in the general population. *Neurology* 1999; **52**: 194–200.

Plazzi G, Corsini R, Provini F, *et al.* REM sleep behavior disorders in multiple system atrophy. *Neurology* 1997; **48**: 1094–7.

Vetrugno R, Provini F, Plazzi G, *et al.* Catathrenia (nocturnal groaning): a new type of parasomnia. *Neurology* 2001; **56**: 681–3.

Wetter TC, Trenkwalder C, Gershanik O, Högl B. Polysomnographic measures in Parkinson's disease: a comparison between patients with and without REM sleep disturbances. *Wien Klin Wochenschr* 2001; **113**: 249–53.

4 Circadian rhythm disorders

Christopher D. Fahey and Phyllis C. Zee

Introduction

Circadian rhythms are physiologic or behavioral cycles which are generated by an internal pacemaker with an oscillatory frequency of approximately 24 hours. The most conspicuous function of circadian rhythms which have evolved in humans is the control of the sleep/wake cycle, with wakefulness commonly promoted during daylight hours and sleep promoted during evening hours. When abnormalities in the phase relationship between the endogenous circadian system and the exogenous light/dark cycle occur, circadian rhythm sleep disorders may ensue. Circadian rhythm sleep disorders are thus defined by this desynchronization and result in a sleep/wake schedule at odds with societal norms or work schedules, with consequent symptoms of excessive daytime sleepiness, insomnia, or an impairment of social, occupational, or academic functioning.

Six currently recognized circadian rhythm sleep disorders exist. The delayed sleep phase type, the advanced sleep phase type, the non-24-hour sleep/wake syndrome, and the irregular sleep/wake rhythm all entail a primary abnormality of an individual's circadian system. The other two circadian rhythm sleep disorders, shift work sleep disorder and jet lag disorder, involve an alteration in the light/dark or social-activity cycles of the surrounding environment which conflicts with the individual's intrinsic circadian timing. Considerable advances in the understanding of the genetic, physiologic, and anatomic basis of circadian rhythms have led to new insights into the pathophysiology of these disorders. This chapter will discuss circadian rhythms and the known factors which influence them as well as provide an update on the evaluation and treatments of the six circadian rhythm sleep disorders. Table 4.1 provides an overview of the clinical presentation and therapeutic options for these disorders. Figure 4.1 provides a graphic representation of each of the six.

Properties of circadian rhythms

The anatomic location of the mammalian master clock is the suprachiasmatic nucleus (SCN), a paired structure located in the anterior hypothalamus. The SCN regulates both the sleep/wake cycle and other important physiological parameters,

Sleep Medicine, ed. Harold R. Smith, Cynthia L. Comella, and Birgit Högl. Published by Cambridge University Press. © Cambridge University Press 2008.

Table 4.1. *A guide to the clinical features, diagnostic workup, and practical therapeutic options for the circadian rhythm sleep disorders. Listed bedtimes and wake times represent those times when the individual is allowed to sleep at his or her desired times. Melatonin is not approved by the US FDA, and there are no established clinical practice parameters for its use.*

Type	Clinical features	Diagnostic evaluation	Therapeutic options
Delayed sleep phase type	Key clinical concept: a delay in bed and wake times Bedtime: 02:00–06:00 Wake time: 10:00–13:00 Symptomatology: morning sleepiness, evening insomnia	Sleep log or actigraphy for at least 1 week DLMO and core body temperature minimum may be useful to verify a delayed endogenous phase	Bright light: 1–3 hours of 2000–10 000 lux upon habitual wake time Melatonin: 0.3–3 mg 5 hours before habitual bedtime Chronotherapy: progressively delay bedtimes by 3 hours every 2 days Sleep hygiene
Advanced sleep phase type	Key clinical concept: an advance in bed and wake times Bedtime: 18:00–21:00 Wake time: 02:00–05:00 Symptomatology: early morning awakenings, early evening sleepiness	Sleep log or actigraphy for at least 1 week DLMO and core body temperature minimum may be useful to verify an advanced endogenous phase	Bright light: 1–3 hours of 2000–10 000 lux before habitual bedtime Chronotherapy: progressively advance bedtimes by 3 hours every 2 days Sleep hygiene
Non-24-hour sleep/wake syndrome	Key clinical concept: a progressive delay in bed and wake times Symptomatology: sleepiness or insomnia which may wax and wane with time Generally seen in blind individuals	Sleep log or actigraphy for at least 1 week to verify a progressive delay in bed and wake times; strong consideration of longer monitoring should be given to clearly establish a progressive delay of circadian phase	Melatonin: 10 mg 1 hour before desired bedtime, 0.5 mg maintenance dose Structured physical and social activity Sleep hygiene

Table 4.1. (*cont.*)

Type	Clinical features	Diagnostic evaluation	Therapeutic options
Irregular sleep/wake rhythm	Key clinical concept: the presence of at least 3 irregular sleep bouts throughout the 24-hour day Total sleep time over 24 hours is age-appropriate Generally seen in individuals with underlying neurological disease	Sleep log or actigraphy for at least 1 week to verify the presence of at least 3 irregular sleep bouts	Bright light: 2 hours of 3000–5000 lux in the morning; increase bright light exposure throughout the day Create a favorable nighttime sleep environment: reduce noise, reduce light, improve continence care Structured physical and social activity Sleep hygiene
Shift work sleep disorder	Key clinical concept: a work schedule (either rotating or permanent) at odds with the individual's endogenous sleep/wake cycle which leads to symptoms of sleepiness and/or insomnia Symptomatology: insomnia symptoms which typically predominate during the newly desired sleep time; sleepiness which typically predominates during the work shift	Sleep log or actigraphy for at least 1 week demonstrates a disrupted sleep/wake pattern PSG may be helpful to rule out comorbid sleep disorders (e.g., sleep-disordered breathing)	Bright light: continuous or intermittent exposure to 1200–10 000 lux bright light during 3–6 hours of the work shift; light should be avoided in the 2 hours prior to the end of the shift; avoid light with use of sunglasses on commute home Melatonin: 3 mg before desired bedtime Behavioral strategies: create a favorable sleep environment, good sleep hygiene, therapeutic napping

| | | | Stimulants: modafinil 200 mg or caffeine to be used at the beginning of the work shift |
| | | | Treat comorbid sleep disorders, if present |

Jet Lag Disorder	Key clinical concept: a self-limited disorder associated with jet travel across at least 2 time zones	Further diagnostic evaluation is generally not indicated	Bright light: strategic exposure to light to either phase advance or phase delay depending on direction of travel; measures can be adopted both before and during travel
	Symptomatology: varies based on direction of travel and number of time zones crossed		Melatonin: 2–5 mg for the initial 4 days after arrival
			Behavioral strategies: good sleep hygiene, avoidance of alcohol and caffeine, sufficient hydration
			Short-acting hypnotic: may be appropriate for the first several days after travel

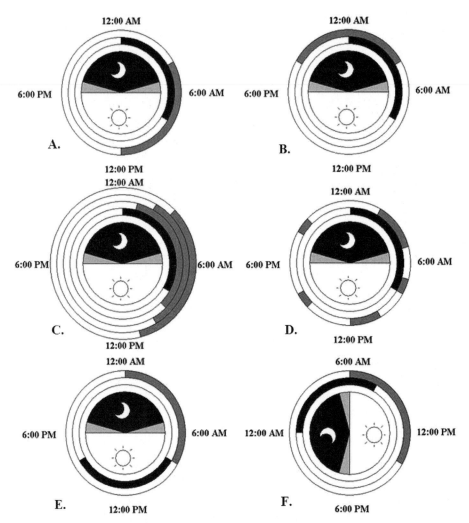

Fig. 4.1. A graphic representation of the circadian rhythm sleep disorders. Black arcs represent the conventional sleep/wake cycle appropriate for a typical work schedule. Gray arcs represent the endogenous sleep/wake cycle of the individual. (A) Delayed sleep phase type. (B) Advanced sleep phase type. (C) Non-24-hour sleep/wake syndrome. (D) Irregular sleep/wake rhythm. (E) Shift work sleep disorder. (F) Jet lag disorder with eastward travel across six time zones.

including temperature and the levels of various endocrine factors. The period of human circadian (Latin for "about a day") rhythms, are, as the name implies, approximately 24 hours. However, when humans are sheltered from time-giving cues, the precise period of their circadian rhythms has been found to be slightly longer than the 24-hour day, with an average of 24.2 hours. The difference between the 24-hour light/dark cycle and the 24.2-hour period of human circadian rhythms necessitates a means through which these rhythms can be synchronized. This synchronization comes about through the input of a wide variety of internal, behavioral, and exogenous temporal cues, termed zeitgebers (German for "time givers"). The most prominent zeitgeber in humans is the light/dark cycle. The SCN receives information on the presence of light through specialized ganglion cells present in the retina which transmit directly to the SCN through the retinohypothalamic tract. These cells have been found to be particularly responsive to light within the short-wave (blue) spectrum.

Light and other zeitgebers

As zeitgebers such as light are entraining agents of the circadian system, and the manipulation of zeitgebers can be used as a therapeutic tool for the circadian rhythm sleep disorders, a brief discussion of their specific effects on circadian rhythms is presented. When the SCN receives input on the presence of light in the evening hours, a phase delay tends to result, wherein a later onset of sleep times, wake times, and other circadian rhythms occurs. On the other hand, light received in the morning hours tends to result in a phase advance, wherein the phase of the various circadian rhythms is shifted to earlier times. These differing responses based on the timing of the exposure of light can be plotted on a phase response curve (PRC), where the circadian timing of the light exposure is presented on the x-axis and the magnitude and direction of subsequent response is presented on the y-axis (Fig. 4.2). Maximal phase shifts occur after light is delivered either directly before or directly after the core body temperature minimum, resulting in a phase delay or phase advancement, respectively. The practical aspects of phototherapy, including dosing, duration, and timing of light therapy, are presented under the circadian rhythm sleep disorders section below.

Melatonin is a hormone produced by the pineal gland, and it is a second critical zeitgeber of the circadian system. Its production and ultimate secretion into the systemic circulation is under the influence of the SCN, while its release is suppressed by exposure to light. Levels of melatonin are lowest during daylight hours and begin to rise several hours before habitual bedtime, reaching a maximum at approximately the time of core body temperature minimum. Melatonin acts to advance circadian rhythms, when delivered at night, as well as facilitating sleep onset. The PRC of melatonin can be envisioned as the body's "dark signal," resulting in the opposite effects to that seen to the PRC of light. Specifically, melatonin exposure in the evening hours leads to a phase delay, and exposure in the morning hours leads to a phase advance. However, the ability of melatonin to phase-delay the circadian system may be of a lesser degree than its ability to produce a phase advancement. Further, relative to light, melatonin likely results in a lesser magnitude of phase shift regardless of delivered time in non-blind individuals.

In addition to melatonin and light, physical activity also appears to be an additional circadian entraining agent, and when exercise is performed in the evening hours it results in a phase delay. Other possible entraining agents include social contact, bedtime and other social cues, mealtimes, and listening to music.

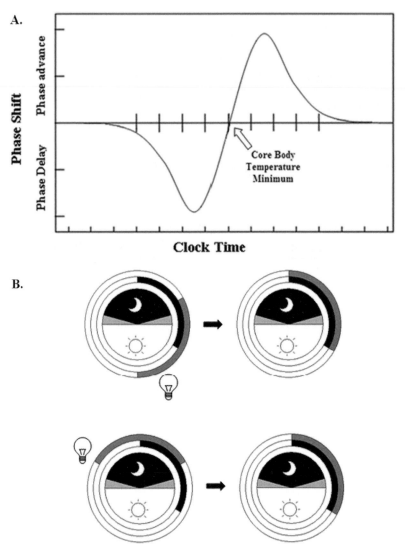

Fig. 4.2. (A) A schematic representation of the light phase response curve. Light delivered before the core body temperature minimum results in a phase delay, whereas light delivered after the minimum results in a phase advance. Light delivered closer to the core body temperature minimum results in a greater magnitude of phase shift. (B) Light given in the morning at awakening, after core body temperature minimum, results in a phase advance. Light given in the evening, before core body temperature minimum, results in a phase delay. The black arcs represent a customary sleep/wake schedule, and the gray arcs represent the endogenous sleep/wake schedule of a patient with delayed sleep phase type (above) or advanced sleep phase type (below).

Tools for the assessment of circadian timing in humans

For the purposes of research and clinical evaluation, it is often important to assess the timing of the endogenous circadian pacemaker and its relationship to the external physical environment (circadian phase). Measurements of circadian phase can be obtained through various surrogate markers of circadian rhythms, including the core body temperature minimum and the dim light melatonin onset (DLMO). Core body temperature reaches its nadir at around 2 hours prior to habitual wake time, whereas the DLMO occurs around 2–3 hours prior to the habitual sleep time (Fig. 4.3). Core body temperature minimum is typically assayed through the use of a rectal thermistor, which may prove unacceptable to some individuals.

In the past, melatonin could be measured either directly from plasma samples or through its major metabolite, 6-sulfatoxymelatonin, in the urine. However, plasma sampling requires an indwelling intravenous line, whereas urinary samples can only be collected every 1–2 hours, limiting the use of either technique. Melatonin is also present within the saliva, primarily in an unbound form. The development of more accurate techniques of salivary melatonin concentration has led to a convenient and relatively inexpensive means of estimating endogenous melatonin production and thus circadian phase. Regardless of the assay, it is critical to collect specimens in dim light conditions (30–50 lux) as melatonin production is suppressed by light.

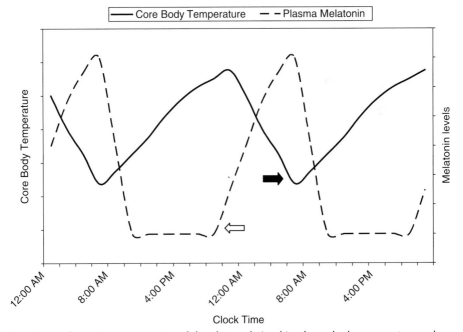

Fig. 4.3. A schematic representation of the phase relationship of core body temperature and melatonin levels over time in an individual with a habitual bedtime of 00:00 and a habitual wake time of 08:00. The open arrow indicates the dim light melatonin onset (DLMO), which typically occurs approximately 2–3 hours prior to habitual bedtime. The closed arrow indicates core body temperature minimum, which typically occurs 2 hours before habitual wake time.

CIRCADIAN RHYTHM SLEEP DISORDERS AND THEIR TREATMENTS

Delayed sleep phase type (also known as delayed sleep phase syndrome)

Clinical presentation

The delayed sleep phase type (DSPT) is typified by a stable propensity towards delayed (later) sleep onset and wake times (Fig. 4.1). When freed from societal constraints, individuals will generally initiate sleep between 02:00 and 06:00 and will awaken between 10:00 and 13:00. If an attempt is made to alter the sleep/wake schedule to correspond to societal norms, sleep-onset insomnia will often result, coupled with excessive daytime sleepiness in the morning hours. Subsequent impairment in daytime functioning as a result of the above symptoms may ensue. In addition to the subjective delay in sleep phase and otherwise normal sleep, the *International Classification of Sleep Disorders* (ICSD-2) has a criterion for diagnosis requiring that the stable delay in the habitual sleep period be confirmed objectively by a sleep log or actigraphy used over at least seven days. Other objective confirmations including a delay in DLMO or core body temperature minimum may be useful, but are not required for the diagnosis. The sleep disorder should not be better explained by an alternative disorder, whether it be medical, psychiatric, or related to the use of medications or other substances.

On questionnaires such as the Horne and Ostberg scale, a person with DSPT will score as an "evening" type, although most who score as "evening" types do not have DSPT. The key to differentiating "evening" types or "night owls" from those with DSPT is to recognize that "evening" types, while indeed preferring later sleep and wake times, retain their ability to conform to more conventional sleep/wake times without complaints of insomnia, sleepiness, or impairments in function. When sleeping at their preferred schedule, individuals with DSPT have sleep which has generally been described as normal when evaluated by polysomnography.

Epidemiology

Within the general population, the prevalence of DSPT has been reported to range between 0.13% and 3.1%. The male-to-female ratio has been reported to be as high as 10:1. Adolescents may be particularly affected, with a prevalence of between 7% and 16% reported. Of those presenting for evaluation for chronic insomnia at a sleep disorders clinic, between 5% and 16% have been estimated to be suffering with DSPT. Delayed sleep phase may also be seen after mild traumatic brain injury.

Pathophysiology

Although several theories as to the underlying cause of DSPT exist, both genetic and behavioral factors undoubtedly play a role. One particular theory holds that the circadian rhythm period of patients with DSPT is longer than the 24.2 hours seen in normal subjects. Over time, in the presence of an otherwise normal ability to entrain to exogenous stimuli, this longer period may result in a persistently delayed phase.

However, others have posited that an abnormality in the master clock's ability to entrain to light may lead to a DSPT-like phenotype. For example, an enhanced sensitivity to evening light or a diminished sensitivity to morning light may both result in an end result of phase delay. Behavioral factors, whereby patients remain active in the evening and stay indoors in the morning, may result in exposure to more light in the evening and less in the morning, worsening their already delayed phase. In addition to the circadian influences, homeostatic factors have also been recognized as a potentially important contributor to the pathophysiology of DSPT. There is evidence that following a period of sleep deprivation, people with DSPT have poorer recovery sleep relative to controls. Genetic differences between selected individuals with DSPT and those with a more normal sleep phase also play a role in the pathophysiology of the disorder. An autosomal mode of inheritance has been described for the DSPT phenotype, and circadian gene polymorphisms have also been linked with DSPT such as human *PER3*, *PER1*, 3111 *CLOCK*, and the arylalkylamine N-acetyltransferase gene, as well as a higher prevalence of HLA-DR1.

Treatment

The various standard approaches to the treatment of DSPT are directed at realigning the circadian phase of the afflicted individual towards a phase more consistent with societal norms. The principal therapeutic options, light and melatonin, take advantage of their respective PRCs to accomplish this goal through phase advancement (wherein light is delivered in the morning and melatonin given in the evening). Other therapeutic options, described below, may also be considered. An individualized treatment approach based on a person's individual circumstances and needs, as well as response and tolerance to therapy, is advised.

Light

Given light's robust ability to shift the circadian phase, the manipulation of a person's exposure to light represents a potentially important part of any treatment plan in DSPT (Fig. 4.2). Light's capability to advance the phase in those with DSPT is now well established. Most of the studies demonstrating effective phase advancement of light have used a lux range of 2500–9500 lux. The precise dosing of light needed for an individual remains uncertain, although a dose-response curve has been demonstrated. In clinical practice, light is typically delivered through the use of a light box using 2000–10 000 lux light. Perhaps, just as important as light therapy, the avoidance of bright light in the evening, either through behavioral strategies or through the use of dark glasses, should also be recommended.

There are several important practical considerations when using light therapy for the treatment of DSPT and other circadian rhythm sleep disorders. Although light delivered in the immediate period after core body temperature minimum results in the greatest magnitude of phase shift, the precise determination of this time point may be difficult outside of an academic sleep center, and awakening someone at this time may be particularly burdensome. Further, if individuals are instructed to wake too early without firm knowledge of their individual core body temperature minimums, light may be delivered upon the phase-delaying portion of the light PRC, exacerbating the problem. Therefore, in clinical practice, light is typically delivered upon awakening for 1 to 3 hours, both for convenience and to avoid the phase-delay portion of the light PRC.

Light boxes can be expensive, with usual costs of at least $200, with many models being considerably more expensive. If light therapy is to be used for a finite period of time, rental units are available. Ultraviolet rays are filtered by light boxes, and they are typically thought of as safe. However, side effects of hypomania, mild headache, nausea and vomiting, and self-limited visual problems have all been reported. People with ophthalmologic disease should be evaluated by an ophthalmologist before beginning light therapy, in order to determine appropriateness for therapy. Additional caution is advised in subjects with pre-existing mania, retinal photosensitivity, and migraine. In sum, although the exact length of treatment and dosing needed have yet to be clearly established, light therapy represents a potentially important instrument in the manipulation of circadian phase. The American Academy of Sleep Medicine also has confirmed the potential usefulness of light therapy on the basis of current level II and level III evidence. Finally, because light within the blue spectrum (at around 460 nm) is more effective than other wavelengths in shifting phase in young adults, short-wavelength light may potentially be more powerful than the commonly used broad-spectrum light sources. Therefore, blue–green enriched light emitters have become available commercially. However, it is important to note that there are very limited clinical data regarding long-term safety with these higher-energy short-wave light sources.

Melatonin

Nighttime melatonin is another useful tool in the treatment of DSPT, and its phase-advancing properties have been extensively studied. Although the optimal dosing and timing have yet to be established, doses of 0.3–3 mg given 5 hours before habitual bedtime are often used in clinical practice and appear effective. After cessation of therapy, many individuals return to their previously delayed sleep phase, perhaps arguing for the importance of maintenance dosing. Melatonin may represent a useful adjunct to light therapy, as the combination of the treatments appears to be more effective than light therapy used in isolation. Melatonin is not approved for the treatment of DSPT or other circadian rhythm sleep disorders by the US Food and Drug Administration (FDA), and the treatment thus represents "off label" use. Melatonin does have soporific effects, and subjects should be told not to drive in the hours after its use. Melatonin also possesses effects on the endocrine system as well as vasoconstrictive effects, and should be prescribed with caution to children or those with cardiovascular disease. In addition, melatonin may aggravate asthma. Finally, as safety data are lacking, caution should be exercised with patients who are breast-feeding or pregnant, as well as with those who are taking medications like anticonvulsants or warfarin. The use of melatonin receptor agonists, such as ramelteon, has yet to be studied, but may represent a therapeutic option in the future.

Other therapeutic approaches

Chronotherapy involves a progressive further delay of bed and wake times until the desired sleep/wake times are reached. That is, instead of advancing the phase, which represents a shorter but more difficult "distance" to the desired sleep/wake schedule, a person delays his or her sleep and wake times by 3 hours every 2 days. Although success has been reported, the length of time required for successful treatment and the need for rigid compliance may preclude the use of this treatment modality in subjects who have occupational or social demands. Further, once the ideal sleep/wake times have been obtained, maintenance of this new schedule may be difficult for some individuals. Finally, development of the non-24-hour sleep/wake syndrome, with continuing progressive delay of sleep and wake times, has been reported following chronotherapy. If used, close follow-up with an emphasis on strict adherence to the chronotherapy regimen must be employed. Vitamin B_{12} was initially reported as an effective treatment in several case reports and series, but a randomized controlled trial did not demonstrate efficacy. Combination therapy, using several of the above-described therapeutic options, has also been shown to be effective.

It is also important to stress behavioral strategies in the management of DSPT. The maintenance of a regular sleep/wake schedule, once the desired sleep and wake times are obtained, is critical. In order to augment homeostatic drive, a regular exercise program and the avoidance of daytime napping may be useful. Even in the absence of formal phototherapy, subjects should be advised to avoid bright light in the evening and to maximize exposure to light in the morning upon awakening. Finally, if present, psychiatric disorders should be appropriately treated and the presence of various life stressors should be assessed.

In children and adolescents with DSPT, behavioral strategies are of particular importance. This population may be especially tempted to "sleep in" on the weekends, which may be an obstacle to successful phase realignment. As in adults, light should be avoided in the evening hours. In addition, melatonin has been reported to be effective in advancing sleep onset times, increasing total sleep, and decreasing school performance difficulties in children aged 10–18. However, melatonin is not approved by the US FDA within this age population, nor for the treatment of DSPT.

Advanced sleep phase type (also known as advanced sleep phase syndrome)

Clinical presentation

The defining characteristic of the advanced sleep phase type (ASPT) is an earlier sleep and wake time compared to conventional or desired sleep and wake times (Fig. 4.1). Sleep times of 18:00 to 21:00 are common, and excessive sleepiness may begin at earlier times, leading to impairment in functioning. Earlier than desired wake times between 02:00 and 05:00 occur, often even if the person attempts to delay his or her sleep times. Sleep is otherwise normal when subjects are permitted to sleep on their typical sleep/wake schedule. As with DSPT, the ICSD-2 diagnostic criteria require verification of the advanced sleep/wake phase through the use of at least one week of actigraphy or sleep log. Additionally, the sleep disturbance should not be better explained by other sleep, medical, mental, or substance-use disorders or medication use. As to be expected, an earlier onset of DLMO and core body temperature minimum are seen, which can be used to confirm the diagnosis. Not all subjects with an advanced sleep phase have ASPT. In fact, many are not particularly bothered by their sleep phase at all and have no consequent impairment in functioning characteristic of the circadian rhythm sleep disorders. As such, these individuals can be considered "morning types" or "larks" rather than ASPT patients in need of treatment.

Epidemiology

The prevalence of ASPT is uncertain, but it appears to be much less common than DSPT. In middle-aged adults, a prevalence of 1% has been estimated. A more recent estimate of prevalence within the middle-aged (40–64 years old) was closer to 7%. Within the general population, ASPT may be much less common. Thus, the prevalence of ASPT appears to increase with advancing age, although rare cases in the young have been reported.

Pathophysiology

As in DSPT, the pathogenesis of ASPT may be heterogenous, with behavioral and genetic factors contributing. By succumbing to their sleepiness at earlier times, individuals may deprive themselves of light that would otherwise delay their sleep phase. This lack of exposure to evening light may be compounded in older subjects with ophthalmologic conditions such as glaucoma, cataracts, or senile miosis. Other circadian factors such as a shortened circadian period have been demonstrated in a person with familial ASPT. In addition to a decreased sensitivity to evening light, those with ASPT may alternatively possess enhanced sensitivity to morning light, resulting in a greater magnitude of phase advancement. Homeostatic factors may also be an important causative factor in ASPT, particularly in older individuals. A mutation of the *PER2* gene has been described in familial ASPT, with resultant hypophosphorylation of the gene product. Finally, an autosomally dominant mode of inheritance has been described in several reports.

Treatment

In contrast to DSPT, the major goal of therapy of ASPT is phase delay. The use of evening light within the phase-delay portion of the light PRC represents an important therapeutic option. Chronotherapy has also been successfully employed, and behavioral adjustments are central to the treatment of the disorder.

Light

Light therapy used in the delay portion (i.e., the evening) of the light PRC may help normalize circadian rhythms in people with ASPT. Successful phase delay with the use of evening light therapy has been reported in several studies, and light may additionally improve sleep efficiency and total sleep time. Tolerance of light therapy may be problematic in older subjects and close follow-up is advised. Unfortunately, light at lower intensities may not be effective in delaying sleep phase. Additionally, relative to their younger counterparts, older individuals appear to have a reduced response to the generally superior phase-shifting properties of short-wavelength light, raising the question of the usefulness of light within this spectrum in the treatment of older people with ASPT.

Melatonin

Melatonin delivered in the morning should result in a delay in sleep phase based on the melatonin PRC, and, as such, it may be expected that melatonin may be a useful treatment tool in ASPT. However, data supporting the efficacy of melatonin in ASPT are lacking. Additionally, melatonin has soporific effects which may make morning usage impractical.

Other therapeutic approaches

Chronotherapy has been used successfully in ASPT, with progressive phase advancement of sleep and wake times by 3 hours every 2 days until the desired sleep/wake schedule is reached. However, the need for rigorous compliance, the length of the treatment, and the necessity for close follow-up again limit the utility of chronotherapy. Behavioral strategies also are important considerations in the treatment of ASPT. Once the desired sleep/wake schedule is obtained, maintenance of this schedule is essential. Further, bright light should continue to be avoided in the morning, and light exposure should be maximized in the evening.

Non-24-hour sleep/wake syndrome

Clinical presentation

The non-24-hour sleep/wake syndrome involves an endogenous period which free-runs relative to the 24-hour day, relatively unencumbered by many of the traditional entraining agents. As the circadian period is generally longer than 24 hours, people with non-24-hour sleep/wake syndrome experience progressively later sleep and wake times (Fig. 4.1). As time moves forward, these individuals will possess a sleep phase which may for a brief time be in sync with that of the 24-hour light/dark cycle, before inevitably delaying further. In fact, a key feature of the disorder is symptoms of excessive daytime sleepiness, insomnia, and daytime impairment which wax and wane as the sleep/wake pattern moves in and out of phase with the desired schedule. Other diagnostic criteria defined by the ICSD-2 consist of confirmation of a progressive delay in sleep and wake times through at least seven days of actigraphy or sleep log (Fig. 4.4), as well as the exclusion of other disorders which may better explain the sleep disturbance.

Epidemiology

Most of those with non-24-hour sleep/wake syndrome are non-cortically blind, as they have lost the capacity to entrain the circadian rhythm with light. Sleep disturbances are extremely common in the blind, with 70% complaining of some degree of

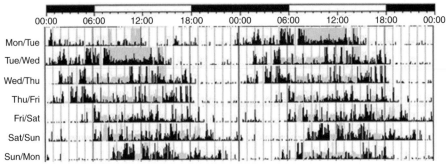

Fig. 4.4. Actigraphy from an individual with non-24-hour sleep/wake syndrome. The areas of higher amplitude represent periods of increased activity (that is, wakefulness), whereas those of lower amplitudes represent quiescence (that is, sleep). Note the progressive delay of sleep onset and wake times.

abnormal sleep and 50% suffering from non-24-hour sleep/wake syndrome. That being said, not all blind individuals have lost their ability to respond to bright light, as the specialized retinal ganglion cells transmitting information to the SCN may still be intact. Rare cases involving individuals with intact vision have been reported, including one posttraumatic case.

Pathophysiology

In someone who is blind, non-24-hour sleep/wake syndrome likely represents the absence of the entraining effects of light on the SCN. Circadian rhythms thus revert to the endogenous period, slightly longer than 24 hours. The pathophysiology within sighted individuals may be related to either a decreased responsiveness to the entraining effects of light or an exceptionally long endogenous period which falls outside of the range of entrainment.

Treatment

Successful treatment of non-24-hour sleep/wake syndrome is dependent upon the entrainment of the free-running endogenous circadian period. The use of light in the treatment of the disorder is generally not feasible and, as such, alternative means of entrainment must be sought. This is typically accomplished with the use of higher-dose exogenous melatonin, but the concurrent use of behavioral entraining agents is also important.

Light

As most people with the disorder are blind and incapable of entraining to light, non-24-hour sleep/wake syndrome is the one circadian rhythm sleep disorder where light therapy is generally not useful. Light therapy can be attempted in sighted individuals, given in a manner similar to that in DSPT (i.e., light delivered upon awakening). That being said, if the cause of the disorder in a sighted person is a diminished sensitivity to the phase-shifting effects of light, then results may be disappointing.

Melatonin

Melatonin, given at higher doses of 10 mg and lower doses of 0.5 mg, is an effective treatment for the disorder in blind people. In clinical practice, melatonin at a dose of 10 mg given 1 hour before the desired bedtime is often given as an initial dose, with lower dosages used as maintenance therapy. Particular import should be given to the timing of melatonin dose in relation to the individual's current sleep/wake cycle. Melatonin therapy initiated when the desired bedtime is within the phase-advance portion of the melatonin PRC may be more successful than when it is initiated during the phase-delay portion of the PRC. Melatonin can also be used to maintain a 24 hour schedule in sighted individuals.

Other therapeutic approaches

The establishment of regular exercise and social cues, as well as proper sleep hygiene, is an important step in effective treatment of the disorder. Another pharmacological option which has been reported in the literature is vitamin B_{12}. When given both with and without a concurrent hypnotic, vitamin B_{12} has been reported effective in non-24-hour sleep/wake syndrome. However, these reports are yet to be confirmed with randomized controlled trials.

Irregular sleep/wake rhythm

Clinical features

The distinguishing feature of the irregular sleep/wake rhythm is the absence of any discernible regular sleep/wake cycle. Although the total amount of sleep obtained over a 24-hour period is generally normal, sleep is broken into at least three different variable sleep periods (Fig. 4.1). The day is marked by erratic napping, whereas nighttime sleep is severely fragmented and shortened. Consequent symptoms of chronic insomnia and/or daytime sleepiness ensue. The ICSD-2 also requires the exclusion of other disorders which may better explain the irregular sleep, as well as at least one week of actigraphy or the use of a sleep log demonstrating three or more sleep bouts within the 24-hour day.

Epidemiology

It is thought that the prevalence of irregular sleep/wake pattern is rare. The disorder may be more common in those with dementia, particularly those who are institutionalized. Other disorders of the central nervous system, including traumatic brain injury and mental retardation, can also lead to an irregular sleep/wake pattern.

Pathophysiology

The pathogenesis of the disease may be related to a loss of neurons or other deleterious changes within the SCN or the hypothalamus. In fact, a marked diminishment in the number of neurons present within the SCN is seen in those with Alzheimer's disease. Also likely contributing to the disorder is the lack of appropriate light or daytime activity, which may result in circadian rhythms with lower amplitudes. Lower daytime light levels are predictive for an increase in nighttime awakenings, even when controlling for the level of dementia.

Treatment

The primary goal of treatment of an irregular sleep/wake rhythm is the consolidation of the sleep/wake cycle. To this end, measures aimed at restoring some degree of normalcy to exposure to the various zeitgebers are critical. Individuals with the disorder should be exposed to bright light during the day, and light should be avoided in the evening. Daytime physical and social activities should also be strongly encouraged. A combination approach using a variety of the available treatment options may be particularly effective.

Light

As many afflicted people suffer from a decrease in daytime light exposure, a keystone of therapy for the irregular sleep/wake pattern is increasing both the duration and intensity of exposure to light throughout the day. Bright light exposure delivered for 2 hours in the morning at 3000–5000 lux over the course of 4 weeks has been found to decrease daytime napping and increase nighttime sleep in demented subjects. Light may further help consolidate nighttime sleep, decrease agitated behavior, and result in stronger amplitudes of the circadian rhythm.

Melatonin

As opposed to the successful reports of the use of light in the irregular sleep/wake pattern, studies evaluating the use of melatonin in the disorder have been conflicting. As such, use of melatonin in the irregular sleep wake schedule is not currently recommended.

Other therapeutic approaches

Structured physical activity and social activity may help provide temporal cues to allow for more regularity in the sleep/wake schedule. Allowing for a favorable sleep environment by reducing nighttime noise and improving incontinence care may reduce awakenings caused by these issues. Other "common sense" measures of keeping a darkened evening room and keeping a comfortable temperature within the room can be considered. The use of a multidimensional, nonpharmacological approach including an increase in sunlight exposure and social activity during the day and a decrease in daytime in-bed time and nighttime noise may be particularly effective.

Shift work sleep disorder

Clinical presentation

Shift work sleep disorder affects either permanent or rotating shift workers who have consequent symptoms of sleepiness or insomnia, with insomnia symptoms generally predominating during the desired sleep time in the daylight and sleepiness predominating during working hours in the evening (Fig. 4.1). The ICSD-2 criteria for the disorder further require these symptoms to be present for at least one month in association with the work schedule, the exclusion of other disorders which may better explain the sleep complaints, and the use of actigraphy or sleep log to verify a disturbance in circadian rhythm or sleep-time misalignment.

After starting a work shift out of phase with their typical nocturnal sleep times, circadian rhythms adjust very gradually, at a pace of approximately 1.5 hours per 24-hour day, and many workers never successfully realign their circadian rhythms with their new shift work schedule. Further compounding the problem is that many shift workers sleep at their previously preferred "normal" sleep and wake times on days free from work. Over time, insufficient sleep may develop, as shift workers have been reported to accrue approximately 10 hours less sleep per week than those with more conventional work times. Sleep may be relatively deficient in REM and stage 2 sleep. It should be noted that the majority of studies of the disorder and its treatment have involved permanent night-shift workers.

Epidemiology

An estimated 20% of workers in industrialized nations work at non-traditional hours, and between 40% and 80% of these workers have at least some complaints of difficulty with sleep. The annual incidence of shift work sleep disorder among this population has recently been estimated to be about 10%. As such, shift work sleep disorder may be one of the more common circadian rhythm sleep disorders. Several factors appear to be important in successful re-entrainment to the new sleep/wake schedule. Those with a greater degree of domestic responsibilities, an older age, a morningness preference, and a longer commute time all appear to have a greater difficulty in adjusting to shift work.

Pathophysiology

Unlike the previously described circadian rhythm sleep disorders, shift work sleep disorder represents a change in the desired sleep times despite an otherwise normally working circadian clock. The consequences of shift work may extend beyond symptoms of insomnia or sleepiness. In fact, shift work has been associated with an increased rate of accidents, as well as depression, cardiovascular disease, gastrointestinal disease, and reproductive disorders. Additionally, shift work appears to result in an increased risk of the development of metabolic syndrome and certain inflammatory markers, independent of age or physical activity.

Treatment

The treatment of shift work sleep disorder is three-pronged in nature and involves the realignment of circadian rhythms, the promotion of alertness during the work shift, and an increase in sleep duration and quality. The realignment of circadian rhythms can be accomplished through the use of light manipulation or melatonin. Alertness during the shift can be addressed pharmacologically through the use of modafinil or caffeine and nonpharmacologically through the use of therapeutic napping. If insomnia is a prominent complaint, sleep can be consolidated with the stressing of appropriate sleep hygiene and/or through the use of sleep aids. Further, alternative causes for the symptoms of both insomnia and sleepiness should be explored. Finally, consideration of the safety of the afflicted individual, as well as his or her coworkers and the general population, is essential in all cases.

Light

Phototherapy delivered to the nighttime shift worker during the work shift has been demonstrated in multiple studies to facilitate daytime sleep and result in a quicker adjustment to the newly desired circadian phase. Light used during the work shift between 1200 and 10 000 lux has been reported successful when used both continuously and in an intermittent fashion. In addition to realigning their circadian rhythms, shift workers who undergo bright light therapy have improved alertness and superior cognitive performance. Light should typically be given during the first half of the work shift and should be avoided in the two hours before the end of the shift. In addition to exposure to light during the night shift, avoidance of light during the day, particularly in the morning drive home, may also be critically important in successful phase re-entrainment in shift work sleep disorder.

Melatonin

Placebo-controlled study of the use of melatonin in improving daytime sleep and expediting phase shifts has led to mixed results. Although an earlier study demonstrated improvement in evening alertness and daytime sleep with the use of melatonin at the desired bedtime, several subsequent studies were negative. That being said, melatonin at a dose of 3 mg before the desired bedtime remains a reasonable therapeutic option.

Other therapeutic approaches

For those individuals complaining of prominent sleepiness during the work shift, additional methods to promote wakefulness can be used. Modafinil at a dose of 200 mg taken at the start of each shift has been reported to reduce attention lapses and accidents or near-accidents in the commute home after a night shift. Importantly, this benefit may come without disruption of subsequent daytime sleep. The FDA has recently approved modafinil in the use of shift work sleep disorder. Caffeine at doses between 250 and 400 mg may also help improve alertness. Brief napping may also be helpful in promoting wakefulness when feasible. If daytime insomnia predominates, traditional hypnotic agents may be used to improve sleep initiation and maintenance, but these agents lack the potential phase-shifting properties of other agents. Healthy sleep hygiene is also important in the treatment of the insomnia associated with shift work sleep disorder. The reduction of disruptive factors towards a good sleep environment, including the elimination of noise and the lessening of domestic burdens, should be put into practice if possible. Given the array of available treatments and the number of social, behavioral, and occupational factors which can lead to difficulty in adjustment to shift work, an individualized and multifaceted treatment strategy should be pursued.

Jet lag disorder

Clinical presentation

Jet lag disorder is a commonly experienced disorder amongst individuals who traverse at least two time zones by air (Fig. 4.1). As the external environment light/dark cycle is now out of phase with the individual's endogenous circadian system, consequent symptoms of daytime sleepiness and insomnia may result. Additional complaints within 1–2 days of travel such as generalized malaise, somatic symptoms such as gastrointestinal disturbances, or impairment in functioning are also required for the diagnosis under ICSD-2 criteria. Eastward travel requires a phase advance, whereas westward travel requires a phase delay. Consequently, eastbound travelers often complain of trouble initiating sleep as well as awakening (similar to the complaints seen in DSPT). Westbound travelers, on the other hand, may have sleepiness in the evening, along with early morning awakenings (similar to the complaints seen in ASPT).

Epidemiology

The prevalence of the disorder is uncertain, but as it is generally self-limited, incidence assuredly exceeds prevalence. As the endogenous circadian period of humans is greater than 24 hours, phase delay is often easier than phase advancement, and travelers often report less difficulty with westward than with eastward travel. Additional to the direction of travel, an increased number of time zones crossed will lead to more severe symptoms.

Pathophysiology

Jet lag disorder involves a relatively sudden change in the surrounding light/dark cycle on the background of an otherwise normally functioning endogenous clock. Frequent jet travel may have more consequences than merely disrupted sleep, as a recent mouse model of "chronic" jet lag demonstrated an increased mortality in those mice exposed to frequent phase advancement.

Treatment

The successful treatment of jet lag disorder can involve strategic use of entraining agents when a traveler arrives at the destination, as well as anticipatory strategies in preparation for the upcoming jet travel. Maximizing and minimizing exposure to light at appropriate times can facilitate circadian phase realignment. Melatonin may also be effective when appropriately used. Finally, good sleep hygiene should be used, and hypnotics may be considered.

Light

With eastward travel, the core body temperature minimum will occur several hours later than it normally would in the new time zone. Consequently, avoidance of bright light (e.g., with use of sunglasses) in the morning hours, which could coincide with the phase-delay portion of the light PRC, is essential. Further, maximizing exposure to light in the late afternoon, after core body temperature minimum has passed, can accelerate the desired phase advancement. Rational use of light in the period leading up to eastward travel can also be helpful in achieving phase advancement. Here, the desired phase advancement should be achieved in the typical manner (i.e., bright light delivered in the morning). Westward travel results in a core body temperature minimum occurring hours earlier than would normally be seen in the new time zone. Therefore, staying awake and maximizing light exposure in the early evening (at the point of phase delay on the light PRC) is crucial.

Melatonin

Melatonin has demonstrable efficacy in treating the symptoms of jet lag, when given at a proper dose and timing. A Cochrane review, based upon 10 randomized controlled trials, concluded that melatonin was effective in reducing jet lag symptoms and that dosages between 2 and 5 mg when taken at the desired bedtime seemed to be beneficial.

Other therapeutic approaches

Hypnotics such as zolpidem can be used to improve sleep quality and length when given over the first few nights after air travel. A slow-release formulation of caffeine may be useful in improving alertness during the day after eastward travel, but subsequent sleep quality may suffer. Behavioral strategies such as good sleep hygiene, a regular eating schedule, and engaging in stimulating rather than sedentary activities during the day may also be helpful.

Summary

Circadian rhythm sleep disorders are commonly underrecognized in clinical practice and should be a part of the differential diagnosis of people who present with symptoms of insomnia and daytime sleepiness. The circadian rhythm sleep disorders are a diverse group unified by an intrinsic circadian rhythm which is out of phase with the external light/dark cycle. This desynchronization can be the result of a primary abnormality of the internal clock, internal desynchronization of circadian rhythms, or a change in the external environment in the background of an otherwise normally functioning internal clock. Resultant symptoms of insomnia and sleepiness may impair functioning at the occupational, social, or academic level. As agents which can demonstrably shift circadian rhythms, light and/or melatonin are effective treatments in nearly all of the circadian rhythm disorders. Behavioral strategies and other pharmacological options may be beneficial as well. Effective management of circadian rhythm sleep disorders thus requires a multimodal approach that combines sleep hygiene education, timed exposure to light, social and physical activities, and, in specific conditions, pharmacologic therapies.

FURTHER READING

Alessi CA, Martin JL, Webber AP, *et al.* Randomized, controlled trial of a nonpharmacological intervention to improve abnormal sleep/wake patterns in nursing home residents. *J Am Geriatr Soc* 2005; **53**: 803–10.

American Academy of Sleep Medicine. *The International Classification of Sleep Disorders: Diagnostic and Coding Manual,* 2nd edn (ICSD-2). Westchester, IL: American Academy of Sleep Medicine, 2005.

Barion A, Zee PC. A clinical approach to circadian rhythm sleep disorders. *Sleep Med* 2007; **8**: 566–77.

Bellingham J, Foster RG. Opsins and mammalian photoentrainment. *Cell Tissue Res* 2002; **309**: 57–71.

Burgess HJ, Crowley SJ, Gazda CJ, Fogg LF, Eastman CI. Preflight adjustment to eastward travel: 3 days of advancing sleep with and without morning bright light. *J Biol Rhythms* 2003; **18**: 318–28.

Czeisler CA, Allan JS, Strogatz SH, *et al.* Bright light resets the human circadian pacemaker independent of the timing of the sleep-wake cycle. *Science* 1986; **233**: 667–71.

Czeisler CA, Johnson MP, Duffy JF, *et al.* Exposure to bright light and darkness to treat physiologic maladaptation to night work. *N Engl J Med* 1990; **322**: 1253–9.

Dagan Y, Yovel I, Hallis D, Eisenstein M, Raichik I. Evaluating the role of melatonin in the long-term treatment of delayed sleep phase syndrome (DSPS). *Chronobiol Int* 1998; **15**: 181–90.

Dijk DJ, Lockley SW. Integration of human sleep-wake regulation and circadian rhythmicity. *J Appl Physiol* 2002; **92**: 852–62.

Eastman CI, Stewart KT, Mahoney MP, Liu L, Fogg LF. Dark goggles and bright light improve circadian rhythm adaptation to night-shift work. *Sleep* 1994; **17**: 535–43.

Fahey CD, Zee PC. Circadian rhythm sleep disorders and phototherapy. *Psychiatr Clin North Am* 2006; **29**: 989–1007; abstract ix.

Herxheimer A. Jet lag. *Clin Evid* 2005; **13**: 2178–83.

Lu BS, Zee PC. Circadian rhythm sleep disorders. *Chest* 2006; **130**: 1915–23.

Manthena P, Zee PC. Neurobiology of circadian rhythm sleep disorders. *Curr Neurol Neurosci Rep* 2006; **6**: 163–8.

Rosenthal NE, Joseph-Vanderpool JR, Levendosky AA, *et al.* Phase-shifting effects of bright morning light as treatment for delayed sleep phase syndrome. *Sleep* 1990; **13**: 354–61.

Sack RL, Brandes RW, Kendall AR, Lewy AJ. Entrainment of free-running circadian rhythms by melatonin in blind people. *N Engl J Med* 2000; **343**: 1070–7.

Shochat T, Martin J, Marler M, Ancoli-Israel S. Illumination levels in nursing home patients: effects on sleep and activity rhythms. *J Sleep Res* 2000; **9**: 373–9.

Weitzman ED, Czeisler CA, Coleman RM, *et al.* Delayed sleep phase syndrome: a chronobiological disorder with sleep-onset insomnia. *Arch Gen Psychiatry* 1981; **38**: 737–46.

Wyatt JK. Delayed sleep phase syndrome: pathophysiology and treatment options. *Sleep* 2004; **27**: 1195–203.

Wyatt JK, Dijk DJ, Ritz-De Cecco A, Ronda JM, Czeisler CA. Sleep-facilitating effect of exogenous melatonin in healthy young men and women is circadian-phase dependent. *Sleep* 2006; **29**: 609–18.

Zee PC, Manthena P. The brain's master circadian clock: implications and opportunities for therapy of sleep disorders. *Sleep Med Rev* 2007; **11**: 59–70.

5 Excessive somnolence disorders

Geert Mayer

Introduction

Excessive somnolence is characterized by the inability to stay awake during the desired wake period resulting in falling asleep in monotonous situations or developing unintended naps. Excessive somnolence can be a consequence of lifestyle, environmental and circadian influences, medical disorders, drugs or substances. When persisting for several weeks it is considered to be pathological, whereas it is a normal condition when occurring for a few days only, such as after sleep deprivation.

Excessive daytime sleepiness (EDS) is the term used for pathological states, defined as falling asleep in inappropriate situations and which cannot be controlled voluntarily. Between 4% and 9% of the general population are affected by EDS. The consequences on quality of life, performance, and concentration are dependent on the severity of EDS. The high socioeconomic costs of EDS have fostered efforts for early diagnosis and treatment. The underlying cause of EDS is determined by an assessment of multiple factors involved in the sleep/wake system. These may include environmental factors, lifestyle, genetics, inflammation, trauma, or tumor.

Sleep disturbances with EDS as the primary symptom have been classified by the *International Classification of Sleep Disorders* 2nd edition (ICSD-2) as "hypersomnias of central origin." EDS may also be a prominent but not primary feature in other sleep disorders that are classified according to their main features, e.g., sleep-disordered breathing or sleep-related movement disorders. Since the discovery of REM sleep, enormous scientific progress has taken place in the understanding of sleep/wake disorders, giving rise to modern treatment options. The recognition and improved classification of sleep disorders has led to a better understanding of specific clinical syndromes, allowing clear comparison among different studies.

Disorders of excessive somnolence are shown in Table 5.1. This chapter focuses on hypersomnias of central origin and arising from insufficient sleep. Other disorders that may result in daytime sleepiness are presented elsewhere in this book.

Diagnostic methods

Disorders of excessive somnolence can be classified in severity by subjective tests such as the Epworth Sleepiness Scale and/or by objective tests such as the multiple

Sleep Medicine, ed. Harold R. Smith, Cynthia L. Comella, and Birgit Högl. Published by Cambridge University Press. © Cambridge University Press 2008.

Table 5.1. *Disorders of excessive somnolence.*

Insufficient sleep
Narcolepsy
Idiopathic hypersomnia
Recurrent hypersomnia
Hypersomnia associated with
Neurological disorders
Psychiatric disorders
Internal disorders

sleep latency test (MSLT) or the maintenance of wakefulness test (MWT). Subjective and objective tests do not correlate well with each other. Clear cutoff scores have been defined within different ranges, and for the MSLT the ICSD-2 has defined mean sleep latencies of < 8 minutes as cutoff scores for narcolepsy and idiopathic hypersomnia. These pathological cutoff scores can also be found in sleep-deprived healthy subjects, however, underlining the necessity to perform these tests strictly according to the published guidelines. One of the purposes of performing the MSLT is the detection of sleep-onset REM periods (SOREMP). The ICSD-2 indicates that two SOREMPs support the diagnosis of narcolepsy, but other disorders associated with sleep deprivation may also result in > 2 SOREMP.

The diagnosistic certainty of hypersomnia associated with narcolepsy is highest when CSF hypocretin-1 levels are assessed. Narcolepsy with and without cataplexy has low hypocretin-1 levels. In contrast, most of the other hypersomnias of central origin have normal hypocretin-1 levels.

Narcolepsy

The term narcolepsy was coined by Gélineau in 1880. The symptoms of EDS, cataplexy, hypnagogic/hypnopompic hallucinations, and sleep paralysis were called the "narcoleptic tetrad" by Yoss and Daly in 1957. The symptoms of EDS and cataplexy are essential features. EDS in narcolepsy fluctuates throughout the daytime and is characterized by involuntary but refreshing naps of seconds to minutes. EDS generally is the first manifestation of narcolepsy, with cataplexy following after months to years. Cataplexy is a characteristic symptom of classical narcolepsy, with sudden loss of muscle tone without change of consciousness lasting seconds to minutes and triggered by personally relevant emotions. Associated features including sleep paralysis, automatic behavior, hypnagogic hallucinations, and nighttime sleep disturbance are common, affecting 40–60%, but these features are nonspecific.

Frequent complaints in narcolepsy

Cataplexy – "I was so excited about shooting the ball straight into the goal that my muscles went limp and I could not shoot the ball." (see also Fig. 5.1)

EDS – "I was so tired that I fell asleep eating with the fork in my mouth."

Sleep paralysis – "I wanted to turn around in bed on falling asleep and could not move or speak. I was getting terribly afraid this immobility would last forever. I could only move again after my wife noticed my condition and gave me a short slap on my back."

Hypnagogic hallucination – "When I was falling asleep, I saw decapitated animals entering by the open window – this has happened several times, and appears so real, that I have to get up every time to make sure the window is closed and everything OK."

There are several physical consequences of narcolepsy. Many people gain weight after the onset of narcolepsy, resulting in obesity, diabetes mellitus, and hypertension.

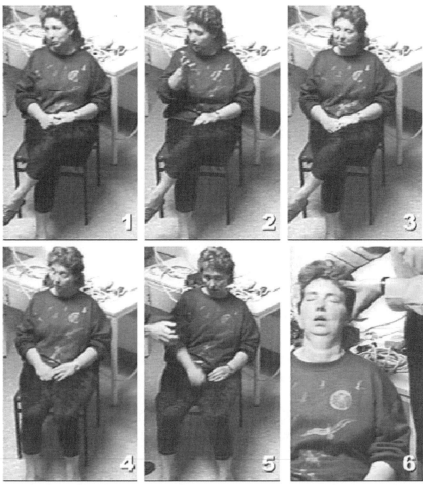

Fig. 5.1. 45-year-old female narcolepsy patient having a cataplexy episode: (1) talking; (2) describing an emotional situation; (3) eyes closing; (4) atonia of legs (cannot keep them crossed any more); (5) atonia of right hand (starting to drop); (6) atonia of neck muscles (head falling back).

The most striking comorbidity is the association with the parasomnias, especially nightmares, REM sleep behavior disorder and sleepwalking. These sleep disturbances highlight the disturbed motor control during sleep in narcoleptic patients.

Epidemiology and pathophysiology

The ICSD-2 categorizes three forms: narcolepsy with cataplexy, narcolepsy without cataplexy, and symptomatic narcolepsy. Narcolepsy generally begins in adolescence, but may manifest at any age. Men and women are equally affected. Narcolepsy is a lifelong disease with important psychosocial consequences for individuals with symptoms of moderate to marked severity. These people have to cope with familial, educational, and professional problems often leading to loss of relationships, social isolation, unemployment, or early retirement.

The risk of narcolepsy in first-degree relatives is 1–2%, compared to 0.02–0.18% in the general population. The risk for partial narcolepsy in family members is 5%. Narcolepsy has the highest HLA association among all medical diseases, with the association of haplotype DRB1*1501, DQA1*0102, DQB1*0602 being the most prominent. This haplotype is located on the short arm of chromosome 6. Two recent studies have revealed a locus on chromosome 21q just a few kb apart from each other.

In addition to the strong genetic component, an autoimmune cause has been theorized to be important in narcolepsy because of loss of hypocretin neurons in the laterodorsal hypothalamus. Thus far no specific antibodies have been consistently demonstrated, however. The cerebrospinal fluid (CSF) of patients reveals almost undetectable hypocretin-1 concentrations, and postmortem examination of the brain shows the loss of hypocretinergic neurons. Functional brain imaging has shown some areas of hypothetical brain damage. Spectroscopy has been more consistent, showing clear signs of thalamic neuronal degeneration.

Narcolepsy without cataplexy seems to be a phenotypic variant with a weaker association with the HLA haplotype and low CSF hypocretin-1 levels. In some cases symptomatic narcolepsy has been reported after head trauma, inflammation of the central nervous system, and brain tumors.

Diagnosis

The diagnosis of narcolepsy when all symptoms are present, including cataplexy, is based on the clinical findings. However, if there is uncertainty in the diagnosis, or if cataplexy is not present, a referral to the sleep laboratory for polysomnography followed by MSLT is necessary. The MSLT criteria include a mean sleep latency of 8 minutes or less with at least two sleep-onset REM periods (Fig. 5.2). The diagnosis may be supported by HLA typing, which is only specific in the presence of low CSF hypocretin-1 levels (< 110 pg/ml). Evaluation of attention and vigilance should also be performed in order to establish baseline values and to evaluate the effect of drug treatment. Different types of neuropsychometric tests assessing severity of the different symptoms may be employed. Brain imaging is required if ruling out symptomatic forms of narcolepsy.

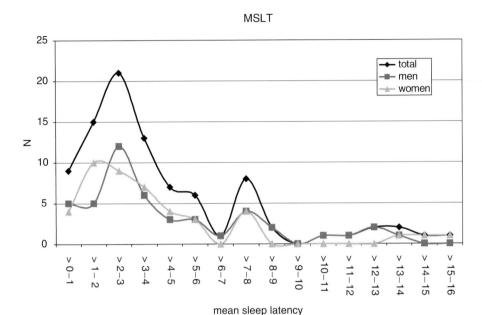

Fig. 5.2. Distribution of sleep latencies in 136 German narcolepsy patients.

The differential diagnosis of excessive daytime sleepiness and narcolepsy is extensive, as shown in Table 5.2. Many of these disorders may also present with two or more sleep-onset REM periods (SOREMP). In particular, these disorders should be considered in individuals suspected of having narcolepsy who do not have cataplexy. Because some of these may coexist with narcolepsy, a complete assessment is recommended.

The delay between symptom onset and diagnosis is prolonged when only EDS is present and short when cataplexy is present (Fig. 5.3).

Therapeutic options

Narcolepsy treatment should always include behavioral components. Few studies have focused on these nonpharmacologic approaches, which include scheduled napping, good sleep hygiene, and the development of support networks. Napping during the day may transiently improve alertness in those with EDS. Most individuals use nap strategies prior to driving or other performance that requires a high level of alertness. A regular sleep/wake rhythm seems to help people to cope better with EDS and nocturnal sleep problems. Other coping strategies include education of family and friends or establishing support systems through attending meetings of self-help groups. Behavioral therapy should always be considered alongside drug therapy.

Until a few years ago, each major narcoleptic symptom potentially had to be treated with different drugs. With the introduction of sodium oxybate, treating several symptoms with one drug became possible. Different recommendations

Table 5.2. *Disorders that may cause EDS and sleep-onset REM periods.*

Kleine–Levin syndrome
Idiopathic hypersomnia
OSA (obstructive sleep apnea syndrome)
PLMD (periodic limb movement disorder)
Restless legs syndrome
Chronic fatigue syndrome
Fibromyalgia
Infections, e.g., mononucleosis
Prader–Willi syndrome
Circadian sleep rhythm disorders (shift work etc.)
Psychophysiologic insomnia
Affective disorders
Depressive disorders
Psychoses
Sleep deprivation
Abuse of benzodiazepines, antidepressants, beta-blockers, neuroleptics, barbiturates
Alcohol abuse
Neurological disorders: epilepsy, Parkinson's disease, Huntington's chorea, myotonic dystrophy

and guidelines have been published on the treatment of narcolepsy. The following therapy options are based on these recommendations.

Stimulants

The most widely used stimulant is modafinil, followed by methylphenidate in most European countries or the USA. Modafinil is a compound with α-1 adrenergic effects and direct and indirect interactions with the dopaminergic system. It significantly reduces EDS, reduces sleep latency on the MWT, and improves the ESS and SF-36 (quality of life) scores. Four class I evidence-based studies have been published. Modafanil is usually taken twice a day at doses of 200–400 mg. The side effects include mood changes, irritability, palpitation, sweating, tremor, nausea, nervousness, headache, and insomnia. Abuse and tolerance have not been reported. Modafinil is an inducer of cytochrome P450 enzymes, and increases the metabolism of oral contraceptives such that effective contraception requires at least 50 µg ethinylestradiol. It is not recommended for use during pregnancy.

Methylphenidate induces dopamine release and has no effect on monoamine storage. Its elimination half-life is 2–7 hours, requiring two or three daily doses. There are five evidence-based studies with class II–III evidence showing improvement in sleep latency on the MWT, and improvements in the Digit Symbol Test and the Wilkinson Addition Test.

Gamma hydroxybutyrate (sodium oxybate) is an endogenous metabolite of GABA with an elimination half-life of 90–120 minutes. It is a neuromodulator of GABA,

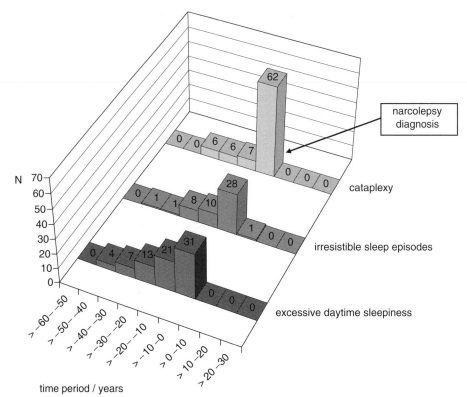

Fig. 5.3. Diagnosis depending on symptom onset in 98 German narcolepsy patients.

serotonin, dopamine, and endogenous opioids. One class I evidence-based study showed improvement of all parameters of sleepiness with two doses of 30 mg/kg. With sodium oxybate, 2.25–4.5 g given twice a night resulted in a dose-dependent reduction in cataplexy of up to 90%, improvement in EDS on MSLT, MWT, and ESS, as well as improvement of disrupted nocturnal sleep, with significant reduction in awakenings and wake after sleep onset, and increased slow-wave sleep. In Europe, sodium oxybate is only approved for the treatment of narcolepsy with cataplexy. In the United States, sodium oxybate is approved for cataplexy, EDS, and disrupted night sleep in narcoleptics. Sodium oxybate is well tolerated (side effects: headache, nausea, dizziness, gait problems when waking up). In combination with modafinil, sodium oxybate is more efficacious in EDS than when given alone. Abuse and tolerance in narcolepsy patients are not known. It has no known interactions with other stimulants or anticataplectic drugs. The dose has to be reduced in those with hepatic problems and carefully monitored in those with congestive heart failure due to the sodium load.

Mazindol has been withdrawn from the market in several countries. It is an imidazolidine derivative that causes a weak release of dopamine, blocks dopamine and norepinephrine reuptake, and has an elimination half-life of 10 hours. One class I and four class IV evidence-based studies have shown a reduction of sleepiness in 50–75%

of narcolepsy patients. In rare cases, mazindol may cause pulmonary hypertension and cardiac valvular abnormalities.

Selegiline, a selective monoamine oxidase B (MAO-B) inhibitor, at doses no greater than 10 mg per day, is metabolized to amphetamine and metamphetamine and may provide some improvement in EDS. Two class I evidence-based studies have shown a reduction in irresistible sleep attacks and EDS at 20–40 mg and a dose-dependent REM reduction. However, at these higher doses, the MAO selectivity may be lost, leading to potential sympathomimetic adverse effects and interactions with other medication (tryptans, serotonin).

Phenelzine is a rarely used nonselective MAO inhibitor that improves irresistible sleep at 60–90 mg. Its side effects are hypertensive crisis if a tyramine-restricted diet is not followed.

In Europe, the first-line stimulant for narcolepsy is modafinil, followed by methylphenidate and sodium oxybate. In the absence of reliable data, none of the stimulants is indicated during pregnancy.

Anticataplectic medication

The effect of anticataplectic drugs correlates with their ability to inhibit norepinephrine uptake, thereby inhibiting REM phenomena. This mechanism may also account for the potential of these agents to improve sleep paralysis and hallucinations.

Among the monoamine uptake inhibitors, clomipramine is the most widely used drug. It is rapidly metabolized into desmethyl-clomipramine, an active metabolite with adrenergic reuptake inhibition. One class I and four class IV evidence-based studies have shown complete suppression or decrease in frequency and severity of cataplexy with 7 mg/day. Adverse effects are dry mouth, sweating, constipation, tachycardia, weight increase, hypertension, difficulty urinating, and impotence. It has to be withdrawn slowly in order to prevent severe rebound cataplexy or status cataplecticus. Tolerance may occur. Teratogenicity is low, but there is a risk of atropine intoxication in infants.

Selective serotonin reuptake inhibitors (SSRIs) are more selective than tricyclic antidepressants. Higher doses than tricyclics are required. Two class I evidence-based studies have demonstrated a reduction in cataplexy on femoxetine at 60 mg/day. There is class II evidence for the use of fluoxetine (20–60 mg/day) and fluvoxamine, which are active in cataplexies. One study has shown citalopram to be effective in three cases of intractable cataplexy. The side effects include CNS excitation, gastrointestinal upset, movement disorders, and sexual difficulties. Tolerance has not been reported.

Treatment adherence issues

Most people with narcolepsy prefer to take one drug during the day, targeted to the symptom that impairs their lives the most. When multiple medications are prescribed, compliance is low as most of them are afraid of side effects, tolerance, and addiction. Addiction is not common in narcolepsy. Tolerance may develop in some individuals, but there is no evidence that regular drug holidays will reduce tolerance. Stimulants can be taken as needed. Anticataplectic medication has to be taken regularly, since sudden withdrawal may cause "rebound cataplexies" or even status cataplecticus. There is a need for careful education concerning drug programs and the need to adhere to therapy and monitor adverse events. Acceptance of the disorder is essential for compliance with medication.

Idiopathic hypersomnia

Idiopathic hypersomnia (IH) was described by Roth in the 1970s. He identified the subtypes oligosymptomatic and monosymptomatic, both forms being characterized by EDS. The oligosymptomatic form included prolonged night sleep with sleep drunkenness upon awakening and EDS. The ICSD-2 replicated this classification, renaming it
(1) IH with long sleep times
(2) IH without long sleep times.
The long sleepers have a sleep period longer than 10 hours at least once a week, with mean sleep latency in the MSLT of < 8 minutes and < 2 SOREMP. The daytime naps are usually unrefreshing, and sleep drunkenness may occur in one-fourth of individuals. In IH with normal sleep time, naps can be either refreshing or unrefreshing. Nighttime sleep may be restless with frequent arousals in half of those with this form of IH. The macrostructure is characterized by an excess of sleep stage 1 and a decrease of stages 3 and 4. Hypnagogic hallucinations and sleep paralysis are as frequent as in narcolepsy without cataplexy. Many IH patients suffer from psychiatric disorders including anxiety, irritability, fatigue, and depression. Whether depression is an associated feature or a consequence of IH remains unresolved. Half of the patients report migraine headache, syncope, orthostatic hypotension, and Raynaud-like symptoms, suggesting a change in the autonomic nervous system. As in narcolepsy, EDS can be stronger after alcohol intake, heavy meals, and intense exercise.

Examples of IH with long sleep times

"My mother wakes me up at least three times. I always answer her, but never get up unless she comes in and shakes me awake. By then I have forgotten about her prior efforts to wake me up."

"During my holidays I went to bed at 10 pm and woke up at 2 pm feeling tired. This went on for days in the same manner without me feeling more awake."

Epidemiology and pathophysiology

IH is a rare disease, with an estimated prevalence of 0.005–0.01% of the population. There is no gender predominance. Familial forms have been reported, with an apparently autosomal dominant mode of inheritance. Symptom onset is mainly in the second and third decade. Generally the disorder persists, although spontaneous remissions have been reported. Since clearcut classifications are missing for those individuals without long sleep episodes, phenotyping is difficult. The psychosocial consequences, although not systematically studied, are likely similar to those in narcolepsy.

The underlying pathophysiology has been addressed in only a few studies. The most comprehensive spectral analysis explains prolonged sleep and EDS by a reduction of slow-wave activity in all sleep cycles, especially in the first two cycles. Another study by Montplaisir found reduction in REM and slow-wave sleep. The permanent lack of slow-wave activity apparently causes long nocturnal sleep periods and EDS. The decrease of REM and slow-wave sleep could be the result of a dampening of the circadian rhythm. A significantly lower nocturnal concentration of melatonin and a phase delay of melatonin and cortisol by more than one hour support this hypothesis. The high number of arousals with increased REM density during nighttime sleep may add to the need for slow-wave activity via sleep fragmentation. CSF hypocretin-1 levels are normal and there is no HLA association, although there are conflicting data. Early studies found a change in the dopaminergic transmission with decrease of dopamine and indoleacetic acid in the CSF, but a reanalysis found a malfunction of the monoaminergic system. No animal model has been developed for IH. During sleep drunkenness, cerebellar signs such as ataxia and impaired motor coordination and proprioceptive hyporeflexia may be found. Neuropsychological testing during sleep drunkenness shows impairments that return to normal when the sleep drunkenness improves. During the time of sleep drunkenness, microsleeps may be recorded on polysomnography.

Diagnosis

The diagnosis of IH is based on clinical features. Medical history often reveals very nonspecific symptoms of EDS. Therefore IH requires completion of polysomnography, MSLT, and sometimes a 24-hour EEG to document long nocturnal sleep. If the MSLT is done without assessing the previous night's sleep, it may not provide sufficient evidence for diagnosis. Billiard (1996) therefore recommends performing the MSLT following a 24-hour polysomnography. HLA typing normally does not help with diagnosis. Neuropsychological tests should be done to exclude psychiatric disorders with hypersomnia. Brain imaging using MRI may be helpful if trauma or structural brain lesions are suspected. CSF analysis should be performed if narcolepsy is suspected. To rule out an upper airway resistance syndrome resulting in EDS, esophageal pressure manometry should be recorded during polysomnography in unclear cases.

Differential diagnosis includes:
- narcolepsy without cataplexy
- insufficient sleep syndrome
- sleep-disordered breathing
- PLMD (periodic limb movement disorder)
- circadian sleep rhythm disorders
- OSA (obstructive sleep apnea)
- hypersomnia associated with dysthymia and mood disorders
- chronic fatigue syndrome

- hypersomnia after viral infection
- posttraumatic hypersomnia
- long sleepers
- isolated sleep drunkenness.

Because of the similarity of the symptoms of IH and narcolepsy without cataplexy, it is not possible to accurately differentiate these disorders on a clinical basis alone, especially if the results of the MSLT are not conclusive. In these cases CSF hypocretin-1 levels should be obtained. Comparison of subjective clinical data in small numbers of individuals with narcolepsy and IH found more often a history of fever in the 6-month period to onset of EDS, less refreshing naps, significantly fewer awakenings, and lower BMI in people with IH. Discriminant analysis revealed two factors which correctly classified 86% of individuals: number of awakenings and reported change in sleepiness since EDS onset. Age at onset, duration of the diseases, and association with parasomnias did not differ. Of note is the observation that people with IH may be able to resist falling asleep during the day for a longer time than those with narcolepsy.

Sleep drunkenness is also found in healthy individuals after sleep deprivation, drug (neuroleptics, antidepressants) or alcohol consumption, and in those with sleepwalking and the Kleine–Levin syndrome.

Therapy

There are no evidence-based studies of treatment for IH. There are no medications for IH that have been approved, although stimulants may be effective in approximately 75% of the patients. Stimulants given at nighttime have been suggested by Roth, apparently relieving sleep drunkenness. Some individuals seem to respond to antidepressants. Based on the finding of reduced slow-wave activity during nighttime, we have used gamma hydroxybutyrate in IH and found it to provide a more normal wake process, reduced sleep time, improved sleep quality, and complete relief of sleep drunkenness. However, the associated EDS did not improve, requiring additional treatment with stimulants during daytime. Based on the hypothesis of a reduced circadian activity, melatonin may be efficacious. Behavioral therapy, such as allowing long sleep periods for several nights, did not result in improved wakefulness, but may reduce sleep drunkenness.

Recurrent hypersomnia

The ICSD-2 classifies two phenotypes with the main symptom of recurrent hypersomnia with asymptomatic intervals:

(1) Kleine–Levin syndrome (KLS)
(2) menstrual-related hypersomnia.

Episodes may occur up to 10 times a year and last a day to several weeks. They end abruptly with one night of insomnia and they return to normal sleep/wake and psychosocial behavior. The menstrual-related hypersomnia starts a few months after menarche. Hormonal imbalances during the menstrual cycle may play a role.

Frequently viral infections are reported prior to the onset of recurrent hypersomnia. Other triggers such as alcohol consumption, head trauma, and sleep deprivation are less frequently reported triggers. The episodes may be preceded by fatigue and headache, followed by prolonged sleep episodes during which a person remains in bed for most of the day, leaving the bed only to eat, drink, and go to the toilet. Hypersomnia is the key symptom, followed by cognitive dysfunction, which is present in almost all cases. Derealization with hallucination and delusion is frequently found and considered to be the most disabling symptom. Most sufferers retrospectively report to perceive their environment as unreal. Irritability, aggressiveness, sexual disinhibition, and binge eating with fast weight gain may occur and are reported in more than half the cases. The full combination of all symptoms is not the rule. At the end of the symptomatic phase, a sleepless night announces the return to normal behavior and sleep.

> *Example* – "When it started I felt exhausted and had to go to bed. The next days I did not feel like I was myself, but as though life was going on behind a thick glass window and having nothing to do with me in any way."

Epidemiology and pathophysiology

An association with parasomnias is reported in 7%, and below normal range of intelligence in 17%. Kleine–Levin syndrome is a rare disorder with a male-to-female ratio of 2 : 1. A systematic review by Arnulf and colleagues found a mean of four newly reported cases a year, but the prevalence and incidence are not known. Clinical symptoms typically begin in the second decade, with a peak age of onset at 16 years. However, onset up to the age of 60 years has been reported. In a few long-term studies, the duration is 0.5–41 years. Since classification criteria in the past decades have not been very strict, it remains unclear if the late-onset cases are idiopathic hypersomnias or hypersomnia caused by lesions of the central nervous system. Recurrent hypersomnia may be very disabling. Depending on the length and frequency of the symptomatic phases, individuals may fail in their education or professions, and offend others by their behavior.

The etiology of recurrent hypersomnia is unknown. Due to the recurrent symptoms, intermittent dysfunction at diencephalic and hypothalamic level has been suggested by some authors. This theory is based on the resemblance of this disorder to symptoms reported in hypothalamic and III ventricle tumors. Several studies have focused on the hypothalamic–pituitary axis by measuring hormone levels during symptomatic periods, and a few during both symptomatic and asymptomatic phases. The results remain discordant, with little if any evidence for hypothalamic and/or circadian dysfunction. Abnormalities in serotonin and dopamine metabolism have been reported in a few KLS cases with increased CSF levels of 5-hydroxytryptamine and 5-hydroxyindoleacetic acid suggesting a neurotransmitter imbalance in the serotonergic and/or dopaminergic pathway.

In one person with additional Prader–Willi syndrome, hypocretin-1 in the CSF was normal (221 pg/ml) in the asymptomatic phase and pathological in the symptomatic phase (111 pg/ml). In two other people, CSF hypocretin-1 levels during the symptomatic phases were normal in one, and intermediate in the other. CSF hypocretin-1 may be a state-dependent marker in this disorder.

Postmortem neuropathological KLS case report studies have not revealed any abnormality in the hypothalamus, but have shown infiltrates of inflammatory microglia in the thalamus, diencephalon, and midbrain. In only one case report, abnormalities in the hypothalamus, the amygdala, and the gray matter of the temporal lobes were reported. In these studies, the finding of focal encephalitis implicates a possible viral infection. This is supported by the frequent association of the periodic clinical symptoms and infections at the onset of symptoms. Both autoimmune and genetic mechanisms have also been proposed.

With the onset during adolescence and typical history of a preceding viral infection, an autoimmune origin is possible. The analysis of gene polymorphism of *HLA-DQB1* revealed a significant increase of frequency of *HLA-DQB1**0201 compared to non-affected controls. Three out of 30 patients and two affected family members were homozygous for *DQB1**0201. Out of 17 heterozygous parents 11 (64.7%) had transmitted the allele to the affected relative, suggesting a preferential transmission.

Diagnosis

The diagnosis is difficult to establish when the first symptoms occur. Continuous sleep logs help to document the recurrent changes in sleep and behavior. In some cases, 24-hour polysomnography (Fig. 5.4) plus videometry during the symptomatic and asymptomatic phases may be helpful to document the changes in sleep and behavior. During the symptomatic phases, motor activity is increased during sleep. Sleep efficiency remains unchanged, stage shifts are increased, REM sleep is increased without shortened REM latencies, whereas slow-wave sleep is decreased (Fig. 5.5). The sleep cycles are preserved.

To rule out symptomatic hypersomnias in stroke, head trauma, or inflammation of the CNS it is recommended to perform a brain MRI and lumbar puncture. The lumbar puncture may include the measurement of hypocretin-1 levels, which may be lowered in the symptomatic phase.

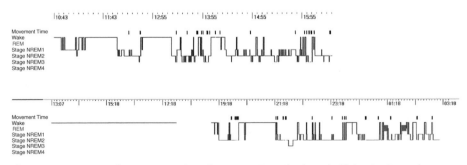

Fig. 5.4. Hypnogram of a symptomatic and an asymptomatic phase in Kleine–Levin syndrome.

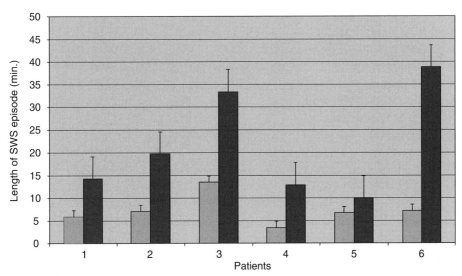

Fig. 5.5. Slow-wave sleep (24-hour PSG) in six Kleine–Levin patients during symptomatic (pale gray) and asymptomatic (dark gray) phases.

Therapeutic options

So far only 186 cases of Kleine–Levin syndrome have been reported in the literature, and there are few reports on the treatment. Of 75 patients treated, stimulants decreased somnolence in 40%. Lithium had a response rate of 41% and was also capable of stopping relapses. Other drugs such as antiepileptics, antidepressants, and neuroleptics were of poor benefit.

Behaviorally induced insufficient sleep syndrome

This disorder is caused by lifestyle-induced sleep deprivation, with nocturnal sleep shorter than individually needed, and shorter than that of a comparable age- and sex-matched population without sleep problems. In children, behavioral abnormalities resulting in sleepiness may be prominent. The abnormal sleep pattern must be present almost daily for at least three months. The insufficient sleep may be caused by lifestyle, work, and social pressure. The actual need for sleep and the amount of sleep taken differs. The ability to initiate and maintain sleep is not disturbed, and there is no underlying medical and rarely psychological pathology. The sleep debt can be easily made up by longer sleep periods.

Depending on their ability to tolerate the permanent sleep deficit, individuals develop daytime sleepiness, problems with concentration, exhaustion, and depression. Their work and driving performance may be impaired, resulting in accidents.

Polysomnography reveals short sleep onset and high sleep efficiency. Sleep cycles are preserved. In the MSLT short sleep latencies of < 8 minutes and even more than two SOREMP may occur.

The differential diagnosis has to exclude all hypersomnias with short night sleep:

- environmental sleep disorder
- psychophysiological insomnia
- affective disorder
- narcolepsy
- sleep-disordered breathing
- long and short sleeper
- PLMD
- sleep phase delay syndrome in children.

Therapeutic options focus on adherence to the individual's sleep need.

Secondary hypersomnias

Hypersomnia may be caused by an underlying medical or neurological disease. Hypersomnia is variable, and long nighttime sleep may be present. Nonspecific symptoms such as hypnagogic hallucinations, sleep paralysis, or automatic behavior may occur. Cataplexy is an exclusion criterion. The MSLT may show short sleep latency, but never more than one SOREMP. Polysomnography may reveal sleep-disordered breathing, PLMD, movement disorders, and parasomnias. It is essential to clarify that the latter are associated with, but not the cause of, the hypersomnia, to which they can contribute. Frequent medical disorders causing hypersomnia are outlined below.

Parkinson's disease

Sleep disorders are one of the most common non-motor symptoms in Parkinson's disease (PD). Both excessive daytime sleepiness and nocturnal sleep disruption can occur. The occurrence of EDS tends to increase with disease progression and medications used to treat PD. Sudden sleep attacks during daytime occur about seven times more frequently compared with healthy elderly persons, and have been associated with the use of dopaminergic drugs. EDS in PD may be intrinsic to the disease process, or may be secondary to other factors, including medications and nocturnal sleep disturbances such as sleep apnea. A recent review by Happe and Trenkwalder provides more details on possible causes. Polysomnography may show sleep fragmentation, decrease of slow-wave sleep, reduced sleep efficiency, or sleep apnea.

Posttraumatic hypersomnia

Hypersomnia has been reported in some cases following head trauma. Diagnosis should only be established after ruling out other causes for hypersomnia, i.e., sleep apnea, PLMD, etc.

Brain tumors, infections, vascular or other CNS lesions

Brain lesions of different origins, especially those involving the hypothalamus, may cause hypersomnias of central origin.

Genetic disorders

Nieman–Pick type C, Norries disease, Moebius syndrome, Smith–Magenis syndrome, and fragile X syndrome are frequently associated with EDS of central origin. Some of the syndromes may resemble narcolepsy. People with autosomal dominant spino-cerebellar ataxias type SCA III frequently suffer from EDS and nocturnal wakenings. Myotonic dystrophy and Prader–Willi syndrome are associated with both EDS and sleep apnea.

Endocrine disorders

Endocrinological dysfunctions may induce hypersomnia, most frequently in hypo-thyroidism, menopause, or dysfunctions of the adrenocortical axis.

Toxic and metabolic conditions

Multiple chemical substances, especially organic solvents with chronic exposure, may cause hypersomnia. Pancreatic, adrenal or renal insufficiency, and hepatic encephalopathy are other causes.

Substance abuse

In these disorders, hypersomnia is due to substance abuse (hypnotics, sedatives, stimulants) or withdrawal from the abused substance. The classification should not be used in individuals using drugs to treat a sleep disorder with hypersomnia of central origin such as narcolepsy. The polysomnographic and MSLT findings depend on the time of last substance intake and state of intoxication or withdrawal.

Adverse drug effects

Hypersomnia may occur as a side effect of many drugs, due either to the soporific effects of the drug or to the effect of the drug on reducing nighttime sleep. The drugs that are frequently implicated include antidepressants, antihistamines, anti-inflammatory substances, antiparkinsonian compounds, antiphlogistics, analgesics, cardiovascular medication, stimulants. Polysomnography is not needed, since the effect on sleep is known in many compounds.

Psychiatric disorders

Excessive daytime sleepiness may be caused by an underlying psychiatric disorder. The disturbed nighttime sleep results in nonrestorative sleep and EDS. Concentration and performance are reduced, social withdrawal and occupational problems are common. Polysomnography reveals fragmented night sleep, reduced sleep efficiency, and increased frequency of awakenings.

Hypersomnias can occur in major depression, seasonal affective disorder, and somatoform disorder. Successful treatment of the underlying psychiatric disorder will improve EDS.

Therapeutic options

In the secondary hypersomnias, treatment is focused on treating the underlying disease. In the case of substance abuse, this means withdrawal of the substance; in the case of toxic conditions, detoxification and avoidance of exposure.

Conclusion

The pathophysiology of disorders of excessive somnolence is not entirely understood, although major scientific efforts have been and continue to be implemented in narcolepsy. The disorders may not directly cause severe physical disability, but they are responsible for major lifelong psychosocial impairment. As most of the disorders are rare, their symptoms often are not recognized by the medical community, and they therefore frequently remain underdiagnosed. With symptom onset often at a young age, the psychosocial consequences of an undiagnosed disorder definitely has a severe negative impact on the future life of a person. Hopefully the information provided may contribute to improved diagnosis and treatment of disorders of excessive somnolence, and in consequence improve the quality of life of these individuals.

FURTHER READING

American Academy of Sleep Medicine. *International Classification of Sleep Disorders: Diagnostic and Coding Manual*, 2nd edn (ICSD-2). Westchester, IL: American Academy of Sleep Medicine, 2005.

Arnulf I, Zeitzer JM, File J, *et al*. Kleine–Levin syndrome: a systematic review of 186 cases in the literature. *Brain* 2005; **128**: 2763–76.

Bassetti C, Aldrich MS. Idiopathic hypersomnia. *Brain* 1997; **120**: 1423–35.

Billiard M. Idiopathic hypersomnia. *Neurol Clin* 1996; **14**: 573–82.

Billiard M. Hypersomnias. In: Billiard M, ed. *Sleep: Physiology, Investigations and Medicine*. New York, NY: Kluwer/Plenum, 2003: 333–6.

Billiard M, Bassetti C, Dauvilliers Y, *et al*. EFNS guidelines on management of narcolepsy. *Eur J Neurol* 2006; **13**: 1035–48.

Bruck D, Parkes JD. A comparison of idiopathic hypersomnia and narcolepsy–cataplexy using self report measures and sleep diary. *J Neurol Neurosurg Psychiatry* 1996; **60**: 576–8.

Dauvilliers Y, Montplaisir J, Molinari N, *et al*. Age at onset of narcolepsy in two large populations of patients in France and Quebec. *Neurology* 2001; **57**: 2029–33.

Dauvilliers Y, Mayer G, Lecendreux M, *et al*. Kleine–Levin syndrome: an autoimmune hypothesis based on clinical and genetic analyses in thirty unrelated patients. *Neurology* 2002; **59**: 1739–45.

Dauvilliers Y, Baumann CR, Carlander B, *et al*. CSF hypocretin-1 levels in narcolepsy, Kleine–Levin syndrome, and other hypersomnias and neurological conditions. *J Neurol Neurosurg Psychiatry* 2003; **74**: 1667–73.

Dodel R, Peter H, Walbert T, *et al*. The socioeconomic impact of narcolepsy. *Sleep* 2004; **27**: 1123–8.

Dolenc L, Besset A, Billiard M. Hypersomnia in association with dysthymia in comparison with idiopathic hypersomnia and normal controls. *Eur J Physiol* 1996; **431** (suppl): R303–4.

Faull KF, Guilleminault C, Berger PA, *et al*. Cerebrospinal fluid monoamine metabolites in narcolepsy and hypersomnia. *Ann Neurol* 1983; **13**: 258–63.

Gélineau J. De la narcolepsie. *Gaz des Hôp* 1880; **53**: 626–8; **54**: 635–7.

Goldberg MA. The treatment of Kleine–Levin syndrome with lithium. *Can J Psychiatry* 1983; **28**: 491–3.

Guilleminault C, Yuen KM, Gulevich MG, *et al*. Hypersomnia after head–neck trauma: a medico-legal dilemma. *Neurology* 2000; **54**: 653–9.

Happe S, Trenkwalder C. Parkinson's disease. In: Ebadi M, Pfeiffer R, eds. *Sleep Disorders in Parkinson's Disease*. Boca Raton, FL: CRC Press, 2005: S217–27.

Honda Y, Juji T, Matsuki K, *et al*. HLA-DR2 and Dw2 in narcolepsy and in other disorders of excessive somnolence without cataplexy. *Sleep* 1986; **9**: 133–42.

Hublin C, Kaprio J, Partinen M, *et al*. Daytime sleepiness in an adult, Finnish population. *J Intern Med* 1996; **239**: 417–23.

Kanbayashi T, Inoue Y, Chiba S, *et al*. CSF hypocretin-1 (orexin-A) concentrations in narcolepsy with and without cataplexy and idiopathic hypersomnia. *J Sleep Res* 2002; **11**: 91–3.

Kawashima M, Tamiya G, Oka A, *et al*. Genomewide association analysis of human narcolepsy and a new resistance gene. *Am J Hum Genet* 2006; **79**: 252–63.

Littner M, Johnson SF, McCal WV, *et al*. Practice parameters for the treatment of narcolepsy: an update for 2000. Standards of Practice Committee. *Sleep* 2001; **24**: 451–66.

Mayer G, Blanke J. Moebius syndrome, narcolepsy and parasomnias: report on two patients. *Somnologie* 2004; **3**: 110–14.

Mayer G, Leonhardt E, Krieg J, Meier-Ewert K. Endocrinological and polysomnographic findings in Kleine–Levin syndrome: no evidence for hypothalamic and circadian dysfunction. *Sleep* 1998; **21**: 278–84.

Mayer G, Kesper K, Ploch T, Peter H, Peter J. The implications of gender and age at onset of first symptoms in narcoleptic patients in Germany: results from retrospective evaluation of hospital records. *Somnologie* 2002; **6**: 13–18.

Montplaisir J, de Champlain J, Young SN, *et al*. Narcolepsy and idiopathic hypersomnia: biogenic amines and related compounds in CSF. *Neurology* 1982; **32**: 1299–302.

Montplaisir J, Poirier G. HLA in disorders of excessive daytime sleepiness without cataplexy in Canada. In: Honda Y, Jui T, eds. *HLA in Narcolepsy*. Berlin: Springer, 1988: 186.

Nevsímalova S, Blazejová K, Illnerová H, *et al*. A contribution to pathophysiology of idiopathic hypersomnia. *Suppl Clin Neurophysiol* 2000; **53**: 366–70.

Ohayon MM. Prevalence and correlates of nonrestorative sleep complaints. *Arch Intern Med* 2005; **165**: 35–41.

Perlis ML, Pigeon WR, Riemann D. State-of-the-science for the treatment of chronic insomnia. *Sleep Med Rev* in press.

Riemann D, Fischer J, Mayer G, Peter HJ. The guidelines for "non-restorative sleep": relevance for the diagnosis and therapy of insomnia. *Somnologie* 2003; **7**: 66–76.

Rogers AE, Aldrich MS, Berrios AM, Rosenberg R. Compliance with stimulant medications in patients with narcolepsy. *Sleep* 1997; **20**: 28–33.

Roth B. *Die Narkolepsie und die Hypersomnie vom Standpunkt der Physiologie des Schlafs*. Berlin: VEB Volk und Gesundheit, 1962.

Roth B, Nevsímalova S, Rechtschaffen A. Hypersomnia with sleep drunkenness. *Arch Gen Psychiatry* 1972; **26**: 456–62.

Roth B, Nevsímalova S, Sagova V, *et al*. Neurological, psychological and polygraphic findings in sleep drunkenness. *Arch Suisse Neurochirurgie Psychiatrie* 1981; **129**: 209–22.

Rye DB, Bliwise DL, Dihenia B, Gurecki P. Daytime sleepiness in Parkinson's disease. *J Sleep Res* 2000; **9**: 63–9.

Schöls L, Haan J, Riess O, *et al*. Sleep disturbance in spinocerebellar ataxias: is the SCA3 mutation a cause of restless legs syndrome? *Neurology* 1998; **51**: 1603–7.

Schweitzer PK. Drugs that disturb sleep and wakefulness. In: Kryger MH, Roth T, Dement WC, eds. *Principles and Practice of Sleep Medicine*, 4th edn. Philadelphia, PA: Saunders, 2005: 499–518.

Sforza E, Gaudreau H, Petit D, Montplaisir J. Homeostatic sleep regulation in patients with idiopathic hypersomnia. *Clin Neurophysiol* 2000; **111**: 277–82.

Standards of Practice Committee. Practice Parameters for the treatment of narcolepsy: An update for 2000. *Sleep* 2001; **24**: 451–66.

Vanková J, Nevsímalová S, Sonka K, Spacková N, Svejdová-Blazejova K. Increased REM density in narcolepsy–cataplexy and the polysymptomatic form of idiopathic hypersomnia. *Sleep* 2001; **24**: 707–11.

6   Insomnias

James K. Wyatt and M. Isabel Crisostomo

Introduction

Insomnia is one of the most common complaints seen in medicine. Incidence and prevalence estimates vary slightly depending on the methodology, but commonly cited figures are that approximately one-third of Americans have symptoms of acute or intermittent insomnia, and that approximately 10% have chronic insomnia. Over the past several decades, there have been great strides in understanding the pathophysiology of insomnia as well as documenting the efficacy of pharmacologic and nonpharmacologic treatments. There are now sufficient data to allow for meta-analyses to be conducted in insomnia, which help compare effect sizes across studies. This chapter provides an overview of the development of insomnia, information required to make a diagnosis of insomnia, the various recognized insomnia diagnoses, and the pharmacologic, cognitive, and behavioral treatments available.

Pathophysiology of the insomnias

As with certain other sleep disorders, there are cases where insomnia is thought to be a primary condition, times when it is thought to have come about entirely secondary to a medical or psychiatric condition, and times when it may be comorbid with other significant illnesses. There are many theories for the development of insomnia itself, including theories relying on cognitive styles, psychiatric vulnerabilities, and physiological sensitivity or over-reactivity. In 1986 Spielman proposed a particularly useful model of the development of chronic insomnia that allows for multiple etiologies – the "3 P model."

Spielman's model assumes that certain individuals have a *predisposition* (the first P) to develop insomnia. This predisposition could come in the form of slow accumulation of homeostatic sleep drive during the day, an increased basal level of physiological arousal, proneness to cognitive styles of worrying or rumination, or other factors. This may be at the heart of idiopathic insomnia (see below), where insomnia is a lifelong complaint. With the occurrence of a *precipitating* event (the second P), the predisposed individual develops acute insomnia. Factors that could precipitate an

---

Sleep Medicine, ed. Harold R. Smith, Cynthia L. Comella, and Birgit Högl. Published by Cambridge University Press. © Cambridge University Press 2008.

episode of insomnia include pharmacologic changes such as starting a medication with an intended effect or a side effect of CNS activation, occurrence of an acute psychosocial stressor such as a job change or marital discord, or acute onset of a new medical condition producing pain or discomfort such as spraining a limb. With resolution of the precipitating factor through action or simply the passage of time, acute insomnia would be expected to resolve. However, many people with insomnia go on to modify their behaviors, thoughts, and even pharmacology in response to an acute episode of insomnia, providing conditions whereby this short-term condition is *perpetuated* (the third P) into a chronic condition. Classic perpetuating factors could consist of behaviors, such as the person who intentionally naps during the daytime or sleeps late on weekends to make up for sleep lost at night. Maladaptive cognitive styles resulting from insomnia include overestimating the degree of next-day cognitive or motor impairment that may result from intermittent suboptimal sleep. Pharmacologic changes include use or abuse of alcohol to try to initiate sleep and/or overuse of caffeine or nicotine during the daytime to compensate for reduced nightly sleep time.

This predisposing–precipitating–perpetuating model of chronic insomnia provides a helpful structure to understand the remainder of this chapter: the workup of a patient presenting with a complaint of insomnia, the current classification scheme for insomnia contained in the *International Classification of Sleep Disorders* 2nd edition (ICSD-2), the differential diagnosis of insomnia, and the pharmacologic and nonpharmacologic treatment options.

Data gathering

The sleep history and physical examination

The most important component involved in the diagnosis of insomnia is a thorough and in-depth sleep history. The sleep history has the same structure as a medical history with emphasis on the sleep problem, which in this instance is insomnia. The history will give information on the evolution of the insomnia. The sleep history will also identify the medical, psychological, behavioral, circadian, cognitive, and pharmacologic factors contributing to the sleep complaint. Table 6.1 shows components of an insomnia intake history.

The past medical history will reveal whether the person has a medical disease which could be causing, contributing to, or worsening the sleep difficulty. Normal sleep would require that a person be free of any other condition which would result in sleep being interrupted such as breathing difficulty, reflux, pain, and limitations in mobility. Symptoms of lung disease including wheeze and cough significantly increase the likelihood of having insomnia; diagnosis of obstructive lung disease and asthma may be associated with awakenings and difficulty with sleep initiation due to dyspnea. Chronic pain syndromes are often associated also with insomnia symptoms. Acute pain will certainly impact on sleep quality. Certain neurological disorders are associated with fragmented sleep patterns and disruptions of the sleep/wake cycle, including Parkinson's and Alzheimer's diseases. Symptomatic reflux

Table 6.1. *Components of an insomnia intake history (reprinted with permission from Summers MO, Crisostomo MI, Stepanski EJ. Recent developments in the classification, evaluation, and treatment of insomnia.* Chest *2006;* **130***: 276–86).*

Sleep pattern

(1) What is the problem – difficulty initiating sleep, difficulty maintaining sleep, waking up too early, feeling poorly rested despite adequate sleep?
(2) When did the problem begin? What was its course (severity, remissions)?
(3) Was there a precipitating factor associated with the onset of the insomnia?
(4) What time does the patient go to bed? How long does it take him to fall asleep?
(5) Does he have awakenings? What wakes him up (see other components of sleep intake such as reflux, dyspnea, choking, nightmares, uncomfortable leg sensations, urination, pain, noise, uncomfortable environmental conditions such as the bed or temperature)?
(6) What time does he wake up? Does he do it spontaneously or with an alarm or bed partner? What time does he eventually get out of bed?
(7) How long does he think he was asleep? How long does he think he needs to sleep to feel better?
(8) How does he feel in terms of sleepiness, alertness or fatigue?

Behavioral factors

(1) Does he do anything else in bed other than sleep, such as watch TV, read, work, or eat?
(2) Is he awakened by noise or light or bed discomfort?
(3) Does he sleep better away from home or more easily in anything other than his bed such as a couch?
(4) Does he nap during the day?
(5) Does he look at the clock?

Cognitive factors

(1) Does the patient feel tense when he sees the bedroom?
(2) Does he think about his sleep problems during the day?
(3) Is he afraid of sleeping?
(4) What does he perceive are the consequences of his poor sleep?

Medical disorders

(1) What other medical conditions does the patient have which can potentially affect sleep (asthma/COPD/congestive heart failure, awakenings with shortness of breath, pain conditions, reflux, neuropathy, etc.)?
(2) What medications is the patient taking that can potentially affect sleep (diuretics, stimulants, beta-blockers, etc.)?

Psychiatric disorders

(1) Has the patient been treated for emotional or psychological problems? Has the patient seen a mental health provider (therapist, psychologist, psychiatrist, social worker)?
(2) Has the patient felt depressed? How is the patient's appetite? Has the patient's weight fluctuated? Does the patient have panic attacks or phobias?
(3) How is the patient's marriage or relationships? Does the patient have an active sex life? Does he have any personal/familial stress?
(4) Does the patient have any work/school-related stress?

Table 6.1. (*cont.*)

Alcohol and medications

(1) Does the patient drink alcohol? At what frequency and amount, and how long?
(2) Does he take any sedative or hypnotic agent, prescribed, OTC, or herbal?
(3) Does he take any illicit/recreational drugs which either stimulate or sedate the patient?
(4) Does he drink any caffeinated beverages? How much and how often? How late during the day does he drink this beverage?

Other sleep disorders

(1) Does the patient have uncomfortable sensations in his legs that prevent him from sleeping or wake him up? Has the bed partner noted leg movement during sleep? (Restless legs syndrome)
(2) Does the patient snore loudly and frequently? Does he awaken gasping for breath? Does the bed partner note any breathing irregularity or pauses in his breathing? Does the patient have a dry mouth in the morning or problems breathing through his nose? (Obstructive sleep apnea)
(3) Does the patient experience difficulty waking up in the morning? Does he sleep later on weekends? Does he work shifts?

occurring at night can cause disruption of sleep. Sleep disturbances are commonly seen during and following perimenopause and menopause.

The history may reveal other sleep disorders that could affect sleep. If snoring is found to be present, there is a possibility of sleep-disordered breathing, which can be the cause of insomnia or contribute to its manifestation. If there is a complaint of uncomfortable leg sensations or repetitive leg movements that have been witnessed by others, then restless legs or periodic limb movement disorder should be considered. Parasomnias should be in the differential diagnosis if the person complains of unusual behaviors or movements during sleep.

A thorough medication list and history is also important. The medications used to treat the medical disorders mentioned earlier, along with other medications that may be taken for other medical indications, can disrupt sleep. Medications with the unintended side effect of contributing to insomnia include anticonvulsants, antidepressants, beta-blockers, bronchodilators, decongestant medications, steroids, and stimulants. Caffeine is a common stimulant which can cause difficulty with sleep initiation and maintenance if consumed during the later portion of the day or in excessive amounts. Stimulants such as amphetamines and cocaine will also cause difficulty with sleep, resulting in insomnia at night and sleepiness during periods of withdrawal of the substance. Alcohol and sedatives can also potentially result in insomnia. Alcohol is commonly used as a sleep aid by the general population, and insomniacs seem particularly susceptible to reinforcing effects of alcohol. Rebound insomnia may develop from withdrawal of alcohol and sedative medications.

A crucial component of the sleep history is a review of the individual's psychiatric history. Insomnia due to a mental disorder is the most common diagnosis among people presenting to a sleep center with a complaint of insomnia. Mood disorders such as depression, dysthymia, bipolar disorder, as well as anxiety disorders, can be associated with a complaint of insomnia. Insomnia may also be the earliest symptom manifested in the course of recurrence of an episode of major depression. As mentioned previously, medications, especially psychotropic medications, are notorious for side effects that can result in difficulty with sleep.

A complete or focused physical examination may be done as suggested by the initial information in the history, for example to examine the possibility of obstructive sleep apnea, restless legs syndrome, or Parkinson's disease. The exam may reveal supporting findings such as a narrowed posterior oropharynx or obstructed naso-pharynx, which may suggest obstructive sleep apnea. There may be evidence for a neuromuscular disorder from the neurological examination. Limitation of joint mobility and pain may also be elicited, which would indicate the presence of a chronic pain or a rheumatologic condition. The pulmonary exam may reveal prolonged expiratory airflow or frank wheezing, thus suggesting obstructive lung disease or asthma.

Measurement of sleep

A prospective, daily sleep diary (also called a sleep log) is an accurate means of tracking a person's sleep/wake schedule. It may help reveal a pattern or set of behaviors which contribute to the insomnia. An example is the finding of increased sleep latency or awakenings associated with intake of caffeine late into the wake period. Sleep logs have been found to correlate modestly or poorly between subjective complaints and objective findings, but they may be better indicators of an individual's own perception of the sleep disturbance.

A wrist actigraph is a watch-sized motion sensor worn by the subject which records rest and activity data. Some models can even collect data on ambient light exposure. The data obtained from actigraphy are coupled with data from the sleep diary to increase its accuracy in estimating the sleep/wake schedule or pattern. The Standards of Practice Committee of the American Academy of Sleep Medicine (AASM) concluded in 2003 that the use of actigraphy is not indicated in the routine diagnosis, assessment, or management of sleep disorders. But actigraphy may serve as a useful adjunct to the evaluation of other disorders such as insomnia, circadian rhythm disorders, or disorders of sleepiness. Recent data reveal its utility in following up treatment evaluation and complementing the use of sleep diaries.

The AASM Standards of Practice Committee also concluded in 2003 that polysom-nography is not indicated for the routine evaluation of transient insomnia, chronic insomnia, or insomnia associated with sleep disorders. However, it may be appro-priate if there is a valid indication and a clear rationale, such as suspicion of sleep-disordered breathing or periodic limb movement disorders. It may also be indicated if initial diagnosis is uncertain or initial treatment fails.

Additional evaluations can be done as indicated by the history, such as struc-tured clinical interviews for psychiatric disorders. In addition, sleep and insomnia symptoms can be diagnosed with a variety of questionnaires, but there is a need for standardization of this methodology.

Diagnostic testing can also be done as indicated from the initial evaluation, such as obtaining ferritin levels in the setting of restless legs syndrome, thyroid levels for suspicion of hypothyroidism or hyperthyroidism, or toxicology screens for suspicion of drug abuse.

Diagnosis

Primary versus secondary versus comorbid insomnia

Primary insomnia refers to insomnia when no other coexisting disorder is identified. Insomnia, however, is often comorbid with other conditions. These have been classified historically as *secondary insomnias*, but there is a concern that labeling these cases as secondary may minimize their importance and foster undertreatment of the sleep problem. In addition, the current limitation of knowledge regarding insomnia precludes firm conclusions about causality. Given these concerns, the term *comorbid insomnia* has been proposed as more acceptable. Examples of comorbid conditions often observed with insomnia include pulmonary disease (obstructive lung disease and asthma), cardiac diseases (congestive heart failure), chronic pain disorders (arthritis and fibromyalgia), neurologic disorders (Parkinson's disease and dementias), psychiatric disorders (depression, bipolar disorder, anxiety disorders), and primary sleep disorders (obstructive and central sleep apnea, restless legs syndrome, periodic limb movement disorder).

International Classification of Sleep Disorders 2 (ICSD-2)

The general criteria for the diagnosis of insomnia include a complaint of difficulty initiating or maintaining sleep, awakening too early, or a sleep that is felt to be nonrestorative. The sleep complaint must persist despite an adequate duration of time allowed to sleep and reasonable conditions for sleep to occur. Finally, the criteria include one or more of a list of daytime symptoms occurring as a consequence of the sleep complaint: fatigue or malaise; attention, concentration, or memory impairment; social or vocational dysfunction or poor school performance; mood disturbance or irritability; daytime sleepiness; motivation, energy, or initiative reduction; proneness for errors or accidents at work or while driving; tension, headaches, or gastrointestinal symptoms in response to sleep loss; concerns or worries about sleep.

The formal insomnia diagnoses as classified in ICSD-2 include:

(1) *Adjustment insomnia* – In adjustment insomnia, there is a link between the onset of the insomnia and a known stressor. The insomnia is short-term in nature, typically lasting days to weeks but no more than three months.

(2) *Psychophysiological insomnia* – This form of insomnia is characterized by physiological hyperarousal and/or learned "sleep-preventing associations" linked to the bed or bedroom environment. There could be worry or anxiety regarding sleep, difficulty falling asleep during planned sleep times such as bedtime or

naps, a lack of difficulty falling asleep when not intending to fall asleep, remitting of symptoms in a different sleep environment such as on a vacation, heightened activation noted in bed such as an inability to control a racing mind or to relax a tense body.

(3) *Paradoxical insomnia* – This was previously called sleep state misperception. In this form of insomnia there is a significant disparity between the individual's account of sleep and the objective sleep recording with polysomnography.

(4) *Idiopathic insomnia* – A person with this type of insomnia has never remembered or been told by a parent about a time he or she did not have insomnia, even as a young child or infant. No significant remission of sleep symptoms is notable.

(5) *Insomnia due to mental disorder* – This applies when the sleep complaint is found exclusively within the context of a co-occurring mental disorder, such as a mood or anxiety disorder. The sleep complaints typically improve or worsen in parallel with changes in the mental disorder.

(6) *Inadequate sleep hygiene* – This subtype of insomnia often accompanies other diagnoses of insomnia. It is characterized by behaviors under voluntary control that are counterproductive to sleep initiation and maintenance. This includes behaviors such as engaging in stimulating activities (e.g., exercise, arguments) or consuming CNS stimulants (e.g., caffeine, nicotine) too close to bedtime, using the bed or bedroom as a location to engage in non-sleep purposeful activities (e.g., television watching, eating, homework), and napping during the daytime.

(7) *Behavioral insomnia of childhood* – This form of insomnia was previously called limit-setting sleep disorder or sleep-onset association disorder. In the "sleep-onset association type" the infant or child comes to associate the presence of certain people or conditions with falling asleep, and hence requires this to initiate sleep or to return to sleep after an awakening. In the "limit-setting type" the parent or caregiver allows too much flexibility in allowing the child to delay bedtime, often leading to the child stalling or refusing to go to bed.

(8) *Insomnia due to drug or substance* – This type of insomnia is diagnosed when the sleep complaint is temporally associated with the use or abuse of a food, chemical, or drug known to impede sleep initiation or to fragment sleep.

(9) *Insomnia due to medical condition* – In this form of insomnia, the comorbidity of a medical condition is thought to be responsible for the sleep complaint. Improvement or worsening of the medical condition brings about parallel changes in the sleep complaint.

In addition, insomnia may be the presenting complaint for people with environmental sleep disorder. In this sleep disorder, the complaint of insomnia or daytime fatigue is thought to result from sleep disruption attributable to an objectively verifiable external stimulus present during sleep episodes, such as noise disruption from motor vehicle or airplane traffic. In the circadian rhythm sleep disorders, misalignment or malfunction of the brain's circadian timekeeping system results in complaints of insomnia and impaired alertness during wakefulness. This category of sleep disorders includes delayed sleep phase type, advanced sleep phase type, irregular sleep/wake type, free-running type, jet lag type, and shift work type.

Differential diagnosis

Individuals with obstructive sleep apnea (OSA) and/or central sleep apnea (CSA) may experience symptoms of insomnia. Sleep apneics can have difficulty with sleep initiation, with a prolonged sleep-onset latency, if apneic events at the initiation of sleep preclude the consolidation of sleep. It is not uncommon for these people to have been inadvertently prescribed sleep aids instead of having been evaluated for the underlying cause of the sleep difficulty. Apneas occurring during the sleep period may also cause arousals and awakenings resulting in sleep fragmentation. The person will then perceive sleep as unrefreshing and may manifest with fatigue and sleepiness during the day. Typically, it is those with central sleep apnea who present with insomnia, more so than those with obstructive sleep apnea, who present typically with fatigue or sleepiness.

Periodic limb movement disorder (PLMD) is characterized by repetitive periodic stereotypic limb movements occurring during sleep along with a complaint of a sleep disturbance that cannot be accounted for by another sleep disorder. It is commonly found in the setting of restless legs syndrome (RLS), REM sleep behavior disorder (RBD), and narcolepsy. PLMD can result in sleep fragmentation and lead to complaints of insomnia or hypersomnia. Its diagnosis requires the demonstration of the periodic limb movements in a polysomnogram.

Restless legs syndrome (RLS) is a sensorimotor disorder characterized by an urge to move the legs due to uncomfortable and unpleasant sensations in the legs. This urge to move begins or worsens during periods of rest or inactivity. Partial or complete relief of this urge to move is achieved by movement such as walking or stretching. The urge to move is worse or occurs only in the evening or at night. Given the sleep-disruptive nature of these symptoms, a common complaint is insomnia.

Pharmacologic treatment

Modern, prescription hypnotic medications are typically those that act as benzodi-azepine receptor agonists (also called BZRAs). The classic benzodiazepine hypnotics include flurazepam (long half-life), temazepam (moderate half-life), and triazolam (short half-life). Due to extreme next-day sedation from an active metabolite with an extremely long half-life, flurazepam is rarely recommended for the routine treat-ment of insomnia. Triazolam is rarely prescribed today, after several well-publicized instances of anterograde amnesia associated with its use (though at a higher dose that is no longer recommended). Newer, non-benzodiazepine BZRAs include the short-half-life medications zolpidem and zaleplon, and the moderate-half-life medi-cations eszopiclone and zolpidem extended release. Relatively new in the arsenal of insomnia treatments is the melatonin receptor agonist ramelteon. This medication has the sole distinction of being the only prescription hypnotic that is not a scheduled drug in the USA, due to data that found no abuse potential or next-day impairment in test subjects. Melatonin is also available in over-the-counter (OTC) form, but this is typically not a first-line treatment recommendation, given the lower production standards for purity and accuracy of dose per pill required of dietary supplements.

In prescribing hypnotics for insomnia, it is helpful to match the type of sleep complaint with the half-life of the medication. For example, a person presenting only with difficulty initiating sleep at the beginning of the night will do well with a short-half-life medication, and have less risk of next-day sedation. Sleep maintenance complaints are typically matched with a moderate-half-life medication, in order to provide sedation further into the sleep episode. Individuals with either type of insomnia paired with significant daytime anxiety may do well with a single, longer-half-life medication that can address both complaints. This is where the anxiolytic medication clonazepam is often used in insomnia treatment.

There is also no consensus in the field of sleep medicine as to whether hypnotics should be used on a nightly or a PRN basis by insomniacs. What is more agreed upon is that hypnotic medications tend not to be used well by individuals with a history of abuse of medication or substances, as they may escalate doses without approval or even against medical advice. The newer hypnotic medications possess much lower risk of respiratory suppression in an overdose scenario, and hence they are safer for people with psychiatric conditions than were the older, barbiturate medications.

As a general rule, the field of sleep medicine is in favor of the short-term use of hypnotic medication for insomnia, in the range of a few nights to three weeks. This is where the consensus ends. Many sleep specialists are uncomfortable pre-scribing hypnotics for insomnia over the long term, due to concerns about the potential for dependence and tolerance. Most hypnotics do not have data to address the concern of possible loss of efficacy over extended use, although a recent study of eszopiclone showed stable efficacy through a 6-month double-blind study and an additional 6-month open-label, extension period. In contrast, other sleep special-ists recognize that some individuals come to clinical attention with fixed beliefs that only a hypnotic medication will work for them, and are not open to alternative treatments. Others may accept only short-term hypnotic use or refuse this route altogether, opting instead for nonpharmacologic treatments.

Curiously, hypnotics are not the sleep aids most commonly prescribed by phys-icians, but rather the antidepressant trazodone. It is perhaps the case that physicians are more comfortable prescribing low doses of sedating antidepressant medications to treat insomnia, though there is a paucity of efficacy data in this area for people who are not depressed but just have insomnia. Insomniacs themselves will commonly opt for OTC sleep aids, which typically contain antihistamines, diphenhydramine, or doxylamine succinate. Alcohol is also frequently used as self-medication for insomnia. While certainly able to help someone fall asleep, alcohol will significantly disrupt sleep later in the night due to rebound CNS activation, it is a potent REM suppressant, and its diuretic properties can also disrupt sleep due to bathroom visits.

Nonpharmacologic treatment

As mentioned above, many people either refuse pharmacologic treatment for insomnia, or their physicians are uncomfortable prescribing hypnotics for long-term use. This certainly increases the need for effective nonpharmacologic treatments. Most of these treatment options can be seen as arising from within the predisposing–precipitating–perpetuating model of Spielman, described above. It is often the case that thoughts and behaviors that came into play in reaction to short-term insomnia are now of sufficient magnitude to sustain the sleep problem over the longer term. These thoughts and behaviors can be made targets for modification, often resulting in significant clinical improvement, if not complete resolution of the insomnia complaint.

Stimulus control

Stimulus control treatment was proposed by Bootzin in 1972, based on the observation that people with chronic insomnia often reported increased arousal in temporal proximity to bedtime and/or in geographical proximity to the bed or bedroom. Based on principles of conditioning theory, repeated attempts to initiate sleep take place in the bed, and hence the bed itself can become a conditioned cue leading to increased physiological and/or mental arousal. Engaging in non-sleep activities in the bed can also make this environment a conditioned cue for arousal instead of relaxation. Thus it was hypothesized that by changing the bed from a conditioned cue for arousal into a cue for relaxation and low arousal, this vicious cycle could be broken. Stimulus control treatment has the best evidence base of any nonpharmacologic insomnia treatment supporting its efficacy.

Stimulus control consists of an extremely simple set of rules that the individual must be taught. The first is to go to bed only when sleepy. Many insomnia sufferers get into bed at a preset bedtime in order to obtain their desired number of hours of sleep, but clearly will not be able to fall asleep if entering the bed when wide awake. Second, the insomniac is not allowed to engage in any non-sleep activities, aside from sex. Third, if the person is not asleep within 20 minutes (a range of 10–20 minutes is typically given), as judged merely by estimation and not by clock-watching, he or she is to leave the bed and ideally also leave the bedroom. A quiet, relaxing activity is to be done until the person feels sleepy enough to perhaps fall asleep, at which point they are to return to the bed to attempt to fall asleep. Fourth, this cycle of leaving the bed after about 20 minutes of wakefulness and returning only when sleepy is repeated as often as necessary, not only for initial sleep onset but also during prolonged mid-sleep awakenings. Fifth, the individual is given a fixed wake time to keep seven days a week, which provides several benefits. It ensures that adequate homeostatic sleep pressure will be present each night to fall asleep since he or she will not sleep in several hours later on any day. It allows for standardization of the time of morning exposure to light, prompting stabilization of circadian phase, which will benefit the individual by correctly aligning the circadian system's sleep- and wake-promoting phases with the desired sleep/wake cycle. Sixth and finally, napping is prohibited, as this will rapidly reduce homeostatic sleep drive, which is needed to facilitate rapid sleep onset at night and consolidation of sleep in the first half of the sleep episode.

Sleep restriction

Sleep restriction was proposed in 1987 by Spielman and colleagues. It is theorized to work due to several possible mechanisms. First, many people who suffer from insomnia increase their time in bed well beyond their possible total sleep time, in order simply to be in bed whenever sleep might occur, since sleep has become unpredictable. Second, the more time is spent in bed awake, the more time is allowed for becoming frustrated and aroused, which obviously will increase wakefulness and maintain the insomnia. Finally, by slightly restricting total sleep time, this increases homeostatic sleep drive, which will help facilitate the onset and consolidation of nocturnal sleep.

Sleep restriction begins by examining sleep-diary data, collected daily, ideally for at least one week or longer. An average total sleep time is calculated based on the sleep diary, which becomes the new duration of time in bed the individual will be allowed for the first week of treatment. Time in bed is rarely set below four and a half hours. A fixed bedtime and wake time are negotiated based on several factors including individual preference and the temporal availability of sufficient activities for the person to engage in prior to bedtime, and perhaps after an early wake time. As an example, someone may self-report an average of five hours of sleep per night based on a week of keeping a sleep diary. Thus, a bedtime of 01:00 and a wake time of 06:00 may be agreed upon for the first week of treatment. The person keeps a daily sleep diary, to be reviewed via fax or at a follow-up appointment with the clinician at the end of that week. If sleep efficiency, the percentage of time in bed spent sleeping versus the total time in bed, is greater than 90%, then the time in bed is increased by 15 minutes for the next week of monitoring. This gradual, data-based increasing of total sleep time and time in bed is continued until sleep efficiency falls below 85%, at which point time in bed is reduced by 15 minutes. If sleep efficiency is maintained between 85% and 90%, total sleep time remains fixed for the next week. As with stimulus control, daytime napping is not permitted as it will sabotage the treatment by decreasing homeostatic sleep pressure.

Sleep hygiene

Originally proposed by Hauri in 1977, and modified innumerable times in the intervening years by other clinicians, sleep hygiene treatment for insomnia targets problem behaviors that likely produce or maintain the difficulty initiating or maintaining sleep. In the original proposal, Hauri set up a simple set of guidelines for improving sleep. The individual was to avoid sleeping more hours than absolutely needed to feel refreshed, to set and adhere to a regular morning wake time, to avoid caffeine and alcohol consumption particularly in the evening hours, to engage in moderate levels of daily exercise, not to go to bed hungry or in an overly warm or noisy bedroom, to engage in a distracting or relaxing activity in the event of trying too hard to fall asleep, and to avoid the chronic use of hypnotics. Intuitively, it seems that sleep hygiene guidelines would be of great benefit in insomnia treatment, and these recommendations are amongst the most frequently utilized insomnia treatments. However, the evidence base is lacking to demonstrate efficacy. Perhaps the greatest problem in demonstrating efficacy of sleep hygiene as a treatment for insomnia is the fact that sleep hygiene is so often used as part of a multi-component treatment in insomnia clinical trials, and hence its independent effect size has not often been the subject of investigation.

Progressive muscle relaxation, diaphragmatic breathing, and mental imagery

There are a variety of nonpharmacologic treatments for insomnia that typically have been used in the treatment for anxiety disorders (e.g., generalized anxiety disorder and panic disorder). These include progressive muscle relaxation, diaphragmatic breathing, and mental imagery. Aside from progressive muscle relaxation, data are lacking to demonstrate efficacy in insomnia treatment. These strategies also require special training, requiring a skilled clinician to deliver them. These approaches are therefore not typically recommended as first-line treatment alternatives, but may be useful for symptom management in specific cases (e.g., teaching diaphragmatic breathing to a person who reports shortness of breath or hyperventilation in bed, perhaps due to anxiety in reaction to not falling asleep).

Paradoxical intention

Perhaps the most intriguing treatment for insomnia is paradoxical intention. In this treatment modality, the symptom is prescribed: the person who reports difficulty falling asleep at night is instructed to get into bed at bedtime and to strive to remain awake as long as possible through mental effort alone. It is hypothesized that since the problem has now been turned into the prescribed behavior, less anxiety will come to the individual when in bed trying to fall asleep, and perhaps the focus of attention on trying to remain awake will prevent rumination on other sleep-preventing and potentially more distressing cognitions. Regardless, some people find that they fall asleep more rapidly under these treatment conditions. Few studies exist testing paradoxical intention treatment for insomnia, but it does appear to have some degree of efficacy.

Cognitive therapy

Cognitive restructuring or cognitive therapy for insomnia is based on the premise that many people with insomnia develop inappropriate or inaccurate fears, worries, or expectations regarding their sleep problem and potential consequences of poor sleep. Just as found by Aaron Beck in those with depression and anxiety disorders, sleep clinicians and researchers have found that insomnia sufferers often fall prey to cognitive errors including but not limited to overgeneralization, personalization, all-or-nothing thinking, and catastrophization. Classic examples of these errors include:

Overgeneralization – "I slept badly last night so I know I'm going to sleep poorly tonight."

All-or-nothing thinking – "I want to be able to sleep perfectly every night to know that my insomnia has been successfully treated."

Catastrophization – "I know I'm going to get yelled at by the boss or maybe even fired, because I only slept four hours last night and I'm going to make bad mistakes at work today."

A very useful, brief screening instrument of great utility in identifying target dysfunctional cognitions in insomnia is the Dysfunctional Beliefs and Attitudes about Sleep (DBAS) developed by Morin in 1993. This short questionnaire asks subjects to mark along a continuum the degree to which they agree or disagree with thirty statements about normal sleep, insomnia, possible consequences of having poor sleep, and behaviors one should engage in after having insomnia. In addition to being very easy to complete, the DBAS greatly simplifies the task of identifying dysfunctional cognitive styles expressed in a given individual. After identifying specific cognitive errors, the clinician names and discusses the types of cognitive errors and alternative ways of thinking (e.g., discussing catastrophic thinking versus the alternative of not being able to accurately predict the future, or the possibility that a wide range of potential consequences may or may not occur). The patient is then assigned the homework task of collecting data that specifically address the identified dysfunctional consequences. An example would be assigning a person who fears next-day consequences of the insomnia to log daily the number of times comments are made by supervisors or coworkers that are critical of his or her work performance. Cognitive treatment thus consists of not merely presenting alternative ways of thinking, but having people collect their own data to challenge the accuracy of their current styles of thinking.

Optimization of treatment for comorbid illnesses

As discussed earlier in this chapter, the field of sleep medicine has evolved from the simplistic notion that insomnia is either a primary condition or entirely secondary to another medical or psychiatric condition. The concept of comorbidity implies not only that insomnia may exist at the same time as other illness, but also that improvement in one condition may have a positive impact on the other. It has been demonstrated that experimentally decreasing total sleep time leads to a decrease in pain thresholds. We know that insomnia is often reported by people with a wide range of pain conditions, including fibromyalgia and rheumatoid or osteoarthritis. Insomnia treatment trials are currently under way examining the potential for improvement in the comorbid medical conditions that may result simply by improving sleep. It is standard practice to recommend to people presenting with insomnia that they work with their other doctors to optimize treatment of their comorbid illnesses. Someone with frequent episodes of nocturnal asthma will obviously experience difficulty maintaining sleep, and may in fact develop anticipatory anxiety prior to falling asleep that will itself increase sleep latency.

Summary

Insomnia is amongst the most frequent complaints seen in medical practice, due to its high prevalence rate as a chronic medical condition and its high incidence as an acute condition. Yet insomnia most often goes undiagnosed and is therefore left untreated. As such, it is important for clinicians, regardless of specialty, to have at least a passing familiarity with the basics of the diagnosis and treatment of insomnia.

Although sleep medicine is a relatively young clinical discipline, research over the past several decades has made tremendous progress in establishing a rigorous diagnostic framework for subtypes of insomnia. Nonpharmacologic treatments have been developed that are relatively easy to deliver and offer efficacy equal to the hypnotics, but they are largely unfamiliar to physicians. Pharmacologic options are certainly plentiful, but focus primarily on the benzodiazepine receptor system. Given the tremendous strides made in understanding the complex pharmacologic regulation of sleep and wakefulness, the coming years should see a diversification amongst hypnotics for target receptors other than benzodiazepine.

FURTHER READING

American Academy of Sleep Medicine. *The International Classification of Sleep Disorders: Diagnostic and Coding Manual,* 2nd edn (ICSD-2). Westchester, IL: American Academy of Sleep Medicine, 2005.

Beck AT. Thinking and depression. I. Idiosyncratic content and cognitive distortions. *Arch Gen Psychiatry* 1963; **14**: 324–33.

Beck AT. Cognitive therapy: a 30-year retrospective. *Am Psychol* 1991; **46**: 368–75.

Bootzin RR. A stimulus control treatment for insomnia. *Proc Am Psychol Assoc* 1972: 395–6.

Bootzin RR, Epstein D, Wood JM. Stimulus control instructions. In: Hauri PJ, ed. *Case Studies in Insomnia.* New York, NY: Plenum, 1991: 19–28.

Buysse DJ, Reynolds CF III, Kupfer DJ, *et al.* Clinical diagnoses in 216 insomnia patients using the International Classification of Sleep Disorders (ICSD), DSM-IV and ICD-10 categories: a report from the APA/NIMH DSM-IV Field Trial. *Sleep* 1994; **17**: 630–7.

Chesson AL Jr, Anderson WM, Littner M, *et al.* Practice parameters for the nonpharmacologic treatment of chronic insomnia: an American Academy of Sleep Medicine report. Standards of Practice Committee of the American Academy of Sleep Medicine. *Sleep* 1999; **22**: 1128–33.

Costa e Silva JA, Chase M, Sartorius N, Roth T. Special report from a symposium held by the World Health Organization and the World Federation of Sleep Research Societies. An overview of insomnias and related disorders: recognition, epidemiology, and rational management. *Sleep* 1996; **19**: 412–16.

Dundar Y, Dodd S, Strobl J, *et al.* Comparative efficacy of newer hypnotic drugs for the short-term management of insomnia: a systematic review and meta-analysis. *Hum Psychopharmacol* 2004; **19**: 305–22.

Fass R, Quan SF, O'Connor GT, Ervin A, Iber C. Predictors of heartburn during sleep in a large prospective cohort study. *Chest* 2005; **127**: 1658–66.

Gjerstad MD, Wentzel-Larsen T, Aarsland D, Larsen JP. Insomnia in Parkinson's disease: frequency and progression over time. *J Neurol Neurosurg Psychiatry* 2007; **78**: 476–9.

Gooneratne NS, Gehrman PR, Nkwuo JE, *et al.* Consequences of comorbid insomnia symptoms and sleep-related breathing disorder in elderly subjects. *Arch Intern Med* 2006; **166**: 1732–8.

Guilleminault C, Eldridge FL, Dement WC. Insomnia with sleep apnea: a new syndrome. *Science* 1973; **181**: 856–8.

Hauri P. *Current Concepts: the Sleep Disorders.* Kalamazoo, MI: Upjohn, 1977.

Irwin MR, Cole JC, Nicassio PM. Comparative meta-analysis of behavioral interventions for insomnia and their efficacy in middle-aged adults and in older adults 55+ years of age. *Health Psychol* 2006; **25**: 3–14.

Johnson MW, Suess PE, Griffiths RR. Ramelteon: a novel hypnotic lacking abuse liability and sedative adverse effects. *Arch Gen Psychiatry* 2006; **63**: 1149–57.

Klink ME, Dodge R, Quan SF. The relation of sleep complaints to respiratory symptoms in a general population. *Chest* 1994; **105**: 151–4.

Kravitz HM, Ganz PA, Bromberger J, *et al.* Sleep difficulty in women at midlife: a community survey of sleep and the menopausal transition. *Menopause* 2003; **10**: 19–28.

Krystal AD, Walsh JK, Laska E, *et al.* Sustained efficacy of eszopiclone over 6 months of nightly treatment: results of a randomized, double-blind, placebo-controlled study in adults with chronic insomnia. *Sleep* 2003; **26**: 793–9.

Littner M, Kushida CA, Anderson WM, *et al.* Practice parameters for the role of actigraphy in the study of sleep and circadian rhythms: an update for 2002. *Sleep* 2003; **26**: 337–41.

Littner M, Hirshkowitz M, Kramer M, *et al.* Practice parameters for using polysomnography to evaluate insomnia: an update. *Sleep* 2003; **26**: 754–60.

Means MK, Edinger JD, Glenn DM, Fins AI. Accuracy of sleep perceptions among insomnia sufferers and normal sleepers. *Sleep Med* 2003; **4**: 285–96.

Morgenthaler T, Kramer M, Alessi C, *et al.* Practice parameters for the psychological and behavioral treatment of insomnia: an update. An American Academy of Sleep Medicine report. *Sleep* 2006; **29**: 1415–19.

Morin CM. *Insomnia: Psychological Assessment and Management.* New York, NY: Guilford Press, 1993.

Morin CM, Stone J, Trinkle D, Mercer J, Remsberg S. Dysfunctional beliefs and attitudes about sleep among older adults with and without insomnia complaints. *Psychol Aging* 1993; **8**: 463–7.

Morin CM, Culbert JP, Schwartz SM. Nonpharmacological interventions for insomnia: a meta-analysis of treatment efficacy. *Am J Psychiatry* 1994; **151**: 1172–80.

Morin CM, Hauri PJ, Espie CA, *et al.* Nonpharmacologic treatment of chronic insomnia. An American Academy of Sleep Medicine review. *Sleep* 1999; **22**: 1134–56.

Morlock RJ, Tan M, Mitchell DY. Patient characteristics and patterns of drug use for sleep complaints in the United States: analysis of National Ambulatory Medical Survey data, 1997–2002. *Clin Ther* 2006; **28**: 1044–53.

National Institutes of Health State of the Science Conference statement on Manifestations and Management of Chronic Insomnia in Adults, June 13–15, 2005. *Sleep* 2005; **28**: 1049–57.

Perlis ML, Giles DE, Buysse DJ, Tu X, Kupfer DJ. Self-reported sleep disturbance as a prodromal symptom in recurrent depression. *J Affect Disord* 1997; **42**: 209–12.

Richardson GS, Malin HV. Circadian rhythm sleep disorders: pathophysiology and treatment. *J Clin Neurophysiol* 1996; **13**: 17–31.

Roehrs T, Vogel G, Roth T. Rebound insomnia: its determinants and significance. *Am J Med* 1990; **88**: 39S–42S.

Roehrs T, Papineau K, Rosenthal L, Roth T. Ethanol as a hypnotic in insomniacs: self administration and effects on sleep and mood. *Neuropsychopharmacology* 1999; **20**: 279–86.

Rybarczyk B, Lopez M, Benson R, Alsten C, Stepanski E. Efficacy of two behavioral treatment programs for comorbid geriatric insomnia. *Psychol Aging* 2002; **17**: 288–98.

Sateia MJ, Doghramji K, Hauri PJ, Morin CM. Evaluation of chronic insomnia. An American Academy of Sleep Medicine review. *Sleep* 2000; **23**: 243–308.

Schweitzer PK. Drugs that disturb sleep and wakefulness. In: Kryger MH, Roth T, Dement WC, eds. *Principles and Practice of Sleep Medicine*, 4th edn. Philadelphia, PA: Elsevier Saunders, 2005: 499–518.

Smith MT, Perlis ML, Park A, *et al.* Comparative meta-analysis of pharmacotherapy and behavior therapy for persistent insomnia. *Am J Psychiatry* 2002; **159**: 5–11.

Spielman AJ. Assessment of insomnia. *Clin Psychol Rev* 1986; **6**: 11–25.

Spielman AJ, Saskin P, Thorpy MJ. Treatment of chronic insomnia by restriction of time in bed. *Sleep* 1987; **10**: 45–56.

Stepanski EJ, Wyatt JK. Use of sleep hygiene in the treatment of insomnia. *Sleep Med Rev* 2003; **7**: 215–25.

Summers MO, Crisostomo MI, Stepanski EJ. Recent developments in the classification, evaluation, and treatment of insomnia. *Chest* 2006; **130**: 276–86.

Sun ER, Chen CA, Ho G, Earley CJ, Allen RP. Iron and the restless legs syndrome. *Sleep* 1998; **21**: 371–7.

Taylor DJ, Mallory LJ, Lichstein KL, *et al.* Comorbidity of chronic insomnia with medical problems. *Sleep* 2007; **30**: 213–18.

Valipour A, Lothaller H, Rauscher H, *et al.* Gender-related differences in symptoms of patients with suspected breathing disorders in sleep: a clinical population study using the sleep disorders questionnaire. *Sleep* 2007; **30**: 312–19.

Wyatt JK. Delayed sleep phase syndrome: pathophysiology and treatment options. *Sleep* 2004; **27**: 1195–203.

Yesavage JA, Friedman L, Ancoli-Israel S, *et al.* Development of diagnostic criteria for defining sleep disturbance in Alzheimer's disease. *J Geriatr Psychiatry Neurol* 2003; **16**: 131–9.

7   Restless legs syndrome and periodic limb movement disorder

Paul Christian Baier and Claudia Trenkwalder

Clinical features

Restless legs syndrome

The most characteristic features of the restless legs syndrome (RLS) are uncomfortable sensations in one or more – usually lower – limbs, associated with an urge to move the affected limbs. Those sensations vary widely in severity from merely annoying to significantly unpleasant. It is occasionally difficult for the individual to express the discomfort that is caused by these sensations. Whereas some individuals with RLS describe them as uncomfortable and inside the leg, others speak of pain, pulling, burning, tearing or creepy-crawly sensations, "like ants crawling" or an electric current. All sensations are accompanied by an irresistible urge to move, described as "focal akathisia."

Symptoms typically begin or worsen during periods of rest or inactivity, such as lying or sitting, e.g., when watching television or trying to fall asleep in bed. Whenever the person is forced to sit still, whether this is at the cinema, in the theatre, or on a long-distance flight, discomfort increases. In moderately and severely affected individuals this may lead them to avoid those precipitating situations, and it significantly influences their quality of life.

Symptoms of RLS demonstrate a circadian pattern, with a maximum of severity in the evening and at night. Disturbance of sleep onset and frequent awakenings at night with difficulty returning to sleep are therefore clinical features of moderate to severe RLS. Many individuals with RLS may initially complain about sleep disturbances or increased daytime sleepiness and report specific RLS symptoms when directly asked. Sleep problems are a common feature of RLS and deserve special consideration when planning treatment. However, as sleep disturbances are not specific for RLS, but are frequent in many diseases, they are not considered essential for the diagnosis of RLS.

In addition to the above-mentioned precipitating circumstances there are other factors that may lead to a worsening of RLS: consumption of alcoholic beverages and caffeine, the intake of neuroleptic drugs and antidepressants, and in some cases vigorous physical activity.

Sleep Medicine, ed. Harold R. Smith, Cynthia L. Comella, and Birgit Högl. Published by Cambridge University Press. © Cambridge University Press 2008.

Table 7.1. *Standards for scoring periodic leg movements in sleep and wakefulness (World Association of Sleep Medicine: Zucconi* et al., Sleep Med, *2006; 7: 175–83).*

Candidate movement (EMG burst)	
Onset	$\geq 8\ \mu V$ above resting baseline
Offset	$< 2\ \mu V$ above resting baseline
Duration	0.5–10 s
PLM event	
Number of candidate movements in sequence	≥ 4
Period	5–90 s

Period is measured from onset to onset. If the interval between two consecutive candidate leg movement events is less than 5 s, then the latter candidate movement is ignored and the period is calculated from the onset of the earlier movement to the onset of the next candidate movement.

Periodic limb movement disorder

Periodic limb movements (PLM) are periodically occurring involuntary movements or jerks of the limbs during wakefulness (PLMW) or sleep (PLMS). They are recorded electromyographically by surface electrodes in polysomnography, or mechanically via actigraphy (Table 7.1). In RLS, both PLMW and PLMS are frequently observed, and are therefore considered to be a supportive diagnostic feature. However, periodic limb movements are rather nonspecific phenomena and can be related to a variety of medical conditions (e.g., narcolepsy, sleep apnea syndrome, Parkinson's disease, and others). They are also reported in otherwise healthy elderly individuals.

In contrast to PLM, the periodic limb movement disorder (PLMD) is defined as the occurrence of PLM, *with* severe sleep disturbance and/or excessive daytime sleepiness, but *without* the typical sensory symptoms of RLS at rest (Table 7.2). PLMD can only be diagnosed when a polysomnographic recording has been performed. Whether pure PLMD represents a singular disease entity or rather is part of the phenotypic spectrum of RLS has not been conclusively elucidated. The treatment of PLMD, if indicated, is assumed to be similar to the treatment of RLS, although there are insufficient treatment trials concerned specifically with PLMD.

Epidemiology

Prevalence studies on RLS had earlier been hampered by the lack of an appropriate and commonly used definition of the syndrome. However, from studies conducted after the International Restless Legs Syndrome Study Group (IRLSSG) had defined minimal diagnostic criteria, a prevalence of about 10% in white populations has been estimated. Women are affected approximately twice as often as men, and the prevalence for all increases with age. The frequency of RLS symptoms varies widely from intermittent occurrence to daily symptoms with severe sleep disorder. The age of onset of RLS ranges from childhood to old age. Early onset of RLS symptoms is more

Table 7.2. *Diagnostic criteria for periodic limb movement disorder (ICSD-2).*

(A)	Polysomnography demonstrates repetitive, highly stereotyped, limb movements that are:

    i. 0.5–5 seconds in duration

    ii. of amplitude greater than or equal to 25% of toe dorsiflexion during calibration

    iii. in a sequence of four or more movements

    iv. separated by an interval of > 5 seconds (from limb-movement onset to limb-movement onset) and < 90 seconds (typically there is an interval of 20–40 seconds)

(B) The PLM index exceeds 5 per hour in children and 15 per hour in most adult cases. *Note: The PLM index must be interpreted in the context of a sleep-related complaint. In adults, normative values higher than the previously accepted value of 5 per hour have been found in studies that did not exclude respiratory event-related arousals (using sensitive respiratory monitoring) and other causes for PLMS. New data suggest a partial overlap of PLM index values between symptomatic and asymptomatic individuals, emphasizing the importance of clinical context over an absolute cutoff value.*

(C) There is clinical sleep disturbance or a complaint of daytime fatigue. *Note: If PLM are present without clinical sleep disturbance, the PLM can be noted as a polysomnographic finding, but criteria are not met for a diagnosis of PLMD.*

(D) The PLM are not better explained by another current sleep disorder, medical or neurological disorder, mental disorder, medication use, or substance use disorder (e.g., PLM at the termination of cyclically occurring apneas should not be counted as true PLMS or PLMD).

---

likely to occur in people with the familial form of RLS. In those with late-onset RLS, i.e., after the age of 50 or 60, secondary causes of the disorder should be considered and excluded.

Pathophysiology

The etiology and pathophysiology of RLS are still not fully understood. However, in the past few decades neuroimaging, neurophysiological, and pharmacological studies have contributed to the development of a variety of hypotheses on the pathogenesis of the disorder. The usually immediate and striking efficacy of treatment with dopaminergic agents, and the observation that dopamine receptor antagonism can clinically worsen RLS symptoms, indicate a central role of the dopaminergic system in RLS pathophysiology. However, compared to Parkinson's disease, the spinal dopaminergic system may be more important in RLS than striatonigral pathways.

Recently attention has turned to brain iron dysregulation as another factor contributing to the pathogenesis of RLS. Several human studies have found a relationship between low serum and CSF ferritin values and RLS symptoms. However, because not all individuals with disturbed iron metabolism develop RLS, some additional factors must contribute to the pathomechanisms. In secondary RLS cases, uremia, iron deficiency anemia and other metabolic disturbances, pregnancy, myelopathy, and peripheral polyneuropathy may enhance the risk for developing RLS symptoms.

Diagnosis

RLS is a clinical diagnosis that usually is based on the individual's history. In order to better define the essential features of RLS, a working group on RLS has presented diagnostic rules that are a further development of the minimal criteria initially published by the IRLSSG. The diagnostic rules include four essential criteria and three supportive clinical features.

Essential criteria

(1) An urge to move the legs, usually accompanied or caused by uncomfortable and unpleasant sensations in the legs. (Sometimes the urge to move is present without the uncomfortable sensations, and sometimes the arms or other body parts are involved in addition to the legs.)

(2) The urge to move or unpleasant sensations begin or worsen during periods of rest or inactivity such as lying or sitting.

(3) The urge to move or unpleasant sensations are partially or totally relieved by movement, such as walking or stretching, at least as long as the activity continues.

(4) The urge to move or unpleasant sensations are worse in the evening or night than during the day, or only occur in the evening or night. (When symptoms are very severe, the worsening at night may not be noticeable but must have been previously present.)

Supportive clinical features

(1) Positive family history.
(2) Response to dopaminergic therapy.
(3) Occurrence of periodic limb movements (during wakefulness or sleep).

Associated features

Features associated with RLS include the following:
- The natural clinical course may be progressive with age, but may also be variable in severity, with periods of improvement.
- Sleep is disturbed, with disrupted nocturnal sleep and/or excessive daytime somnolence.
- The physical examination is generally normal.

Forms of RLS

Restless legs syndrome exists as a primary (idiopathic) disorder – sporadic or familial – or as a secondary disorder associated with a variety of neurological and other medical conditions.

Idiopathic RLS

RLS is idiopathic if it is not due to another medical condition. In approximately half of the idiopathic RLS cases a positive family history can be documented. The familial cases of RLS cannot be distinguished by their clinical presentation, but familial cases may show an earlier age of onset, a higher severity, and more progression with age.

Secondary RLS

End-stage renal disease and uremia – Symptoms of venous diseases, vascular insufficiency, uremic polyneuropathy, pruritus, and chronic pain are common in terminal renal insufficiency, and may confound the diagnosis of RLS. However, RLS is a frequent problem in people with uremia, with the prevalence reported to be at least 20%. Although no clear predictive marker for RLS in uremia has yet been identified, RLS improves after successful renal transplantation. As anemia and iron deficiency are frequent in terminal renal failure, it is possible that there is a concurrence of the pathophysiologies contributing to RLS.

Pregnancy – Prevalence of RLS in pregnant women is estimated to be around 25%. The onset of symptoms is usually in the third trimester. Women who experience RLS symptoms before pregnancy frequently report an increase in severity during pregnancy. In most cases RLS symptoms improve after delivery, but they may reoccur later in life. The cause of RLS in pregnancy is still not known. Changes in the metabolism of iron and folate as well as hormonal changes, are suspected.

Iron deficiency – An association between iron metabolism and storage and the occurrence of RLS has been known for a long time. RLS severity correlates with serum ferritin levels, and even when ferritin is within "low normal" values oral and intravenous administration of iron can improve RLS symptoms. However, the relationship between iron and RLS is complex, as not everyone with disturbed iron metabolism develops RLS. Ferritin levels should be monitored regularly, as they may decrease rapidly after supplementation with iron, possibly as part of the pathophysiology of the disease.

Other disorders associated with RLS – There are various neurological disorders that have been reported to be associated with the secondary forms of RLS. Case reports have been published of an association of RLS with Charcot-Marie-Tooth and other neuropathies, spinocerebellar ataxia, syringomyelia, and spinal cord lesions. In disorders involving the dopaminergic system, such as Parkinson's disease and Tourette's syndrome, an increased prevalence of RLS compared to the normal population has been reported. Although so far not systematically investigated, several drugs seem to be able to, if not induce, at least worsen an existing RLS; these include dopamine-antagonistic medications, such as neuroleptics, and various antidepressant drugs, such as SSRIs and mirtazapine. Caffeine has frequently been noted to aggravate RLS symptoms.

Clinical interview

When taking the medical history of a person who is suspected of suffering from RLS, the above-mentioned diagnostic criteria should be applied. Originally developed to standardize methods for clinical trials but also useful for everyday clinical application is the RLS Diagnostic Index (RLS-DI). This index (Fig. 7.1) is based on the minimal diagnostic criteria and the associated and supportive features, and delivers a score between 0 (no RLS) and 20 (definite RLS). When the diagnosis of RLS has been made, the International RLS Score (IRLS; Fig. 7.2) is useful for determining the severity of the disorder. The IRLS produces scores between 0 and 40. A person with a score > 20 is considered to suffer from severe RLS.

Neurological examination

The medical and neurological examinations in idiopathic RLS are usually normal. However, abnormal findings in the examination such as polyneuropathy (reduced reflexes, sensory deficits) do not exclude RLS, as RLS can occur with comorbid conditions and as a secondary form associated with polyneuropathy and radiculopathy.

Laboratory tests

In idiopathic RLS no pathological findings would be expected in the laboratory tests. However, to exclude secondary forms of RLS the following blood tests could be performed:
- hematology
- iron metabolism, including at least ferritin or soluble transferrin receptor
- renal function (including urea, creatinine)
- vitamin B_{12}
- folate.

Additionally, if there is clinical evidence, thyroid function could be measured.

Clinical neurophysiology

A basic clinical neurophysiologic examination could be performed in the initial evaluation of RLS. In idiopathic RLS, motor and sensory nerve conduction studies are expected to be (age-corrected) normal. If polyneuropathy is present, RLS is considered to be secondary. However, as polyneuropathy and RLS are both common disorders, it can be difficult to decide whether they are independent and concomitant or associated with each other. When the nerve conduction velocity is pathological, a full electromyographic investigation should be performed.

Polysomnography

In individuals with a typical medical history of RLS, polysomnography does not necessarily have to be performed. However, in some cases polysomnography is recommended, specifically in children, in potentially confounding comorbidity, and if official expertise is requested, e.g., regarding working capability. The Motor

Restless Legs Syndrome Diagnostic Index (RLS-DI)

Please interview the patient about the occurrence of complaints typical of RLS or complaints frequently associated with RLS. The period of assessment refers to the past 7 days.
Please make sure to complete all 5 questions.

Essential criteria	Occurs regularly (on ≥ 5 of 7 days)	Occurs occasionally (on 1 to 4 of 7 days)	Not applicable / not present
1. Do you feel an urge to move your legs (arms)?	2	1	-4
2. When feeling an urge to move, do you experience unpleasant sensations in legs (arms) such as itching, stabbing, pulling, pain?	2	1	-1
3. Do your urge to move / unpleasant sensations begin or worsen when you are at rest (lying, sitting) or when you are inactive?	2	1	-4
4. Is there relief of urge to move / unpleasant sensations, partial or complete, by movement (eg, walking or stretching)?	2	1	-4
5. Are urge to move / unpleasant sensations worse in the evening or at night than during the day? (That means, complaints are worse at night than during the day or occur only in the evening or at night). In severe RLS, this criterion must have been previously present.)	2	1	-1

Total "A": Item 1 to 5 ☐ Σ(1+2+3) = ☐ Σ1 + ☐ Σ2 + ☐ Σ3

The following items are to be assessed by the physician interviewing the patient as well as in consideration of medical records and clinical findings. **Please make sure to complete all questions.** In the event the data were not (yet) collected, please tick the column "Not assessable / not done".

Associated and supportive criteria	Definite	Uncertain	No	Not assessable / not done
6. Does the patient suffer from sleep disturbance? (That means: prolonged time to fall asleep, sleep interrupted, sleep duration shortened during the past 7 days)	2	1	-1	0
7. Does a first-degree relative (parents, brothers and sisters, children) suffer from urge to move / unpleasant sensations (item 1-5)?	2	1	0	0
8. Did urge to move / unpleasant sensations improve with dopaminergic therapy? (Treatment with L-dopa or dopamine agonists)	2	1	-4	0
9. Polysomnography findings: Indication of RLS (definite = eg, increased PLM Index>15/h, PLMS Arousal Index>5/h, PLMW)	2	1	-2	0
10. Can urge to move / unpleasant sensations be sufficiently explained by other medical factors/concomitant diseases? Note: Please do **not** consider medical and pharmacological conditions which can cause a "secondary" RLS. Please specify the cause of secondary RLS, if applicable: _____	-4	-1	2	0

Total "B": Item 6 to 10 ☐ Σ(4+5+6) = ☐ Σ4 + ☐ Σ5 + ☐ Σ6

Total 1 to 10 ☐ Σ(total) = ☐ Total "A" + ☐ Total "B"

Probability of diagnosis of restless legs syndrome	
16 – 20	Definitely restless legs syndrome
11 – 15	Probably restless legs syndrome
5 – 10	Possibly restless legs syndrome
1 – 4	Unlikely restless legs syndrome
≤ 0	No restless legs syndrome

© Dr. Heike Benês, somni bene Institut for Medical Research and Sleep Medicine Ltd., Schwerin Germany - heike.benes@somnibene.de

Fig. 7.1. RLS Diagnostic Index (RLS-DI). The RLS-DI is a diagnostic tool that provides a score allowing a statement on the probability of the diagnosis of RLS. Reproduced with the kind permission of Dr. Heike Benês.

International RLS Scale- IRLS

Version as published in Walters et al. 2003

Rate your symptoms for the following ten questions. Unless otherwise instructed, you should rate the average symptoms that you have experienced for the most recent two week period.

(1) Overall, how would you rate the RLS discomfort in your legs or arms?
   (4) Very severe
   (3) Severe
   (2) Moderate
   (1) Mild
   (0) None

(2) Overall, how would you rate the need to move around because of your RLS symptoms?
   (4) Very severe
   (3) Severe
   (2) Moderate
   (1) Mild
   (0) None

(3) Overall, how much relief of your RLS arm or leg discomfort do you get from moving around?
   (4) No relief
   (3) Slight relief
   (2) Moderate relief
   (1) Either complete or almost complete relief
   (0) No RLS symptoms and therefore question does not apply

(4) Overall, how severe is your sleep disturbance from your RLS symptoms?
   (4) Very severe
   (3) Severe
   (2) Moderate
   (1) Mild
   (0) None

(5) How severe is your tiredness or sleepiness from your RLS symptoms?
   (4) Very severe
   (3) Severe
   (2) Moderate
   (1) Mild
   (0) None

(6) Overall, how severe is your RLS as a whole?
   (4) Very severe
   (3) Severe
   (2) Moderate
   (1) Mild
   (0) None

(7) How often do you get RLS symptoms?
   (4) Very severe (This means 6 to 7 days a week)
   (3) Severe (This means 4 to 5 days a week)
   (2) Moderate (This means 2 to 3 days a week)
   (1) Mild (This means 1 day a week or less)
   (0) None

(8) When you have RLS symptoms how severe are they on an average day?
   (4) Very severe (This means 8 hours per 24 hour day or more)
   (3) Severe (This means 3 to 8 hours per 24 hour day)
   (2) Moderate (This means 1 to 3 hours per 24 hour day)
   (1) Mild (This means less than 1 hour per 24 hour day)
   (0) None

(9) Overall, how severe is the impact of your RLS symptoms on your ability to carry out your daily affairs, for example carrying out a satisfactory family, home, social, school or work life?
   (4) Very severe
   (3) Severe
   (2) Moderate
   (1) Mild
   (0) None

(10) How severe is your mood disturbance from your RLS symptoms – for example angry, depressed, sad, anxious or irritable?
   (4) Very severe
   (3) Severe
   (2) Moderate
   (1) Mild
   (0) None

Fig. 7.2. International RLS score (IRSL). The IRLS is a tool that provides a score between 0 and 40 when used on patients diagnosed with RLS. Those who score >20 are considered to suffer from severe RLS. The IRLS can be used to document treatment response. Reproduced with the kind permission of the International Restless Legs Syndrome Study Group.

Disorders study group of the German Sleep Society recommends the performance of polysomnographies:

- in cases of suspected RLS with atypical symptoms and/or with sleep disturbances persisting despite treatment, to confirm the diagnosis.
- in individuals with daytime somnolence as the major morbidity and less pronounced RLS symptoms.
- in young individuals with severe RLS before the start of a dopaminergic or opioid-ergic treatment.
- in individuals with RLS and sleep-disordered breathing.

When polysomnography is indicated, a standard recording should be performed. This should include EEG, EOG, ECG, a recording of respiration, and surface electrodes on both tibialis anterior muscles and chin muscles. The most characteristic features expected in a polysomnography are the increased number of periodic limb movements in sleep and/or wakefulness at night. The sleep profile of individuals with RLS displays increased sleep latency, frequent arousals, and a reduction of slow-wave and REM sleep phases compared to healthy controls.

Actigraphy and movement recordings

Activity monitoring of leg or foot movements by a motion detector system provides an alternative to measuring limb movements with polysomnography. The advantage of this method is that it is much less costly and time-consuming than polysomnography and can be used for at-home recordings over several nights. However, the major disadvantage is that no relation between limb movements and arousals/sleep stages can be determined.

Suggested immobilization test

The suggested immobilization test (SIT) utilizes the fact that an urge to move in RLS increases with the duration of immobilization. The SIT is performed 3–5 hours before normal bedtime in the late afternoon or evening. Individuals are instructed to lie or sit with stretched legs for 60 minutes in a comfortable position. EEG and anterior tibial muscle surface EMG are monitored. Every 15 minutes the individual documents his or her symptoms on visual analogue scales.

Differential diagnosis

There is a broad spectrum of differential diagnoses with RLS, including neurological and primary sleep disorders. Peripheral polyneuropathy, which, similar to RLS, often causes paresthesias and pain in the limbs and tends to worsen at night, is probably the most common differential diagnosis. In contrast to RLS, polyneuropathy is not associated with restlessness, movements do not lead to an improvement, and the circadian variation is not as distinct as in RLS. However, it has to be considered that RLS can occur secondary to and concurrently with peripheral polyneuropathy. Other differential diagnoses include:

- radiculopathy
- vascular insufficiency

- leg cramps
- sleep myoclonus/hypnic jerks
- "painful legs and moving toes" syndrome
- neuroleptic-induced and other akathisias
- arthritic conditions
- chronic pain syndromes of other etiologies.

Allen and Earley in 2001 defined six aspects that may help to distinguish RLS from other disorders. These aspects are based on IRLSSG minimal diagnostic criteria:

(1) RLS is precipitated by rest unrelated to any other prior activity or body position. Although it is not related to body position, it must be described as occurring when resting or lying down, and not typically occurring only when sitting.

(2) RLS is focal, and requires that a person experiences an irresistible sense or feeling that a specific body part – usually one or both lower limbs – must be moved.

(3) The irresistible urge to move the limb is relieved at least partly by movement of the affected limb. The immediacy of the relief distinguishes RLS from many other disorders, particularly those involving pain.

(4) The relief from movement continues as long as the limb is being moved. Persistence of the relief with movement distinguishes RLS from more general pain syndromes. Symptoms may reoccur almost immediately when movement ceases, leading some people to report falsely that they have no relief with movement. The clinician must be careful to ask about temporary relief from symptoms *while* moving.

(5) There should generally be a time of day when RLS symptoms are not present or are much less severe. This time is usually from early morning until afternoon. In that interval, it should be possible to rest for longer, with a reduced intensity of the urge to move. In more severe cases, however, the individual may describe the symptoms as occurring almost constantly without any circadian pattern. These individuals should be able to report a circadian pattern for the symptoms at an earlier time in their life when their RLS symptoms were not as intense.

(6) There are no signs of other disorders in the affected limbs. That is, typically there are no changes in physical appearance of the limbs, including changes of the muscles or dystrophic skin changes.

Treatment

In secondary forms of RLS the treatment of the primary disorder is the initial approach. For people with iron-deficient RLS, iron supplementation to high-normal values should be the aim, as this subgroup of individuals seems to be at higher risk of developing augmentation when treated with dopaminergic agents. Additionally, behavioral measures such as sleep hygiene could be considered. Pharmacological treatment with dopaminergic agents or other medication could be started, as outlined in Fig. 7.3 and summarized in Table 7.3.

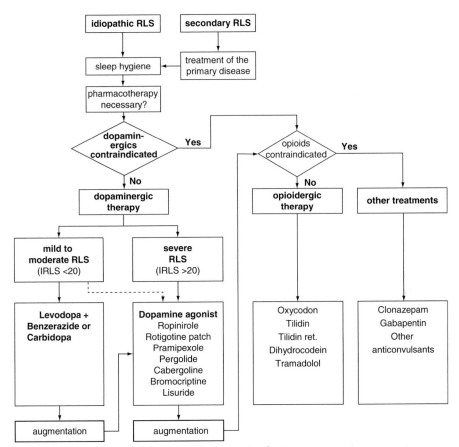

Fig. 7.3. Treatment algorithm for RLS. IRLS, International RLS score.

Pharmacological treatments

Levodopa

Levodopa combined with benserazide is licensed for RLS treatment in Europe but not in the USA. In the USA, levodopa combined with carbidopa can be used off-label. However, studies have only been performed with levodopa/benserazide, not with levodopa/carbidopa. Levodopa is a short-acting medication and effective in treating RLS symptoms. It therefore seems to be an appropriate substance for treating mild and intermittent RLS, although all treatment trials to date have been performed in individuals who suffered from moderate to severe RLS. A combination of slow-release levodopa and standard levodopa has been reported to be superior to standard levodopa alone. Long-term treatment studies on levodopa are still lacking. A few case series and follow-up trials have shown a substantial percentage of patients with augmentation, especially when the levodopa dosage was increased to more than 200–300 mg per night. Other than augmentation there are few side effects from levodopa when used in recommended doses for RLS: nausea and dizziness are mostly transient side effects and disappear after some days.

Table 7.3. *Treatments of RLS.*

Levodopa	Levodopa/benserazide 1–4 × 100/25 mg, combination of slow-release formulation with standard formulation in higher doses	Licensed in Europe, off label in the USA
Non-ergot dopamine agonists	Ropinirole 1 × 0.5 – 1 × 4 mg	Licensed in Europe and USA
	Pramipexole 3 × 0.125 mg – 3 × 0.5 mg (salt; USA) 3 × 0.088 – 3× 0.35 mg (base; Europe)	Licensed in Europe and USA
	Rotigotine patch	Not yet available
Ergot dopamine agonists	Pergolide 1 × 0.25–0.75 mg	Possible valvulopathy. Withdrawn from US market. Restricted off-label use in Europe only with specific monitoring.
	Cabergoline 1 × 1–2 mg	Possible valvulopathy. Restricted off-label use only with specific monitoring.
	Lisuride patch	Not yet available
Opiates	Oxycodone < 11 mg/day	Off label
	Tramadolol < 50 mg/day	Off label, reports of augmentation
	Propoxyphene 50–100 mg/day	Off label
	Methadone 5–40 mg/day	Off label
Benzodiazepines	Clonazepam 0.5–2.0 mg/day	Off label
Others	Gabapentin 100–2000 mg/day	Off label

Non-ergot dopamine agonists

The non-ergot dopamine agonists ropinirole and pramipexole are licensed for the treatment of RLS in the USA and Europe. A significant number of large-scale trials are available for both drugs, proving their efficacy and safety in those with moderate to severe RLS and a baseline IRLS score > 15. For mild RLS, there is seldom a need for these medications.

Ropinirole has been investigated in several controlled studies and the data comprise almost 1000 people with RLS. In a European 12-week study, a mean dosage of 1.90 mg was given once daily 2 hours before bedtime to treat RLS symptoms at night. Individuals with daytime symptoms were excluded in this ropinirole trial program. Recent studies, however, showed that splitting the dosage in the afternoon or early evening and shortly before bedtime can be an alternative regimen for those who suffer from afternoon or evening symptoms. Sometimes 0.5–1 mg ropinirole, two or three times a day, is a sufficient dosage. In a controlled polysomnographic treatment trial, sleep was improved and the PLM index decreased significantly. Sleep efficiency measured by PSG was not improved, whereas sleep adequacy on a subjective scale was significantly improved with ropinirole treatment.

With pramipexole, similar results were obtained for a single dose of 0.25–0.75 mg before bedtime. In polysomnographic studies 0.25–0.75 mg reduced both the PLMS index to normal values and the PLMW index significantly. Further large-scale trials in Europe and the USA revealed a significant improvement in subjective RLS symptoms during both daytime and sleep over a 12-week observation period. In a blinded study, people who had responded well to pramipexole in a 6-month open treatment worsened with RLS symptoms within days when the drug was withdrawn. Long-term observations in a retrospective case series of 60 people with RLS over 2 years provided stable treatment results with a dosage increase from 0.38 to 0.63 mg pramipexole and a rate of mild augmentation in 33%, who were treatable with increased doses earlier in the day. From clinical experience, a low dose of pramipexole (0.25 mg salt, i.e., 0.18 mg base), in split dosages in the afternoon and in the evening, is very effective.

Rotigotine, another non-ergot dopamine agonist, is currently being studied in large trials, with early data suggesting promising results for treating RLS using a patch application. Typical side effects of non-ergot dopamine agonists are nausea, vomiting, and dizziness. The patch application may also lead to local skin reactions.

Ergot dopamine agonists

None of the available ergot-derived dopamine agonists is licensed for the treatment of RLS. Pergolide and cabergoline have proven to be effective in large controlled trials, but the pharmaceutical companies producing these substances have not filed for a license for RLS therapy. Pergolide has been withdrawn from the US market because of possible valvulopathy. Pergolide and cabergoline can be used in Europe and other countries only with specific monitoring and restricted use. Other ergot dopamine agonists such as lisuride (in a patch application) or dihydroergocryptine have been investigated in open trials or case series only. All substances share side effects of nausea and vomiting. A limitation of the use of ergot dopamine agonists is the possibility of valvular and pulmonary fibrosis, which has been described in people with Parkinson's disease treated with ergot agonists. Recent publications have reported the development of valvular fibrosis in up to 38% of those treated with the ergot dopamine agonists cabergoline and pergolide. Monitoring with echocardiography is therefore necessary for all individuals treated with ergot dopamine agonists. For lisuride such side effects have not to date been reported.

Opiates

Opiates were recommended as treatment for RLS by Thomas Willis as early as 1684. Although opiates are reported from clinical experience to be very efficient treatments for RLS, only a few clinical trials have been performed, limiting the scope for making any evidence-based statement concerning efficacy, and especially long-term treatment outcomes. In one open study methadone 5–40 mg/day was administered to individuals in whom dopaminergic treatment had failed for 4–44 months, and a significant reduction in RLS symptoms was observed without the occurrence of augmentation.

However, only for oxycodone and propoxyphene is information available from double-blind studies showing reductions of subjective complaints and PLMS. Long-term observations are available only from a case series. Opioid treatment may result in a minimal risk of dependency, and also worsening of sleep apnea. With tramadolol the occurrence of augmentation has been published in two reports. Opioids should be used as a second choice, when dopamine agonists are not effective enough or when augmentation has occurred.

Gabapentin and other anticonvulsants

Gabapentin is considered to be an effective treatment of primary RLS, reported in two controlled trials with a limited number of patients. It is probably effective in secondary RLS, although this has never been studied formally in any trial. It seems especially helpful in treating RLS with painful symptoms or associated neuropathy. In hemodialysis patients a reduced dosage after each dialysis is recommended (200 mg per day). Other anticonvulsants such as carbamazepine or valproic acid have not been studied in large trials and are no longer used for the treatment of RLS.

Benzodiazepines and other sedative-hypnotics

In contrast to older recommendations, benzodiazepines are not considered as a treatment of first choice for RLS. Even though the efficacy of benzodiazepines, especially of clonazepam, was suggested in some studies, they should only be used when dopaminergic and opioidergic treatments are contraindicated, or when a sleep disturbance persists in spite of suppressed PLMS. Controlled studies have been performed only in people with PLMS, not in clinically defined RLS.

Augmentation

The term augmentation describes an increase in the severity of RLS, a time shift of the start of symptoms to earlier in the day, a shorter latency to RLS symptoms at rest, and/or a spreading of symptoms to other body parts (a development from focal akathisia to almost general akathisia). Apart from substance-specific side effects usually occurring transiently at the start of a new treatment, augmentation is the main complication of long-term pharmacological treatment of RLS. The key features of augmentation are listed in Table 7.4.

The pathophysiological mechanisms leading to augmentation are not known so far. Nevertheless, because there is some evidence that low ferritin values predispose to augmentation, in the case of suspected augmentation iron supplementation should be considered. Although augmentation initially was thought to be an exclusive problem of levodopa treatment, it has been found to develop with other dopaminergic treatments as well. Furthermore there is some evidence from case reports that it also might be a problem of non-dopaminergic treatments.

Physicians not familiar with augmentation are tempted to increase the levodopa dosage to very high levels as soon as the efficacy of dopaminergic treatment weakens, thus inducing a vicious cycle. There is no evidence-based recommendation that can be made for the management of augmentation. However, from clinical experience

Table 7.4. *Key features of augmentation in RLS (Allen RP, et al.,* Sleep Med *2003; 4: 101–19).*

Feature 1 has to be present, or two out of features 2–7.

(1) Augmentation is the shifting of symptoms to a period of time 2 or more hours earlier than was the typical period of daily onset of symptoms before pharmacologic intervention.

(2) An increased overall intensity of the urge to move or sensation is temporally related to an increase in the daily medication dosage.

(3) A decreased overall intensity of the urge to move or sensations is temporally related to a decrease in the daily medication dosage.

(4) The latency to RLS symptoms at rest is shorter than the latency with initial therapeutic response or before treatment was instituted.

(5) The urge to move or sensations are extended to previously unaffected limbs or body parts.

(6) The duration of treatment effect is shorter than the duration with initial therapeutic response.

(7) Periodic limb movements while awake either occur for the first time or are worse than with initial therapeutic response or before treatment was instituted.

one would recommend – in order to avoid augmentation – to start with low dosages and to keep them low in the course of treatment. People who develop augmentation under levodopa treatment should be treated with lower and split dosages in mild cases. In more severe cases, levodopa has to be stopped and treatment switched to a dopamine agonist. If augmentation occurs again with dopamine agonist treatment, treatment should be split into low dosages or changed to opiates (Fig. 7.3).

FURTHER READING

Allen RP, Earley CJ. Restless legs syndrome: a review of clinical and pathophysiologic features. *J Clin Neurophysiol* 2001; **18**: 128–47.

Allen RP, Picchietti D, Hening WA, *et al.* Restless legs syndrome: diagnostic criteria, special considerations, and epidemiology. A report from the restless legs syndrome diagnosis and epidemiology workshop at the National Institutes of Health. *Sleep Med* 2003; **4**: 101–19.

American Academy of Sleep Medicine. *The International Classification of Sleep Disorders: Diagnostic and Coding Manual*, 2nd edn (ICSD–2). Westchester, IL: American Academy of Sleep Medicine, 2005.

Hening W. The clinical neurophysiology of the restless legs syndrome and periodic limb movements. Part I: diagnosis, assessment, and characterization. *Clin Neurophysiol* 2004; **115**: 1965–74.

Hornyak H, Kotterba S, Trenkwalder C. Motor Disorders Study Group of the German Sleep Society. Indications for performing polysomnography in the diagnosis and treatment of restless legs syndrome. *Somnologie* 2001; **5**: 159–62.

Montplaisir J, Nicolas A, Denesle R, Gomez-Mancilla B. Restless legs syndrome improved by pramipexole: a double-blind randomized trial. *Neurology* 1999; **52**: 938–43.

Trenkwalder C, Paulus W. Why do restless legs occur at rest? Pathophysiology of neuronal structures in RLS. Neurophysiology of RLS (Part II). *Clin Neurophysiol* 2004; **115**: 1975–88.

Trenkwalder C, Paulus W, Walters AS. The restless legs syndrome. *Lancet Neurol* 2005; **4**: 465–75.

Trenkwalder C, Garcia-Borreguero D, Montagna P, *et al.* Ropinirole in the treatment of restless legs syndrome: results from the TREAT RLS 1 study, a 12 week, randomised, placebo controlled study in 10 European countries. *J Neurol Neurosurg Psychiatry* 2004; **75**: 92–7.

Walters AS, LeBrocq C, Dhar A, *et al.* Validation of the International Restless Legs Syndrome Study Group rating scale for restless legs syndrome. *Sleep Med* 2003; **4**: 121–32.

Zucconi, M, Ferri R, Allen R, *et al.* The official World Association of Sleep Medicine (WASM) standards for recording and scoring periodic leg movements in sleep (PLMS) and wakefulness (PLMW) developed in collaboration with a task force from the International Restless Legs Syndrome Study Group (IRLSSG). *Sleep Med* 2006; **7**: 175–83.

8   Sleep apnea (central and obstructive)

Kannan Ramar and Christian Guilleminault

Introduction

Sleep-disordered breathing constitutes an important health problem with significant morbidity and mortality. There are two types of sleep apnea: obstructive and central, based on the presence or absence of respiratory effort.

The criteria for the classification of sleep-related breathing events have been established by the American Academy of Sleep Medicine (AASM). According to these criteria, an apnea is defined as cessation of airflow for at least 10 seconds. Hypopnea is defined as a 30% reduction or more in airflow associated with a drop in oxygen saturation of more than 3%. Central apnea is defined by the absence of respiratory effort, while obstructive apnea occurs despite persistent respiratory effort. There may be associated abdominal paradox with obstructive apnea, as illustrated in Fig. 8.1. Mixed apnea is usually a combination of both central and obstructive: an initial central part (lack of respiratory effort) followed by the terminal obstructive part (presence of respiratory effort), as illustrated in Fig. 8.2. Mixed apneas are usually grouped under obstructive apneas. The apnea/hypopnea index (AHI) is the number of apneas and hypopneas per hour of sleep. The respiratory disturbance index (RDI) is defined as the AHI plus the respiratory effort-related arousals (RERA). An illustration of RERA is shown in Fig. 8.3. This chapter will focus on the pathophysiology, clinical features, and management of obstructive and central sleep apnea.

Central sleep apnea

Central sleep apnea (CSA) is characterized by the occurrence of apnea (of 10 seconds or longer) due to a lack of respiratory effort related to loss of ventilatory motor output. Central hypopnea, which is related to central apnea, is a reduction in respiratory effort leading to a reduction in airflow. Central hypopneas may be difficult to differentiate from obstructive hypopneas without the help of an esophageal pressure monitor. Some authors may classify central hypopneas based on the rounded nasal pressure signal. Central apneas and hypopneas stem from the same pathophysiologic mechanisms and are only different with respect to the severity of the phenomenon. Central hypopnea and apnea are discussed together in this chapter.

Sleep Medicine, ed. Harold R. Smith, Cynthia L. Comella, and Birgit Högl. Published by Cambridge University Press. © Cambridge University Press 2008.

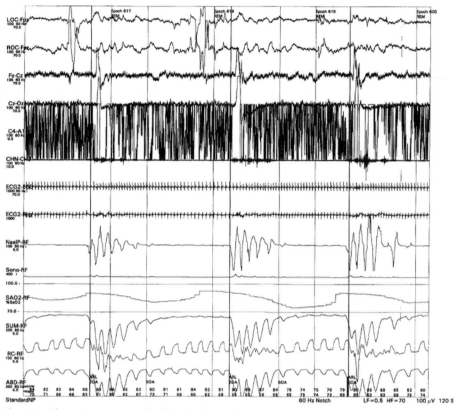

Fig. 8.1. Obstructive apnea with abdominal paradox.

- CSA accounts for less than 15% of individuals with sleep apnea evaluated at sleep disorder centers.
- Though central apneas can occur in people with obstructive sleep apnea, diagnosis of CSA is usually made when more than 50% of the apneic events are central in nature.

Pathophysiology

Central sleep apnea may occur secondary to lesions that affect the sensory component, the integrative and executive neuronal systems, or the motor component (i.e., the lower motor neurons, nerves, and muscles) of the neural systems involved in respiratory control. The sensory component consists of changes in the PCO_2 and PO_2 of the arterial blood, the peripheral and central chemoreceptors where the changes are monitored, and the relay of these changes to the brainstem, where the signals are received and analyzed. After the noted changes of the sensory component (i.e., changes in PO_2 or PCO_2) are received by the integrative and executive neuronal systems in the brainstem, the motor loop is mobilized, which stimulates the muscles of respiration. Instability in any of these components can lead to central sleep apnea. The instability can occur due to:

(1) Increased circulation time, which can delay the transmission of sensory input (from the lungs to the chemoreceptors).

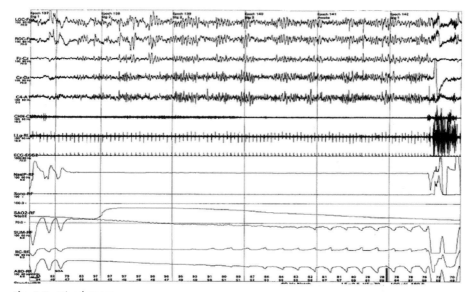

Fig. 8.2. Mixed apnea.

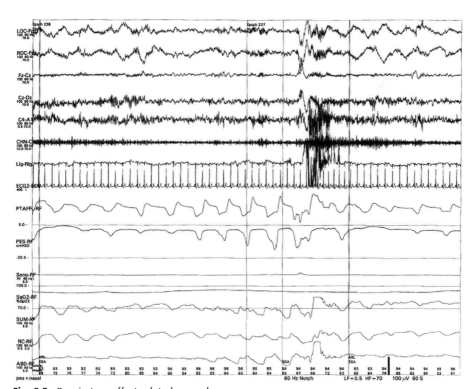

Fig. 8.3. Respiratory effort-related arousal.

Table 8.1. *Common causes of nonhypercapnic central sleep apnea (CSA).*

Idiopathic
Congestive heart failure
Chronic renal failure
Periodic breathing at high altitude
Sleep-onset(transition) central sleep apnea
Nasal CPAP titration

(2) Increased controller gain (sensitivity), which can lead to overcorrection of the physiologic fluctuations in blood gases. The controller gain is synonymous with chemoresponsiveness.

(3) Reduction in the dampening of the system, which can lead to instability.

Central sleep apnea is often classified as hypercapnic (daytime hypoventilation) or nonhypercapnic, based on minute ventilation (product of respiratory rate and tidal volume).

Nonhypercapnic CSA

Nonhypercapnic central sleep apnea is the most common form of CSA. The most frequent causes are listed in Table 8.1. Nonhypercapnic CSA manifests as periodic occurrences of apnea or hypopnea alternating with hyperpnea due to increased chemoresponsiveness.

CSA due to Cheyne–Stokes breathing

The Cheyne–Stokes breathing pattern is a specific type of periodic breathing characterized by recurrent apneas, hypopneas, or both, and with the hypopneas alternating with prolonged hyperpneas in a crescendo/de-crescendo pattern (Fig. 8.1). Arousals tend to occur near the maximum point of ventilatory effort (hyperpneic phase), as illustrated in Fig. 8.4. This can lead to repeated oxygen desaturations and sleep fragmentation. Symptoms may include excessive daytime sleepiness, insomnia, and dyspnea, but some individuals remain completely asymptomatic.

CSA due to Cheyne–Stokes breathing is seen in people with congestive heart failure (CHF), neurological disorders such as stroke, and probably renal failure.

- The prevalence of CSA in individuals with CHF is 30–50%, though this number may be lower now with more effective treatment of CHF.
- The prevalence in those with stroke is approximately 10%.
- Risk factors for CSA are male gender, atrial fibrillation, age greater than 60 years, and hypocapnia ($PCO_2 < 38$ mm Hg) during wakefulness.
- CSA characteristically occurs during NREM sleep (usually stages 1 and 2) and is attenuated during REM and stages 3 and 4 NREM sleep.
- CSA due to Cheyne–Stokes breathing in the setting of CHF is associated with poor prognosis, though its clinical significance in the setting of stroke or renal failure is not known.
- Usually patients have a low PCO_2, less than 45 mm Hg during wakefulness.

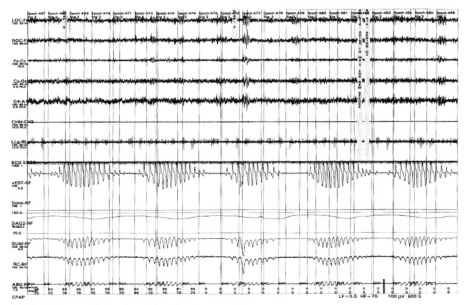

Fig. 8.4. Cheyne–Stokes breathing due to central sleep apnea.

Pathophysiology

The precise mechanism of central sleep apnea due to Cheyne–Stokes breathing is not completely understood. Generally, it arises at the transition of wake to NREM sleep or during stable NREM sleep. It is usually seen in people who hyperventilate chronically during wake and sleep secondary to stimulation of pulmonary vagal irritant receptors. This may lead to apneas since it drives the PCO_2 below the apneic threshold. People with Cheyne–Stokes breathing pattern have PCO_2 closer to the apneic threshold than those without. Though there is conflicting evidence regarding the sustained breathing instability, it is believed to be due to recurrent arousals at the termination of apneas leading to hyperpneas and thereby lowering of the PCO_2 below the apneic threshold, causing apneas. It is therefore post-hyperventilatory in nature. Apart from increased chemoresponsiveness to PCO_2, there is also a prolonged lung-to-chemoreceptor circulatory delay (length of circulation time) resulting in gradual build-up and fall of ventilatory stimulation. The length of the ventilatory phase cycle tends to correlate with the length of circulation time and to be inversely related to cardiac output. The length of the circulation time is usually longer than 45 seconds. Also, the apnea length depends on the amount of hypocapnia at sleep onset.

The length of the circulation time can be calculated on the polysomnogram by estimating the time difference between the end of the apnea and the lowest point of oxygen desaturation.

Treatment

Treatment should focus on optimizing cardiac function. Positive airway pressure can reduce the amount of CSA due to Cheyne–Stokes breathing. An optimal continuous positive airway pressure (CPAP) cannot be identified, but the usual strategy is to start at a lower pressure setting to eliminate the obstructive events and titrate upwards over a month as tolerated to 10–12 cm of water. CPAP is believed to work by increasing oxygen stores (increasing functional residual capacity) and causing a modest increase in PCO_2.

CPAP may improve cardiac function by the following mechanisms:

(1) Increases intrathoracic pressure:
 - decreases venous return
 - decreases afterload and augments cardiac output
 - decreases the negative pleural pressure by reducing the interstitial edema.
(2) Increases pleural pressure, which in turn decreases the transmyocardial pressure and reduces the myocardial oxygen consumption, as shown in the following equations:
 - cardiac wall stress = transmyocardial pressure × radius of curvature of the heart / thickness of the heart (*Laplace's Law*)
 - transmyocardial pressure (determinant of cardiac wall stress and afterload) = intracavitary pressure – pressure outside the heart (which is the pleural pressure).
(3) Eliminates or reduces OSA, if present:
 - individuals with OSA will have increased upper airway resistance, which will increase the negative pleural pressure to generate a breath.

Bilevel positive airway pressure can also be tried, but if inspiratory positive airway pressure (IPAP) is considerably greater than expiratory positive airway pressure (EPAP), this may worsen CSA. Newer modalities of treatment including adaptive servo-ventilators (ASV) help in controlling and reducing the amount of CSA due to Cheyne–Stokes breathing, but long-term data are currently lacking. ASV can be used on the first night of titration rather than needing to wait for a month as with CPAP. ASV can be started at a low EPAP to treat the obstructive events, and the IPAP tends to vary depending on the previous level of ventilation. Oxygen can also be used to lower the CSA events and arousals. Theophylline can do the same, but there is a risk of arrhythmias. The theophylline data are based on a trial that lasted only 5 days.

Short-term pilot studies with CPAP have shown improvement in cardiac function as measured by ejection fraction, a reduction in sympathetic tone, and improvement in exercise tolerance with 3 months of CPAP use. Also, a relative risk reduction of 81% in mortality/transplantation rate was noted at 3 months with CPAP therapy. This was followed by the much-anticipated Canadian positive airway pressure trial (CANPAP), which randomly assigned people with both heart failure and central sleep apnea to receive either CPAP or no treatment in order to test whether intervention improved transplant-free survival. The trial resulted in lower norepinephrine levels, increased ejection fraction, and an early but transient improvement in exercise tolerance, but no mortality benefit. The trial had a few limitations. Despite a careful titration protocol in treatment with CPAP, the AHI was reduced by only 50%, with a substantial residual AHI of about 20 events per hour. There was a lower than expected recruitment rate, with a time-dependent decline in mortality in CHF

Table 8.2. *Therapies for CSA due to Cheyne–Stokes breathing.*

Optimal medical management of congestive heart failure (CHF)
Positive airway pressure therapy
CPAP
Bilevel with spontaneous timed mode
Adaptive servo-ventilator (ASV)
Oxygen
CO_2 inhalation
Medications
Theophylline
Acetazolamide
Hypnotics

patients with CSA, raising the possibility of a role for beta-blockers and spironolactone in the treatment of CHF. Nonetheless, newer approaches such as more effective positive airway pressure devices (e.g., ASV), cardiac resynchronization therapy, and medication (acetazolamide) may enable a more complete resolution of central sleep apnea and improved sleep quality, which may translate into better clinical outcomes. Therapies for CSA due to Cheyne–Stokes breathing are summarized in Table 8.2.

Primary or idiopathic CSA

This is an uncommon disorder (less than 5% of individuals with sleep apnea) with no known etiology. Patients may present with complaints of insomnia, excessive daytime sleepiness, snoring, and occasional episodes of gasping or choking during the night. The polysomnogram is characterized by frequent isolated central apneas, or runs of them. These may occur following arousals due to a non-respiratory stimulus. Individuals with primary or idiopathic CSA have a high ventilatory response to CO_2. They also have low PCO_2 during wakefulness. The other variables that have been proposed as possible predisposing or exacerbating factors are insomnia, nasal obstruction, and certain neurological disorders such as multiple system atrophy and Parkinson's disease (especially when associated with autonomic dysfunction). In some people, a supine position precipitates the CSA, possibly due to triggering of the upper airway reflexes that may inhibit respiration. Apart from recurrent central apneas on the polysomnogram, similar to those of CSA due to Cheyne–Stokes breathing, it is commonly seen during stages 1 and 2 NREM sleep and attenuates during REM sleep. Arousals tend to occur at apnea termination rather than at the hyperpneic phase (as in Cheyne–Stokes CSA). Also, there is a shorter circulation time (time between termination of apnea and lowest point of oxygen desaturation) than in Cheyne–Stokes breathing. Patients usually respond to continuous positive airway pressure (CPAP) therapy (potential mechanism is by increasing PCO_2), though other treatment options (as mentioned in Table 8.3) have been tried with some success.

Table 8.3. *Treatment options for idiopathic CSA.*

CPAP
Position therapy: lying on side rather than supine
Acetazolamide
Oxygen therapy
Benzodiazepines and non-benzodiazepine GABA-A active hypnotics

Sleep-onset or sleep-transition CSA

Central sleep apnea usually occurs at sleep onset or with sleep transition, and resolves with sleep consolidation. This may be a normal phenomenon occurring in subjects who have high ventilatory response to PCO_2. It results in hypocapnia and subsequently apnea at onset of sleep (as the PCO_2 may have fallen below the apneic threshold). The apnea continues until the PCO_2 builds up to reinitiate breathing. This may be seen in individuals who have recurrent arousals from various different causes, such as periodic limb movements (PLM). This may not require treatment in an otherwise asymptomatic person with no other comorbidity. Hypnotics may be tried in selected individuals to decrease the recurrent arousals and thereby the CSA.

CSA following nasal CPAP titration

Nasal CPAP titration may lead to CSA. This may become more pronounced at high altitude, and may be secondary to a reduction in PCO_2 to below apneic thresholds once the upper airway resistance is lowered with CPAP. The treatment is to reduce the CPAP pressure until the central apneas disappear and the obstructive events are eliminated. Increasing the CPAP may not help with eliminating central sleep events, and may in fact worsen it. Increasing CPAP may help with central sleep apnea only when obstructive events have been misclassified as central events. It may not always be possible to distinguish obstructive from central events, especially in an obese individual or where the impedance belt may not be fitting well enough to measure abdominal movements. (Esophageal pressure monitoring [Pes] and a nasal pressure cannula may help to differentiate central from obstructive events). CSA with CPAP titration may also resolve on its own when the CPAP is continued, due to resetting of the apneic threshold in a few months.

Hypercapnic CSA

The common causes of hypercapnic CSA are listed in Table 8.4. Hypercapnic CSA has the following features:

- It is characterized by hypoventilation. The common physiologic abnormality noted is blunted chemoresponsiveness (unlike the increased chemoresponsiveness noted in people with nonhypercapnic CSA).
- The hypoventilation is secondary to reduced ventilatory motor output.
- During REM sleep, more profound arterial oxygen desaturation is noted, especially in individuals with neuromuscular disorders. Measurement of transcutaneous PCO_2 reveals an increase in PCO_2 during NREM, with further increase during REM sleep.

Table 8.4. *Common causes of hypercapnic CSA.*

Congenital central hypoventilation
Cerebrovascular disorders
  Brainstem disease
Chest wall disorders
  Kyphoscoliosis
Neuromuscular disorders
  Amyotrophic lateral sclerosis
  Muscular dystrophy involving thorax or diaphragm (such as maltase deficiency)
  Unilateral or bilateral diaphragmatic paralysis

- Symptoms may include right-sided heart failure (cor pulmonale), morning headache (secondary to PCO_2 retention) that tends to get better as the day progresses, pedal edema, polycythemia, and abnormal pulmonary function tests (mainly a restrictive ventilatory defect). There may also be poor nocturnal sleep, snoring, and daytime sleepiness.

One form of hypercapnic CSA is congenital central hypoventilation, which has the following features:

- Onset in infancy.
- Hypoventilation worse during sleep than wakefulness.
- Occurs due to abnormalities in brainstem integration of afferents from the peripheral chemoreceptors.
- Breathing problems are worse during NREM than REM sleep, unlike other hypercapnic CSA causes.
- Treatment requires the use of noninvasive bilevel, with or without oxygen, during sleep, while some may require ventilatory support via tracheostomy.
- Associated features:
  - Hirschsprung's disease
  - autonomic dysfunction
  - neural tumors: neuroblastoma
  - swallowing dysfunction
  - ocular abnormalities.

Obstructive sleep apnea (OSA)

Obstructive sleep apnea (OSA) is a condition characterized by repeated episodes of upper airway closure during sleep. OSA commonly affects middle-aged men and women. The prevalence of OSA in white adults in the United States has been reported to be 4% in men and 2% in women between the ages of 30 and 60 years, though the actual prevalence may be higher. The prevalence of OSA reported in the literature has a wide range, due to inconsistencies in the definition and sampling biases. On the basis of pooled data from four large prevalence studies that used similar in-laboratory monitoring, diagnostic criteria, and sampling methods, it is estimated that 1 in 5 white adults with a body mass index (BMI) of 25–28 kg/m^2 has an AHI ≥ 5 (mild disease) and 1 in 15 has an AHI ≥ 15 (moderate to severe disease). OSA is a polygraphic pattern observed when performing sleep studies, and it is characterized by sleep fragmentation due to repeated arousals and disruption of normal sleep architecture secondary to partial or complete closure of the upper airway during sleep.

Risk factors

There are many risk factors for OSA, as shown in Table 8.5, with obesity and craniofacial features being by far the most common.

Pathophysiology and pathogenesis

In discussing the pathophysiology of OSA, we will include risk factors and their role in the pathogenesis of OSA. Sleep-disordered breathing (SDB) is due to increased upper airway resistance at one or more sites of the upper airway. Locations of narrowing include the nose, retropalatal region, retroglossal region, or, less commonly, the hypoglossal region.

Table 8.5. *Risk factors for obstructive sleep apnea (OSA).*

Obesity
Fat distribution
Neck circumference
Craniofacial features
Skeletal features
Mandible
Maxilla
Hyoid bone
High and narrow hard palate
Soft tissues of the pharynx
Tonsils
Lateral pharyngeal wall
Soft palate
Uvula
Tongue
Nose
Snoring
Age
Gender
Menopause
Ethnicity
Smoking
Alcohol
Specific diseases
Polycystic ovary syndrome
Conditions causing macroglossia
Neurological conditions like cerebrovascular accidents, neuromuscular disorders
Congenital abnormalities that cause retrognathia

Airway factors

The size of the pharyngeal upper airway is dependent on a balance of forces between the upper airway dilators, maintaining upper airway patency, and the negative pharyngeal intraluminal pressure created during thoracic expansion as a result of inspiration. To prevent upper airway closure, pharyngeal reflexes are normally activated at least 100–500 ms before beginning of inspiration to activate contraction of upper airway dilator muscles to oppose the subatmospheric intrathoracic pressure. A lack of coordination between inspiratory muscles and upper airway dilators will lead to upper airway occlusion during sleep. This was reported as early as 1978 by Guilleminault and Motta in an investigation of people with postpoliomyelitis syndrome treated with a cuirass ventilator. These individuals developed a negative intrathoracic pressure that could not be counteracted by the upper airway dilators, and this led to the development of OSA.

During sleep, many of the upper airway dilator muscles have much less contractile power than the diaphragm. The genioglossus and geniohyoid muscles are particularly affected: their motor activity is abnormal in individuals with OSA, with heightened contraction during the daytime and decreased contraction at sleep. This physiologic change allows the development of abnormal inspiratory upper airway resistance, which may result in partial or complete occlusion. If abnormalities of the upper airway (anatomic, physiologic, or neurologic) reduce size to a level lower than critical, or limit the capabilities of upper airway dilator muscles, a more or less pronounced collapse will occur during sleep in this very flexible region. It has been shown that there is a greater decrease in muscle tone in these groups of muscles in those with OSA than in controls, as measured by EMG.

Skeletal factors

Skeletal factors also play a role by narrowing the upper airways further. Bernoulli's principle dictates that narrowing of any segment while airflow is maintained causes an increased velocity of airflow in that segment. This decreases intraluminal pressure and further narrows the segment, favoring upper airway collapse. There is a constellation of jaw malformations associated with OSA, including a highly arched hard palate and class II dental occlusion (overjet). The position of the mandible relative to the maxilla determines the posterior extension of the tongue. Because the genioglossus muscle inserts on the mandible, with retrognathia or micrognathia the genioglossus originates on a backwardly displaced mandible and thus extends further posterior, predisposing to hypopharyngeal obstruction. During sleep in the supine position, gravity pulls the tongue further into the pharyngeal lumen, and varying degrees of decreased muscle tone additionally relax the tongue dorsally. The position of the hyoid bone is also important, with inferior displacement being a risk factor for OSA. The hyoid bone serves as a central anchorage for the tongue muscles and thereby partly determines the position of the tongue. The hyoid bone is displaced inferiorly in those with OSA, compared with normal subjects. This inferior displacement of the hyoid bone may be accompanied by an inferior displacement of the tongue into the hypopharyngeal area.

Soft tissues

The soft tissues of the pharynx (tonsils, lateral pharyngeal walls, uvula, soft palate, and tongue) also contribute to upper airway narrowing. Obesity and hypothyroidism can predispose to macroglossia. Allergies and recurrent upper respiratory infections can cause hyperplasia and scarring of lymphoid tissue. Snoring renders the uvula more edematous because of suction and trauma, which further compromises the small oropharyngeal space. Nasal obstruction from any cause, including allergic congestion, inflamed lymphoid tissue, or septal deviation can trigger narrowing of the upper airways by converting breathing from the nasal to the oral route. Oral breathing predisposes to backward displacement of the base of the tongue and leads to abnormal airway dynamics favoring pharyngeal collapse. The dilating genioglossus and geniohyoid muscles become mechanically disadvantaged and airway resistance is increased. Enlargement of these tissues can also occur secondary to hereditary and acquired factors, and we will discuss this further below.

Obesity

Obesity is a well-known risk factor for OSA. It plays a significant role by compromising the upper airways. Adiposity compromises the upper airway not only because the "double chin" externally compresses the pharynx in the supine position, but also through internal infiltration of parapharyngeal structures (i.e., the adipose tissue alters and reduces airspace). Pharyngeal dilator muscle mechanics may be compromised by this loading as well. Obesity predisposes to OSA by the following mechanisms:

- change in upper airway structure (e.g., altered anatomy)
- change in upper airway function (e.g., increased collapsibility)
- unstable relationship between respiratory drive and workload
- exacerbation of OSA events via obesity-related reductions in functional residual capacity and increased whole-body oxygen demand.

These hypotheses are supported by studies that have shown that in obese men with OSA, weight loss increases the upper airway cross-sectional area, and thereby decreases the severity of OSA.

Reflex arc

There are other potential factors that play a role in the pathogenesis of OSA. Recent studies have suggested that a potential upper airway stabilizing mechanism may be initiated by the flow of air into the pharynx during inspiration. Although full details of this reflex have not been described, it appears that a reflex loop is activated once inspiration starts the flow of air into the upper airway, with the following sequence of events: (1) sensory neurons in the upper airway are activated, (2) sensory afferents travel to the brainstem, which subsequently activates the efferent hypoglossal nerve that innervates the genioglossus and geniohyoid, and (3) genioglossus and geniohyoid contraction keep the pharynx open during inspiration. This reflex may be altered in OSA because of damage to the muscle and nerves from the vibratory trauma of snoring. This theory is supported by findings of abnormal sensory nerves and nerve function in histological and neurophysiologic studies of upper airway muscles in individuals with OSA.

Hormonal factors

Testosterone may contribute to obstruction by inducing more parapharyngeal muscle bulk and more centripetal fat distribution. This may also explain the gender differences, and why premenopausal women have a lesser prevalence and are more protected from the development of OSA than their male counterparts. The reasons for gender differences in the prevalence and severity of sleep apnea are multifactorial. Some of the most commonly proposed hypotheses include differences in the effect of weight, differences in body fat distribution, abnormalities in upper airway mechanics, control of breathing, and structural differences in upper airway dimensions.

Genetic and developmental factors

The genetic and environmental factors that determine early craniofacial development can also play a role in the pathogenesis of OSA. Several studies have demonstrated familial aggregation of craniofacial morphology (reduction in posterior airway space, increased mandibular-to-hyoid distance, inferior hyoid placement) in people with sleep apnea. The data from these studies indicate that elements of craniofacial structure in those with sleep apnea are inherited. Demonstrating heritability of upper airway structures provides further support for the importance of upper airway anatomy as a risk factor for the development of OSA.

A developmental paradigm should be used to better understand the role of the craniofacial skeleton in the appearance of abnormal breathing during sleep. OSA has been demonstrated in longitudinal studies of children treated with tonsillectomy and adenoidectomy. Children who were considered to have normal breathing post-surgery presented with OSA 10–12 years later. Guilleminault and colleagues linked the reappearance of abnormal breathing during sleep to the presence of unrecognized and untreated modest skeletal changes in early childhood, and the progressive impact over time of these early-life changes on the normal development of the upper airway. This indicates the importance of early craniofacial developmental features as a factor in the development of OSA in adulthood. Understanding the impact of early-life development on enhanced nasal resistance is critical due to the speed of craniofacial growth: by 4 years of age 60% of the adult face is built, and about 90% by 11–12 years of age. Chronic nasal obstruction during childhood that results in oral breathing may induce craniofacial changes predisposing to sleep apnea later in life. This has been shown in rhesus monkeys with experimentally partially occluded nostrils that developed mandibular deficiency relative to paired controls. Oral breathing changed EMG activity in facial muscle groups, leading to altered forces on the developing facial skeleton. Partial improvement in these changes occurred if the obstruction was relieved early enough. Upper airway obstruction from enlarged adenoids in children has been shown to lead to decreased mandibular size and retrognathia, among other craniofacial changes.

The speed of craniofacial growth is an important factor, as the craniofacial skeleton will have reached most of its adult size before the full impact of the pubertal hormonal secretion manifests itself on muscles and soft tissues located in the upper airway. The combined geniohyoid and genioglossus muscles are the largest muscle mass in proportion to the bony cavity that contains them. This large muscle mass may account for lack of adequate development of facial skeletal features, leading to reduced airway lumen. The presence of early-life abnormal nasal resistance, absence of treatment for the causes of this resistance, and neglect of treatment of already induced skeletal abnormalities due to early environmental factors will leave a narrow skeleton that will not be able to appropriately accommodate the soft tissues enlarged under the hormonal pubertal surge. The fact that these changes happen during a fast-growth period means that factors involved in the normal growth of the skeleton interact continuously. Some of these growth factors are under genetic influence, and are thus difficult to act upon. Some of these genetic factors are already obvious at birth, some are associated with ethnicity (for example Far–East Asian versus European), and others are familial, but these genetic factors influence the continuous growth of craniofacial features particularly during the prepubertal years, and will continuously interact with environmental factors, potentially increasing nasal resistance.

Morbidity: cardiovascular system
Hypertension
Obstructive sleep apnea is a well-established independent risk factor for systemic hypertension. There are several mechanisms that contribute to increases in blood pressure:
- intermittent hypoxemia
- large negative fluctuations in intrathoracic pressure
- repetitive arousals from sleep.

Arterial hypoxemia signals the carotid chemoreceptors to trigger vasomotor center-mediated arteriolar constriction, leading to increased systemic vascular resistance. Repetitive hypoxemia associated with apneic and hypopneic events leads to important changes in the autonomic nervous system neuronal network with a resetting of the sympathetic receptors. This resetting leads to continuous discharges, even during the daytime when hypoxemic events are not present. This abnormal sympathetic activity during waking hours leads to vascular changes along with progressive endothelium impairment involving the nitric oxide (NO) system. Endothelium NO system impairment has been strongly implicated in the development of plaques and atherosclerosis, which are responsible for the development of hypertension with OSA.

Large negative fluctuations in intrathoracic pressure occur in individuals with OSA during the apneic phase. This leads to a series of changes. There is a decrease in cardiac output due to decreased venous return, as well as significant bowing of the interventricular septum. There is also an increase in the left ventricular transmural pressure, thereby increasing the afterload. With the termination of apnea and resumption of ventilation, there is an increase in sympathetic discharge, documented by measurement of urinary catecholamines. Peroneal nerve microneurography has shown that individuals with OSA have increased muscle sympathetic nerve activity (MSNA) during wake compared to controls. Pulmonary stretch reflexes induce tachycardia, which increases cardiac output. Changes in preload and afterload due to the repetitive Muller and, at times, Valsalva maneuvers are also factors in the cardiac output changes.

Apart from OSA being an independent risk factor for hypertension, hypertension is a frequent comorbid condition with sleep apnea. Unfortunately, many of the studies are on obese people with OSA, and it is therefore difficult to tease out the role of obesity as a confounder for the development of hypertension. Approximately 30% of people with systemic hypertension have sleep apnea, whereas 50% or more of those with sleep apnea have systemic hypertension. Peppard and colleagues showed a dose–response association between OSA at baseline and the presence of hypertension 4 years later that was independent of known confounding factors, with odds ratios for the presence of hypertension at follow-up of 1.42 for an AHI of 0.1–4.9 events per hour at base line as compared to none, 2.03 for an AHI of 5–14.9, and 2.89 for an AHI of 15.0 or more. Another study reported that 40% of 301 people with congestive heart failure had OSA and systemic hypertension. After controlling for other risk factors, those with OSA were 2.89 times more likely to have systolic hypertension than those without OSA. The degree of systolic blood pressure elevation was directly related to the frequency of hypopneas and apneas.

Hypertension may improve after treatment of apnea. One case–control study reported a drop in blood pressure in 24 people with OSA after 14 months of CPAP therapy, which correlated with a decrease in both plasma renin and plasma angiotensin II concentrations. However, many of those with hypertension and OSA do not go back to normal blood pressure, probably indicating permanent vascular endothelial damage.

Heart failure

Heart failure also appears to occur as a consequence of OSA. The Sleep Heart Health Study reported that OSA is associated with an odds ratio of 2.38 for heart failure, independent of other known risk factors. OSA is also prevalent in people with heart failure, with one study reporting that about 50% of those with isolated diastolic heart failure had an AHI of at least 10.

Whether people with heart failure who have sleep-disordered breathing benefit from CPAP treatment is unclear. Several studies have shown that short-term use of CPAP in heart failure and obstructive sleep apnea improved left ventricular ejection, blood pressure, and ventricular systolic volume. CPAP is recommended in cases of heart failure with clearcut OSA.

Pulmonary hypertension

Moderate to severe increases in pulmonary arterial pressure occur with each apneic episode. Maximal pulmonary pressures coincide with maximal hypoxemic and hypercapnic values, and probably reflect hypoxic pulmonary vasoconstriction. When pressure gradients between the pulmonary artery lumen and thoracic cavity are evaluated, transpulmonary arterial pressure decreases during the first 25 seconds of apnea, then increases until breathing returns and transiently rises more rapidly. Another hemodynamic change consists of reductions in cardiac output of up to one-third of baseline values in apneas longer than 35 seconds.

The development of persistent pulmonary hypertension during wakefulness, and cor pulmonale, may be due to severe hypoxemia during sleep but is more likely a result of daytime hypoxemia. There has again been controversy on the persistence of daytime pulmonary hypertension. Earlier studies estimated the prevalence of pulmonary hypertension in people with OSA to be as high as 20–41%. These studies were small, but there is an agreement that a subgroup of individuals with OSA present with pulmonary hypertension, usually moderate during the day, related to their sleep-related problem. The American College of Chest Physicians recommends that evaluation for OSA should be part of the initial workup in those with pulmonary hypertension. Possible mechanisms thought to cause pulmonary hypertension include hypoxemia-induced endothelial cell dysfunction and pulmonary artery remodeling. The reversal of pulmonary hypertension after treatment for OSA is reported to be poor.

Cardiac arrhythmias

Cardiac arrhythmias that occur exclusively during sleep are common in apneics. Sinus arrhythmia accompanies each obstructive respiratory cycle, in which rate diminishes with the cessation of airflow and accelerates when breathing resumes. These changes can result in repetitive cycles of bradycardia and tachycardia, fluctuating from fewer than 30 to more than 120 beats per minute. Severe sinus bradycardia (fewer than 30 beats per minute) affects approximately 10% of sleep apneics, and is usually seen with severe hypoxemia. These aberrations of rate combined with hypoxemia predispose to conduction defects, malignant arrhythmias, and perhaps sudden death. Asystoles of up to 13 seconds, second-degree atrioventricular (AV) block, premature ventricular contractions, and runs of ventricular tachycardia are among documented apnea-related abnormalities. A prospective study of 147 consecutive patients demonstrated significantly higher prevalence of nocturnal paroxysmal asystole in people with OSA, and increased episodes of bradycardia and pauses, which correlated with the severity of the sleep apnea.

Proposed mechanisms for bradycardia, Mobitz I AV block, and asystole involve vagal nerve activation due to both Muller maneuver and hypoxemic carotid body stimulation. EEG arousal with airway reopening and lung expansion triggers cardiac acceleration. Increased sympathetic tone due to hypoxemia and acidosis may be expressed after vagal influence is withdrawn, leading to premature ventricular contractions (PVC), sinus tachycardia, and ventricular tachycardia. Frequency of PVCs and other ventricular arrhythmias has been shown to correlate with severity of oxygen desaturation, increasing threefold with desaturations lower than 60% (as compared to 90%).

Cardiac ischemia

Various studies have demonstrated that OSA can precipitate cardiac ischemia, especially in people with underlying coronary artery disease. The postulated mechanisms are:

- increased left ventricular afterload
- increased sympathetic drive
- post-apneic tachycardia
- profound bradycardia as the perfusion gradient drops, especially when diastole is prolonged.

From a global perspective, many of these physiologic responses to asphyxia may be viewed as an attempt to preserve perfusion to the critical cerebral and coronary systems. Increased systemic pressure selectively perfuses these critical central vessels, while bradycardia decreases myocardial oxygen consumption. As bradycardia becomes more profound, however, myocardial perfusion may become impaired, because the perfusion gradient drops as diastole is prolonged. Coronary ischemia may result in ventricular arrhythmia. On return of ventilation, cardiac rate and output arise in the setting of sympathetic dominance and decreased systemic resistance. The demand for myocardial oxygen to accomplish this work outweighs the supply of reperfused blood, rendering the myocardium vulnerable to ischemia and malignant arrhythmias.

Stroke

Sleep apnea and even snoring have been epidemiologically linked to increased incidences of stroke. One study of risk factors for stroke in approximately 400 individuals with OSA, matched with controls for sex and age, found an odds ratio of 3.2 for symptoms of snoring. Another study found an increased odds ratio even after adjustment for alcohol use, hypertension, and heart disease. The ratio increased approximately fourfold if obesity, observed apneas, and a subjective sense of excessive daytime sleepiness (EDS) were present. Recently a study of over 1000 people showed an increased hazard ratio in those with OSA of 2.24 for stroke or death from any cause over a several-year period. After adjustment for multiple risk factors (age, sex, race, obesity, hypertension, etc.) the hazard ratio was 1.97 (95% CI 1.12–3.48). A trend analysis indicated that those with more severe OSA were more likely to reach these endpoints. Though this study strongly suggests that OSA increases the risk of stroke or death, it may underestimate its risk in the development of these endpoints, as many of the OSA patients were treated surgically or with CPAP during the study period.

The increased incidence of stroke in OSA is likely secondary to multiple reasons. During apnea there is a greater chance of hypoxemia, hypercapnia, increased frequency of cardiac arrythmias, increased coagulation, and paradoxical embolism through a patent foramen ovale. However, Yaggi and colleagues presented data supporting that OSA is an independent risk factor for stroke.

Stroke and transient ischemic attacks are also a risk factor for OSA. Sixty-nine to ninety-five percent of individuals with acute strokes or transient ischemic attacks have OSA. Stroke patients who have OSA appear to have higher mortality as well. One study has shown that successful treatment of OSA with CPAP was associated with a decreased risk of subsequent strokes.

Metabolic syndrome

Obstructive sleep apnea has been associated with increased levels of leptin, C-reactive protein, homocysteine, and possibly insulin-resistance syndrome. However, some of the abnormalities observed have been determined to be related not to the OSA but to the frequently associated obesity: for example, C-reactive protein is not elevated in people with OSA with a maximum BMI of 25 kg/m^2 despite a mean AHI of 30 events per hour. Abnormal levels of leptin and ghrelin seen in these subjects seems to be more related to the severity of the sleep fragmentation (or total sleep loss) induced by the syndrome than directly from apnea and hypopnea. Leptin and ghrelin levels can normalize once a person's sleep apnea has been treated. Elevated levels of interleukin 6, tumor necrosis factor alpha, and leptin have been demonstrated in sleep apnea, independent of obesity.

OSA may be a predisposing factor in atherosclerosis and plaque formation, due to its action on the arterial endothelium and the NO system. Ultrasonographic examination has shown significantly increased carotid intima-media thickness in men with OSA, compared to habitual snorers. Age and BMI were significantly associated with intima-media thickness, whereas age and respiratory disturbance index (RDI) were most predictive for plaque.

Treatment

There are various treatment options for OSA, as listed in Table 8.6. The treatment is influenced by the severity of OSA, relative efficacy of various treatment options, associated comorbid conditions, and personal preference.

Weight loss

Weight loss in obese people is effective in the reduction of the number of apneas, sleep fragmentation, and the extent and number of oxygen desaturations. Several small studies of surgical or dietary weight loss interventions have shown consistent and substantial decreases in OSA severity following weight loss: an approximate 3% reduction in AHI is associated with each 1% reduction in weight. In overweight people without obvious fixed anatomic considerations such as retrognathia, weight loss may result in eventual cure. For most individuals, nasal CPAP should be instituted along with weight loss measures, whether bariatric surgery, diet with or without pharmacologic intervention, or exercise. When applicable, a program of exercise may be facilitated after daytime somnolence is ameliorated by CPAP. For those who are not completely cured by weight loss, the significant reduction in weight often allows a lower CPAP pressure requirement or increases the likelihood of a surgical cure. Individuals who lose significant weight should undergo retitration to the lowest effective pressure.

Role for bariatric surgery

Significant weight loss has been achieved with bariatric surgery, with significant reduction in AHI and an improvement in oxygen saturations. The studies were carried

Table 8.6. *Treatment options for OSA.*

Weight loss
  Diet
  Exercise
  Medications
  Bariatric surgery
Behavioral modifications
  Alcohol avoidance
  Avoidance of medications that can relax the upper airway muscles, such as sedatives
  Nicotine avoidance
  Avoidance of sleep deprivation
Medications
  TCAs like protriptyline – to suppress REM sleep and to increase the muscle tone
  Progesterone – respiratory stimulant in obese individuals, no impact on obstructed
    airway
  Paroxetine – mild decrease in apneas during NREM sleep
  Modafanil – to treat residual daytime sleepiness
Positional therapy
Oral appliance
Positive airway pressure therapies
  Continuous positive airway pressure (CPAP)
  Bilevel positive airway pressure
  Auto-titrating positive airway pressure
Surgery
  Nose
  Septoplasty, polypectomy, radiofrequency turbinate reduction
  Hyoid and subhyoid myotomy
  Geniotuberle advancement via inferior sagittal osteotomy
  Uvulopalatopharyngoplasty or uvuloflap surgery with tonsillectomy
  Maxillomandibular advancement
  Tracheostomy

---

out on small numbers of patients, however, with no long-term follow-up, so we do not know if the effects of the weight loss and reduction in AHI will be sustained in the long term.

Behavioral modifications and positional therapy

Elimination of central nervous system depressants such as alcohol or sedatives from the bloodstream at bedtime decreases the severity of OSA.

If a strong positional relationship is discovered, recommendation to remain in a lateral or prone position can be made. Though position therapy appears to be a feasible option for some individuals, most still end up lying on their backs in spite of good measures to prevent it.

Pharmacologic therapy

Tricyclic antidepressants such as protriptyline have been used to increase upper airway muscle tone and diminish REM sleep time in cases of mild or REM sleep-related OSA. Progesterone acts as a respiratory stimulant in obese individuals but has no impact on an obstructed airway. Paroxetine has been shown to mildly decrease apneas during NREM sleep. Modafinil has USFDA approval to treat residual daytime sleepiness in those receiving treatment for OSA, and has demonstrated statistical improvements in maintenance of wakefulness (MWT) and Epworth Sleepiness Scale scores compared to controls. To date, pharmacologic approaches to treat sleep-disordered breathing have been largely unsuccessful.

Oral appliances

There are various types of oral appliances, which work by:
- increasing upper airway space by advancing the tongue and soft palate
- providing a stable anterior position of the mandible
- possibly by changing the genioglossus muscle activity.

The upper airway space gained is much less than that obtained with surgical procedures. A recent meta-analysis concluded that oral appliances mildly improved subjective daytime sleepiness and sleep-disordered breathing compared with controls, but less effectively than CPAP. The AASM guidelines state that oral appliances should be used for people with mild to moderate OSA who prefer them to CPAP therapy, or for those who do not respond to CPAP, are not appropriate candidates, or fail treatment attempts with CPAP.

Positive airway pressure therapy

Since the original description of the use of CPAP in five people with severe OSA by Sullivan *et al.* in 1981, there has been an enormous advance in the treatment of OSA using positive airway pressure. CPAP:
- serves as a pneumatic splint to keep the upper airway patent
- increases the functional residual capacity (FRC) and thereby improves oxygenation
- improves ventilation/perfusion (V/Q) mismatch.

The last two mechanisms help to improve oxygenation, especially in individuals who are overweight or obese.

Pressure requirements must be established during sleep for each individual. Optimum pressure is the lowest one that completely eliminates obstructive apneas, hypopneas, and snoring. People who routinely consume alcohol in the evening are most accurately titrated to CPAP after consuming their usual intake, which raises the pressure requirement.

Various studies have shown the effects of CPAP, as follows:
- decreases AHI
- improves sleep efficiency
- decreases the symptoms of excessive daytime sleepiness
- improves neurocognitive performance
- improves quality of life

- improves driving performance on simulators
- reduces overall motor vehicle accidents.

Disadvantages of CPAP

Compliance – Between 25% and 50% of people with OSA abandon CPAP. Tolerance in the first week of use is poor, and abandonment is usually in the first 2–4 weeks. Interestingly, the severity of OSA based on AHI, pretreatment Epworth Sleepiness Score, age, and CPAP pressure (higher vs. lower pressure) do not necessarily predict compliance with CPAP.

Claustrophobia – The use of CPAP may cause people to feel claustrophobic and intolerant of the restriction of their movement, and they may perceive the treatment as an obstacle to intimacy with a bed partner and a reminder of their mortality.

Nuisance – Those traveling frequently may find it inconvenient. Generally, young adults and people who are dating find this treatment to have an unacceptable social impact.

Nose – Common physical difficulties encountered include reactive nasal congestion or rhinitis, sinusitis and epistaxis, or drying of the nasal–oral mucosa, discomfort or skin trauma from a poorly fitting mask, and allergic reaction to (or contact dermatitis with) the mask. Nasal symptoms usually subside after the first few months and can be ameliorated with heated humidification and a nasal steroid inhaler.

Helping people cope with CPAP

Comfort issues and dermatitis should be closely supervised and addressed with trials of various modes of delivery. Psychological distress is minimized by support from the entire sleep laboratory team, with reassurance and understanding at the time of initiation and close follow-up. Sleep apnea support groups exist in many areas to help with coping and compliance. Occasionally, a brief course of bedtime anxiolytics is required. Flow leaks through an open mouth can be minimized by use of a chin strap.

Compliance with CPAP can be improved by a number of strategies, as shown in Table 8.7. Not everyone will find the treatment equally acceptable. Table 8.8 lists characteristics that can be used to predict the likelihood of this form of therapy being accepted and used.

Bilevel positive airway pressure

Bilevel differs from CPAP in using separate inspiratory and expiratory pressures. Bilevel machines time themselves to patient-initiated breathing (S-mode). By reducing the pressure on expiration, it lowers the resistance against which the person must exhale.

Indications for bilevel

- Individuals who cannot tolerate CPAP due to a high pressure requirement (usually > 14 cm of water) leading to persistent mask leak or exhaling against a high pressure.
- Concomitant severe COPD (emphysema and asthma).

Table 8.7. *Methods to improve CPAP compliance.*

Education and encouragement, with good medical personnel support system
RAMP features
C-flex
Addressing claustrophobia through psychosocial support systems, biofeedback, and desensitization techniques
Treatment of nasal discomfort and other nasal issues
Humidification, nasal steroids
Proper fitting masks
Selective nasal surgery to relieve nasal obstruction can reduce pressure requirements and improve CPAP tolerance
Lowering CPAP pressure does not usually help to improve compliance

Table 8.8. *Predictors on who will use CPAP.*

"First night" effect: tolerance of CPAP on initial night during CPAP titration
More severe sleepiness: higher EDS score
Those people who perceive its benefits
More severe hypoxemia
Increased sleep efficiency post-usage
Higher education
Personality trait: ability to cope with new or difficult situations
Healthcare support with easy access to the provider, e.g., to change mask or provide education and support

- Morbid obesity – either because of the high pressure requirement on CPAP or because of concomitant obesity hypoventilation.
- Concomitant sleep-related hypoventilation disorder.
- Concomitant neuromuscular disorder.
- Central sleep apnea (use of S-T mode of bilevel).
- Severe nasal discomfort due to drying of the mucosa from CPAP, as bilevel decreases airflow relative to CPAP.

Bilevel also offers a higher range of inspiratory pressures than CPAP, with maximum pressures of 40 cm H_2O. The newer devices with extended pressure range also have the ability to control inspiratory time (flow) and are thereby more appropriate for persons with isolated neuromuscular disease. Nasal intermittent positive pressure ventilation may be more useful in some individuals with sleep-related hypoventilation who cannot be maintained on bilevel units. Bilevel timed modes (S-T mode) are also available, allowing the respiratory rate to be set to a predetermined value. This is of benefit for people with severe neuromuscular weakness, or for those who have decreased minute ventilation for different causes.

Ideally, titration of CPAP or bilevel pressure should be based on a PSG study, performed over 1–2 nights to allow adequate assessment. By the end of the first night, the optimum pressure is approximated; on the second night, this pressure can be checked for adequacy throughout all stages and positions. It is especially critical to evaluate the individual in the supine position and during REM sleep, when the maximum pressure requirement occurs. Unfortunately, financial constraints, bed availability, and traveling distance increasingly dictate that split-night studies be performed. This method of diagnosis and treatment tends to inaccurately estimate the severity of disease, because treatment takes place in the latter half of the night when apnea is usually at its worst. In severe apneics, a rebound of unusually long REM sleep and SWS that may be out of phase occurs once adequate airway patency is attained. REM sleep rebound shows unusually prominent phasic activity, whereas the SWS episodes may show exceptionally high voltages. Rare but dangerous sequelae of REM rebound have been seen in severe apneics with CO_2 retention under slightly suboptimum pressure. Arousal is suppressed during a long rebound, and if partial upper airway closure persists, dangerous hypoxemia may result.

Auto-titrating positive airway pressure

Auto-titrating positive airway pressure (APAP) devices detect snoring, apneas, hypopneas, flow limitation, and changes in airway resistance or impedance, which are then interpreted by a central processing unit based on specific diagnostic algorithms to determine the resultant voltage for the auto-titrating positive airway pressure blower in response to these signals.

Among the advantages of an auto-titrating system are that it requires a lower pressure than CPAP (mean pressure 2.2 cm of water lower than CPAP); that it may prevent swallowing of air and thereby abdominal bloating; that it may improve compliance (four randomized control trials have shown no difference in compliance, while three studies have shown improved compliance/adherence with APAP). A recent meta-analysis found no differences between CPAP and APAP in compliance, AHI, or EDS. It is possible that APAP may be suitable for people who fail to use CPAP successfully, but there are currently no data on this. The chief disadvantage of APAP is that it is more expensive than CPAP. Studies have also shown significant variability between different auto-titrating devices, with undertreatment of 13–60% of patients using three different devices (residual RDI > 5 during treatment).

The 2002 AASM practice parameters on auto-titrating positive pressure recommend:
(1) Diagnosis of OSA must be established by an acceptable method.
(2) Treatment with these devices is not currently recommended for people with congestive heart failure, significant lung disease (e.g., chronic obstructive pulmonary disease), daytime hypoxemia and respiratory failure from any cause, or prominent nocturnal desaturation other than from OSA (e.g., obesity hypoventilation syndrome). In addition, individuals who do not snore (either due to palate surgery or naturally) should not be titrated with an APAP device that relies on vibration or sound in its algorithm.

(3) Auto-titrating positive airway pressure may be used during attended titration to identify a single effective pressure for use with standard CPAP.

(4) Auto-titrating positive airway pressure may be used in self-adjusting mode for unattended treatment of OSA after an initial successful attended CPAP or APAP titration.

(5) People being treated with fixed CPAP on the basis of an auto-titrating positive airway pressure titration, or being treated with auto-titrating positive airway pressure, require follow-up to determine treatment efficacy and safety.

(6) If symptoms do not resolve, or if auto-titrating positive airway pressure therapy is ineffective, re-evaluation should be performed and, if needed, a standard CPAP titration should be done. Considering the slowness of response, the auto-titrating machine should be set 3 cm H_2O above and below titrated CPAP value.

Treatment with nasal CPAP or bilevel offers advantages of safety and assured efficacy over surgical approaches. They offer immediate and complete treatment for OSA and are less costly than extensive surgery. They can be used temporarily while weight loss is pursued or surgery is contemplated. Positive pressure eliminates risk factors for associated morbidity, along with daytime somnolence.

Surgical approaches

Tracheostomy

The original surgical treatment for OSA was tracheostomy. This bypasses all the three main levels of potential obstruction: nose, soft palate, and base of the tongue. This intervention is rarely needed now, because of the pervasive use of positive pressure therapy. Although used infrequently, tracheostomy provides immediate profound improvement for some individuals with severe OSA. Maintenance of a tracheostomy, however, is associated with morbidity and psychosocial implications.

Other surgical procedures address the three main levels of potential obstruction either sequentially or simultaneously. Anyone contemplating surgery must understand that surgical treatment is a serious step, with greater risks than medical treatment. In addition, surgery carries no guarantee of cure in an individual, with only statistical cure rates available.

Nose

Nasal obstruction can be corrected with septoplasty, polypectomy, and/or radio-frequency turbinate reduction.

Soft palate

Soft palate resection via uvulopalatopharyngoplasty (UPPP) or uvuloflap surgery carries approximately a 50% success rate. Potential postoperative adverse effects include:

- severe throat pain for approximately two weeks (most common)
- transient or permanent nasal reflux
- nasal speech due to palatal incompetence
- minor loss of taste

- tongue numbness
- scarring with retraction leading to palatal stenosis.

Because this procedure ameliorates snoring caused by vibration of the uvula without addressing potential obstruction behind the base of the tongue, a major sign of ongoing residual obstruction may be masked. It is therefore imperative to follow up all surgeries with a postoperative sleep study after 3–6 months.

Geniotubercle advancement via inferior sagittal osteotomy addresses the retroposition of the tongue by advancing the insertion point of the genioglossus. The surgeon makes a small mandibular incision at the geniotubercle, pulls the bone segment through the jaw, and allows the fracture to heal. This is usually performed in conjunction with UPPP. Common complications are usually minor and consist of:

- transient dental nerve anesthesia
- mandibular fracture (may occur if the incision extends into the alveolus).

Hyoidotomy with subhyoid myotomy and anterior superior repositioning with a fascia graft is now commonly performed in association with geniotubercle advancement. Midface advancement involving a Le Fort I mandibular osteotomy and a maxillary osteotomy is reserved for individuals for whom other treatments have failed and who do not want to be treated with nasal CPAP. They will previously have had the other surgeries, discussed earlier, and will have failed to show clear improvement at the 4- to 6-month follow-up, which includes clinical evaluation and polygraphic monitoring. A study of such surgery in 30 patients revealed no significant differences in efficacy as compared to curative treatment with nasal CPAP on indices of oxygen desaturation nadir, RDI, and normalization of sleep architecture. Long-term follow-up of individuals who underwent maxillomandibular advancement showed that most remained cured, but weight gain was associated with the recurrence of OSA.

Isolated radiofrequency reduction of the base of the tongue does not produce a successful long-term treatment outcome for a person with OSA, and possible side effects include pain and tongue abscess.

FURTHER READING

American Thoracic Society. Idiopathic congenital central hypoventilation syndrome: diagnosis and management. *Am J Resp Crit Care Med* 1999; **160**: 368–73.

Atwood CW Jr, McCrory D, Garcia JG, Abman SH, Ahearn GS. American College of Chest Physicians. Pulmonary artery hypertension and sleep-disordered breathing: ACCP evidence-based clinical practice guidelines. *Chest* 2004; **126** (1 Suppl): 72S–77S.

Bady E, Achkar A, Pascal S, Orvoen-Frija E, Laaban JP. Pulmonary arterial hypertension in patients with sleep apnoea syndrome. *Thorax* 2000; **55**: 934–9.

Bassetti C, Aldrich MS. Sleep apnea in acute cerebrovascular diseases: final report on 128 patients. *Sleep* 1999; **22**: 217–23.

Berry RB, Parish JM, Hartse KM. The use of auto-titrating continuous positive airway pressure for treatment of adult obstructive sleep apnea: an American Academy of Sleep Medicine review. *Sleep* 2002; **25**: 148–73.

Black JE, Hirshkowitz M. Modafinil for treatment of residual excessive sleepiness in nasal continuous positive airway pressure-treated obstructive sleep apnea/hypopnea syndrome. *Sleep* 2005; **28**: 464–71.

Bonnet MH, Dexter JR, Arand DL. The effect of triazolam on arousal and respiration in central sleep apnea patients. *Sleep* 1990; **13**: 31–41.

Bradley TD, Logan AG, Kimoff RJ, *et al.* Continuous positive airway pressure for central sleep apnea and heart failure. *N Engl J Med* 2005; **353**: 2025–33.

Franklin KA, Eriksoon P, Sahlin C, *et al.* Reversal of central sleep apnea with oxygen. *Chest* 1997; **111**: 163–9.

Friberg D, Gazelius B, Hokfelt T, Nordlander B. Abnormal afferent nerve endings in the soft palatal mucosa of sleep apnoics and habitual snorers. *Regul Pept* 1997; **71**: 29–36.

Gonzalez MA, Selwyn AP. Endothelial function, inflammation, and prognosis in cardiovascular disease. *Am J Med* 2003; **115** (Suppl 8A): 99S–106S.

Guilleminault C, Motta J. Sleep apnea syndrome as a long-term sequela of poliomyelitis. In: Guilleminault C, Dement W, eds. *Sleep Apnea Syndromes*. New York, NY: Liss, 1978: 309–15.

Guilleminault C, Connolly SJ, Winkle RA. Cardiac arrhythmia and conduction disturbances during sleep in 400 patients with sleep apnea syndrome. *Am J Cardiol* 1983; **52**: 490–4.

Guilleminault C, Motta J, Mihm F, Melvin K. Obstructive sleep apnea and cardiac index. *Chest* 1986; **89**: 331.

Guilleminault C, Partinen M, Hollman K, *et al.* Familial aggregates in obstructive sleep apnea syndrome. *Chest* 1995; **107**: 1545–51.

Guilleminault C, Li K, Chen NH, Poyares D. Two-point palatal discrimination in patients with upper airway resistance syndrome, obstructive sleep apnea syndrome, and normal control subjects. *Chest* 2002; **122**: 866–70.

Guilleminault C, Kirisoglu C, Ohayon MM. C-reactive protein and sleep-disordered breathing. *Sleep* 2004; **27**: 1507–11.

Guilleminault C, Lee JH, Chan A. Pediatric obstructive sleep apnea syndrome. *Arch Pediatr Adolesc Med* 2005; **159**: 775–85.

Hanly PJ, Millar TW, Steljes DG, *et al.* The effect of oxygen on respiration and sleep in patients with congestive heart failure. *Ann Intern Med* 1989; **111**: 777–82.

Horner RR, Mohiaddin D, Lowell S, *et al.* Sites and sizes of fat deposits around the pharynx in obese patients with obstructive sleep apnea and weight matched controls. *Eur Respir J* 1989; **2**: 613–22.

Hyland RH, Hutcheon MA, Perl A, *et al.* Upper airway occlusion induced by diaphragmatic pacing for primary alveolar hypoventilation: implications for the pathogenesis of obstructive sleep apnea. *Am Rev Respir Dis* 1981; **124**: 180–5.

Issa FG, Sullivan CE. Reversal of central sleep apnea using nasal CPAP. *Chest* 1986; **90**: 165–71.

Javaheri S. Acetazolamide improves central sleep apnea in heart failure: a double-blind, prospective study. *Am J Respir Crit Care Med* 2006; **173**: 234–7.

Javaheri S, Parker TJ, Wexler L, *et al.* Effect of theophylline on sleep-disordered breathing in heart failure. *N Engl J Med* 1996; **335**: 562–7.

Kaneko Y, Floras JS, Usui K, *et al.* Cardiovascular effects of continuous positive airway pressure in patients with heart failure and obstructive sleep apnea. *N Engl J Med* 2003; **348**: 1233–41.

Kapsimalis F, Kryger MH. Gender and obstructive sleep apnea syndrome, part 1: clinical features. *Sleep* 2002; **25**: 412–19.

Kapsimalis F, Kryger MH. Gender and obstructive sleep apnea syndrome, part 2: mechanisms. *Sleep* 2002; **25**: 499–506.

Khoo MC, Kronauer RE, Strohl KP, Slutsky AS. Factors inducing periodic breathing in humans: a general model. *J Appl Physiol* 1982; **53**: 644–59.

Kushida CA, Morgenthaler TI, Littner MR, *et al.* Practice parameters for the treatment of snoring and obstructive sleep apnea with oral appliances: an update for 2005. *Sleep* 2006; **29**: 240–3.

Lattimore JD, Celermajer DS, Wilcox I. Obstructive sleep apnea and cardiovascular disease. *J Am Coll Cardiol* 2003; **41**: 1429–37.

Lavie L, Hefetz A, Luboshitzky R, Lavie P. Plasma levels of nitric oxide and L-arginine in sleep apnea patients: effects of nCPAP treatment. *J Mol Neurosci* 2003; **21**: 57–63.

Li KK, Powell NB, Riley RW, Guilleminault C. Temperature-controlled radiofrequency tongue base eduction for sleep-disordered breathing: long-term outcomes. *Otolaryngol Head Neck Surg* 2002; **127**: 230–4.

Linder-Aronson S. Adenoids: their effect on mode of breathing and nasal airflow and their relationship to characteristics of the facial skeleton and the dentition. *Acta Otolaryngol Suppl* 1970; **265**: 1–132.

Marrone O, Bongsignore MR. Pulmonary hemodynamics in obstructive sleep apnea. *Sleep Med Rev* 2002; **6**: 175–93.

Martinez-Garcia MA, Galiano-Blancart R, Roman-Sanchez P, *et al.* Continuous positive airway pressure treatment in sleep apnea prevents new vascular events after ischemic stroke. *Chest* 2005; **128**: 2123–9.

Mayer J, Becker H, Brandenberg U, *et al.* Blood pressure and sleep apnea: results of long term nasal continuous positive airway pressure therapy. *Cardiology* 1991; **79**: 84–92.

Meoli AL, Casey KR, Clark RW, *et al.* Clinical practice review committee: hypopnea in sleep disordered breathing in adults. *Sleep* 2001; **24**: 469–70.

Mezzanotte WS, Tangel DJ, White DP. Influence of sleep onset on upper-airway muscle activity in apnea patients versus normal controls. *Am J Respir Crit Care Med* 1996; **153**: 1880–87.

Miller WP. Cardiac arrhythmias and conduction disturbances in the sleep apnea syndrome. *Am J Med* 1982; **73**: 317–21.

Møller DS, Lind P, Strunge B, Pedersen EB. Abnormal vasoactive hormones and 24-hour blood pressure in obstructive sleep apnea. *Am J Hypertens* 2003; **16**: 274–80.

Naimark A, Cherniack RM. Compliance of the respiratory system and its components in health and obesity. *J Appl Physiol* 1960; **15**: 377–82.

Narkiewicz K, Somers VK. Sympathetic nerve activity in obstructive sleep apnoea. *Acta Physiol Scand* 2003; **177**: 385–90.

Naughton M, Benard D, Tam A, *et al.* The role of hyperventilation in the pathogenesis of central sleep apnea in patients with congestive heart failure. *Am Rev Respir Dis* 1993; **148**: 330–8.

Palomaki H, Partinen M, Juvela S, Kaste M. Snoring as a risk factor for sleep-related brain infarction. *Stroke* 1989; **20**: 1311–15.

Partinen M, Guilleminault C, Quera-Salva MA, Jamieson A. Obstructive sleep apnea and cephalometric roentgenograms: the role of anatomic upper airway abnormalities in the definition of abnormal breathing during sleep. *Chest* 1988; **93**: 1199–205.

Peppard PE, Young T, Palta M, Skatrud J. Prospective study of the association between sleep-disordered breathing and hypertension. *N Engl J Med* 2000; **342**: 1378–84.

Pepperell JC, Davies RJ, Stradling JR. Systemic hypertension and obstructive sleep apnoea. *Sleep Med Rev* 2002; **6**: 157–73.

Powell N, Riley R, Guilleminault C, Troell R. A reversible uvulopalatal flap for snoring and sleep apnea syndrome. *Sleep* 1996; **19**: 593–9.

Redline S, Kump K, Tishler PV, *et al.* Gender differences in sleep disordered breathing in a community-based sample. *Am J Respir Crit Care Med* 1994; **149**: 722–6.

Riley RW, Powell NB, Guilleminault C. Maxillofacial surgery and nasal CPAP: a comparison of treatment for obstructive sleep apnea syndrome. *Chest* 1990; **98**: 1421–5.

Shahar E, Whitney CW, Redline S, *et al.* Sleep-disordered breathing and cardiovascular disease: cross-sectional results of the Sleep Heart Health Study. *Am J Respir Crit Care Med* 2001; **163**: 19–25.

Shiomi T, Guilleminault C, Stoohs R, Schnittger I. Leftward shift of the interventricular septum and pulsus paradoxus in obstructive sleep apnea syndrome. *Chest* 1991; **100**: 894–902.

Sin DD, Fitzgerald F, Parker JD, *et al.* Relationship of systolic BP to obstructive sleep apnea in patients with heart failure. *Chest* 2003; **123**: 1536–43.

Solow B, Siersbaek-Nielsen S, Greve E. Airway adequacy, head posture, and craniofacial morphology. *Am J Orthod* 1984; **86**: 214–23.

Somers VK, Dyken ME, Clary MP, Abboud FM. Sympathetic neural mechanisms in obstructive sleep apnea. *J Clin Invest* 1995; **96**: 1897–904.

Spiegel K, Tasali E, Penev P, Van Cauter E. Brief communication: sleep curtailment in healthy young men is associated with decreased leptin levels, elevated ghrelin levels, and increased hunger and appetite. *Ann Intern Med* 2004; **141**: 846–50.

Stein I, Colapinto N, Rotstein LE, *et al.* Improvement in upper airway function after weight loss in patients with obstructive sleep apnea. *Am Rev Respir Dis* 1988; **138**: 1192–5.

Stoohs R, Guilleminault C. Snoring during NREM sleep: respiratory timing, esophageal pressure behavior and EEG arousal. *Respir Physiol* 1991; **85**: 151–67.

Sullivan CE, Issa FG, Berthon-Jones M, Eves L. Reversal of obstructive sleep apnoea by continuous positive airway pressure applied through the nares. *Lancet* 1981; **1** (8225): 862–5.

Teschler H, Dohring J, Wang Y, *et al.* Adaptive pressure support servo-ventilation: a novel treatment for Cheyne–Stokes respiration in heart failure. *Am J Resp Crit Care Med* 2001; **164**: 614–19.

Tilkian AG, Motta J, Guilleminault C. Cardiac arrhythmias in sleep apnea. In: Guilleminault C, Dement W, eds. *Sleep Apnea Syndromes*. New York, NY: Liss, 1978: 197–210.

Valencia-Flores M, Orea A, Herrera M, *et al.* Effect of bariatric surgery on obstructive sleep apnea and hypopnea syndrome, electrocardiogram, and pulmonary arterial pressure. *Obes Surg* 2004; **14**: 755–62.

Vargervik K, Miller AJ, Chierici G, Harrold E, Tomer BS. Morphologic response to changes in neuromuscular patterns experimentally induced by altered modes of respiration. *Am J Orthod* 1984; **85**: 115–24.

Whittle AT, Marshall I, Mortimore IL, *et al.* Neck soft tissue and fat distribution: comparison between normal men and women by magnetic resonance imaging. *Thorax* 1999; **54**: 323–8.

Xie A, Rankin F, Rutherford R, Bradley TD. Effects of inhaled CO_2 and added dead space on idiopathic central sleep apnea. *J Appl Physiol* 1997; **82**: 918–26.

Xie A, Skatrud J, Puleo D, Rahko PS, Dempsey JA. Apnea-hypopnea threshold for CO_2 in patients with congestive heart failure. *Am J Respir Crit Care Med* 2002; **165**: 1245–50.

Yaggi HK, Concato J, Kernan WN, *et al.* Obstructive sleep apnea as a risk factor for stroke and death. *N Engl J Med* 2005; **353**: 2030–41.

Young T, Palta M, Dempsey J, *et al.* The occurrence of sleep-disordered breathing among middle-aged adults. *N Engl J Med* 1993; **328**: 1230–35.

Young T, Peppard PE, Gottlieb DJ. Epidemiology of obstructive sleep apnea: a population health perspective. *Am J Respir Crit Care Med* 2002; **165**: 1217–39.

Young T, Shahar E, Nieto FJ, *et al.* Predictors of sleep-disordered breathing in community-dwelling adults: the Sleep Heart Health Study. *Arch Intern Med* 2002; **162**: 893–900.

Section 3 – Sleep in specialty areas

9 Sleep and neurologic disorders

Ilonka Eisensehr

Introduction

Sleep is a complex and colorful phenomenon, driven by different activities of the brain. Dysfunctions of the brain can change wakefulness and sleep and cause various sleep disorders. The details of these sleep disorders depend on the localization of the damage in the brain or other parts of the central nervous system. Almost every neurological disease is associated with sleep disorders. This chapter describes only a small selection of neurological diseases, those which are most strongly associated with sleep disorders.

Sleep and Parkinson's disease

The prevalence of sleep disorders in Parkinson's disease (PD) is estimated to be as high as 74–81%. Polygraphic sleep recordings in people with PD found decreased sleep efficiency, increased wake after sleep onset, and sleep fragmentation. Up to 80% of those with PD report having 2–5 awakenings per night. Sleep disorders in PD may be based on the neurodegenerative process, or they may result from nocturnal bradykinesia and rigidity, medication, psychiatric disorders, circadian rhythm disturbance, or REM sleep behavior disorder (RBD).

Parkinson's disease and sleep-disordered breathing

Sleep breathing disorders are common in PD. About half of all individuals with PD show obstructive sleep-disordered breathing. Rigidity, diaphragmatic dyskinesias, failure of autonomic control, and disorder of the mechanisms of breathing control can reduce the function of respiratory muscles and thus cause a restrictive respiratory dysfunction. Furthermore, abnormal movement in glottic or supraglottic structures, for example tremor-like oscillations and stridor during dystonic episodes, can cause intermittent closure of the upper airway. Sleep-disordered breathing in PD may also be promoted by dopaminergic drugs. Excessive administration of dopaminergic agents has been associated with dyspnea and irregular tachypnea. However, obstruction of the upper airway may also be due to withdrawal of dopaminergic drugs. Sleep apnea

Sleep Medicine, ed. Harold R. Smith, Cynthia L. Comella, and Birgit Högl. Published by Cambridge University Press. © Cambridge University Press 2008.

may affect 20% or more of all people with PD. One study showed that 43% of those with PD undergoing polysomnography because of sleep complaints were diagnosed with sleep apnea. Sleep apnea may contribute to daytime somnolence in PD.

Parkinson's disease and periodic leg movement disorder

PLMS is more severe and more frequent in PD than in healthy controls. Restless legs syndrome (RLS), which is often associated with PLMS, occurs frequently in PD, although no clear association has been established. Interestingly, RLS was reported to improve dramatically in six individuals with PD undergoing bilateral subthalamic stimulation. However, RLS was also reported to be unmasked after subthalamic deep brain stimulation in PD, possibly due in part to reduction of antiparkinsonian medication during subthalamic nucleus deep brain stimulation in PD. One major problem of RLS treatment in those with PD occurs with RLS augmentation resulting from the high dosages of dopaminergic drugs needed in PD. In this case, treatment of RLS in PD with opioids may be considered, to overcome augmented RLS.

Parkinson's disease and REM sleep behavior disorder

RBD involves complex motor behavior in sleep due to the absence of skeletal muscle atonia during REM sleep (Fig. 9.1). People often recall violent dreams, and sometimes injure themselves or their bed partner during episodes of RBD. The minimum diagnostic criteria for RBD as defined in the International Classification of Sleep Disorders (ICSD-2) include movements of limbs or body associated with dream mentation and at least one of the following: potentially harmful sleep behavior, dreams that appear to be "acted out," or sleep behavior that disrupts sleep continuity. The underlying cause of RBD is still unknown. Experimental lesions of the dorsolateral pontine tegmentum in animals cause the absence of physiological REM muscle atonia.

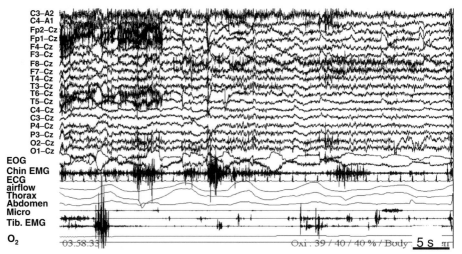

Fig. 9.1. Thirty seconds of the polysomnogram of a person with PD and RBD. One can see REM sleep with increased muscle activity.

[I-123]IPT SPECT in patients and controls

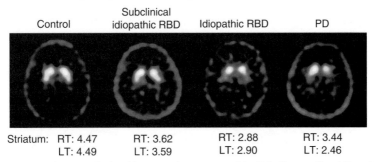

Fig. 9.2. IPT-SPECT images of a healthy control, a person with clinically manifest idiopathic RBD, a person with polysomnographically diagnosed subclinical RBD, and a person with PD.

Findings from experimental lesion studies in animals and MRI studies suggest that degenerated or lesioned brainstem nuclei are the anatomic basis for RBD.

Recent studies have shown that a large number of individuals with RBD eventually develop PD (66%). RBD is frequent in multiple system atrophy (MSA) (90%). The presynaptic dopamine transporters have been demonstrated recently to be reduced in idiopathic RBD as in PD. Clinical symptoms of RBD are reported by 15% of people with PD and their caregivers. Another study, which did not include polysomnography (PSG), showed that clinical symptoms of RBD preceded the onset of MSA by more than 1 year in 44% of those who developed MSA. Idiopathic RBD is associated with decreased striatal dopamine transporter binding, levels of which are in between normal and PD levels (Fig 9.2).

If reduced striatal dopaminergic neurons cause RBD, why do all those with PD not also suffer from RBD? In PD, additional brainstem neurons that play significant roles in behavioral state control, particularly brainstem monoaminergic nuclei, also degenerate. There are two different glutamatergic receptors in the dorsolateral pons and the nucleus magnocellularis: one promotes REM sleep without atonia and with locomotion, the other promotes atonia in REM sleep (Fig 9.3). In PD, additional degeneration of neurons in the brainstem, which promote REM sleep without atonia, might therefore cancel the effect of heightened phasic discharge of the internal segment of the globus pallidus secondary to dopamine cell loss in the substantia nigra. Conversely, additional degeneration of neurons in the brainstem, which promote REM sleep with atonia, might promote RBD. This hypothesis might explain why only some people with PD are affected by RBD, even if reduced striatal dopaminergic neurons without further brainstem lesions might promote RBD. The observation that MSA is frequently associated with RBD also supports the degenerative concept.

Sleep and stroke

Atherothrombotic brain infarcts often occur during sleep in the early morning hours. Snoring has been suggested to be a risk factor for brain infarction. Heavy snoring is associated with obstructive sleep apnea (OSA), which may have several harmful

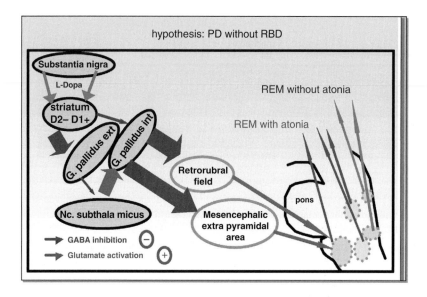

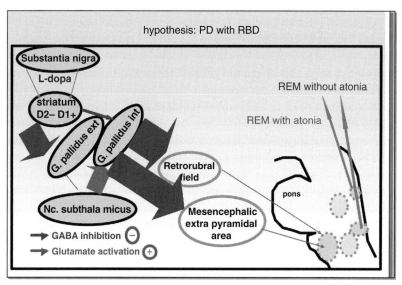

Fig. 9.3. The hypothesis concerning the pathophysiology of idiopathic RBD.

effects on the cardiovascular system. The elevated mortality rate associated with OSA has been attributed to cardiovascular mortality. OSA is also overrepresented among myocardial infarction survivors.

Sleep apnea as a risk factor for stroke

Snoring, which almost invariably accompanies OSA, is reported to be a risk factor for stroke. Considerable evidence is available in support of an independent association between obstructive sleep apnea (OSA) and cardiovascular disease, which is particularly strong for systemic arterial hypertension, and growing in relation to ischemic heart disease, stroke, heart failure, atrial fibrillation, and sudden cardiac death. Almost two-thirds of people with stroke have OSA. Severe OSA (defined as apnea/hypopnea index [AHI] $\geq$ 30 per hour of total sleep time) increases the risk of ischemic stroke in the elderly population, independent of known confounding factors. Besides hypertension, increased BMI, male sex, and advanced age (all very common factors in OSA), other pathophysiological mechanisms possibly involved in high cardiovascular and cerebrovascular morbidity in OSA are increased risk for atherosclerosis due to apnea-induced hypoxemia and altered fibrinolytic and platelet function. In a preliminary study of six individuals, platelet aggregability (measured as P-selectin expression) was increased in those with OSA, and decreased after treatment with CPAP: this suggests that the change in platelet function is secondary to OSA. We found that severe OSA is independently associated with increased platelet activation. While the earlier data were conflicting regarding the absolute causative relationship of OSA to stroke, there is a wealth of information relating OSA to many other vascular conditions and risk factors. Given that OSA is relatively easy to diagnose and treat, and given that the benefits of risk factor modification and improved quality of life are unarguable, appropriate diagnosis and management of OSA become vital. OSA significantly increases the risk of stroke or death from any cause (twice as high as in those without OSA), and the increase is independent of other risk factors, including hypertension.

Sleep apnea as a consequence of stroke

The reticular formation of the medulla oblongata contains the respiratory neurons, which are closely related to motor activity centers of the upper respiratory tract. There are a few published observations of isolated cases with bulbar strokes and sleep apnea. Sleep-disordered breathing is common particularly in elderly men with diabetes, nighttime stroke onset, and macroangiopathy as a cause of stroke. It improves after the acute phase of the stroke and is associated with increased post-stroke mortality. Strokes associated with pharyngeal muscle dysfunction can coincide with initial severe OSA in the acute phase of the stroke, but with decreased OSA indices in the subacute phase coinciding with the recovery of pharyngeal muscle function.

Sleep apnea and the outcome of stroke

A recent study comparing 15 people with stroke and OSA treated with CPAP and a similar group without CPAP treatment found poor compliance in using CPAP and no difference in outcome scores. OSA severity is associated with high 24-hour blood pressure values but only weakly with stroke severity and outcome. However, there is evidence that OSA negatively affects the outcome of stroke. In an earlier small-scale study a higher nocturnal desaturation index was associated with greater mortality and more severe disability in survivors 12 months after the event. More recently, a high AHI during the first night after a stroke was found to be associated with early neurological deterioration, although this did not correlate with disability 6 months later. A clear relationship between OSA (AHI > 10) in the first 24 hours after stroke and length of hospital stay (24 days vs. 43 days) and mortality (25% vs. 45%) could be shown. Another recent study of younger people in a rehabilitation unit also reported that OSA 6 weeks after a stroke was independently associated with longer hospital stay and greater long-term functional impairment. In another study, CPAP acceptance was associated with improved subjective wellbeing and decreased nocturnal blood pressure, which may improve prognosis in those who have suffered a stroke.

Stroke and sleep/wake disorders

About 20–40% of stroke victims have sleep/wake disorders (SWD), mostly in the form of insomnia, excessive daytime sleepiness/fatigue, or hypersomnia (increased sleep needs). Depression, anxiety, sleep-disordered breathing, stroke complications, and medications may contribute to SWD and should be addressed first therapeutically. Brain damage per se, often at thalamic or brainstem level, can be also a cause of persisting SWD. Posterior hypothalamic lesions were associated with hypersomnolence, anterior hypothalamic lesions with hypervigilance. In appropriately selected individuals, hypnotics, dopaminergic agents, or stimulants (e.g., modafinil) may be considered. Figures 9.4 and 9.5 show the hypnogram of an individual with bilateral posterior hypothalamic lesion, and the MR imaging of the lesion.

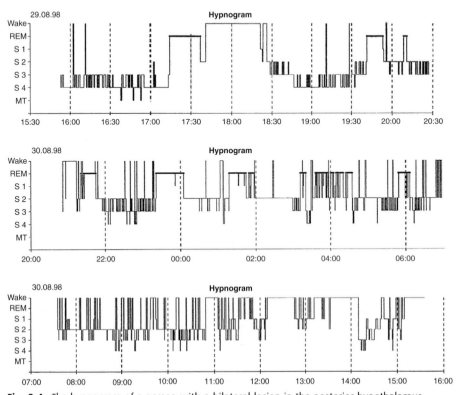

Fig. 9.4. The hypnogram of a person with a bilateral lesion in the posterior hypothalamus.

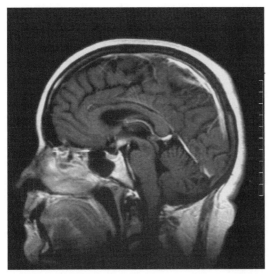

Fig. 9.5. An MRI of the bilateral lesion in the posterior hypothalamus causing hypersomnia (the same individual as in Fig. 9.4).

Sleep and neuromuscular diseases

Breathing abnormalities during sleep, with associated disrupted sleep and daytime fatigue, are common in neuromuscular diseases such as amyotrophic lateral sclerosis, muscular dystrophies, myotonic dystrophy, myopathies, Guillan–Barré syndrome, and myasthenia gravis. Respiratory muscle weakness causing apneas and hypopneas may contribute to nocturnal desaturation and sleep disruption, even before daytime ventilatory failure occurs.

Breathing physiology during normal NREM sleep

At sleep onset ventilation falls instantly and is associated with a more rapid, shallow, and regular breathing pattern. Upper airway resistance increases abruptly at sleep onset due to reduced activity of the pharyngeal dilator muscles. Changes in ventilation during sleep probably result primarily from a reduction in ventilatory drive due to reduced chemosensitivity and loss of the wakefulness drive to breathe.

Breathing physiology during normal REM sleep

During REM sleep the tone of skeletal muscles is generally reduced, except for the diaphragm and extraocular muscles. The breathing pattern during REM sleep is more irregular. REM sleep in healthy subjects is associated with a shift from predominantly ribcage to diaphragmatic breathing. During bursts of rapid eye movements breathing is more irregular, rapid, and shallow, with a fall in ventilation.

Sleep architecture in neuromuscular diseases

Total sleep time and sleep efficiency are reduced in people with respiratory muscle weakness. Sleep is fragmented, and complete suppression of REM has been reported in association with severe diaphragmatic weakness. The quality of life in those with amyotrophic lateral sclerosis correlates with both daytime respiratory muscle function and polysomnographic indices of nocturnal sleep-related respiratory disturbances.

Sleep-disordered breathing is common in neuromuscular disease, irrespective of the primary disorder. The classification of respiratory events as "central" or "obstructive" using non-invasive sleep monitoring is complicated in neuromuscular disease. Obstructive apnea may be misclassified as central when respiratory muscles are too weak to move the chest wall against the closed pharynx. Furthermore, severe diaphragmatic weakness causes paradoxical movement of the chest and abdomen even without narrowing of the upper airway; this may cause misclassification of central hypopneas as obstructive. An increasing phase difference between chest and abdominal movements, increasing submental EMG, and snoring provide strong supportive evidence of an obstructive etiology. Studies in which esophageal pressure was recorded to determine the central or obstructive nature of respiratory events during sleep in individuals with amyotrophic lateral sclerosis have reported predominantly central events. The degree of desaturation is related to the severity of diaphragmatic weakness. Interestingly, in neuromuscular disease indices of daytime lung function (vital capacity and maximal inspiratory pressure) are better predictors of survival than overnight oxygen saturation. Daytime somnolence is very sensitive in predicting nocturnal desaturation, and regularly improves when the sleep breathing disorder is treated with non-invasive ventilation.

Amyotrophic lateral sclerosis (ALS)

The most common cause of nocturnal desaturation in ALS is hypoventilation during sleep. Usually there is only a moderate increase in the AHI to values between 10 and 20 events per hour total sleep time. Nocturnal desaturations in ALS are mainly due to diaphragmatic weakness and hypoventilation rather than to obstructive events due to bulbar weakness.

Duchenne muscular dystrophy

Sleep architecture in Duchenne muscular dystrophy seems to be better preserved than in ALS. Most studies including monitoring of esophageal pressure reported predominantly central events. Similar to other neuromuscular diseases, the correlation between daytime neurologic function and sleep-disordered breathing is poor. Daytime function, particularly if vital capacity is less than 1 liter, is a more powerful prognostic predictor than any nocturnal index.

Myotonic dystrophy

The severity of sleep-disordered breathing in myotonic dystrophy is greater than in nonmyotonic neuromuscular disease with a similar degree of respiratory muscle weakness. Moreover, daytime somnolence and hypercapnia is a common phenomenon in myotonic dystrophy. Myotonic dystrophy is associated with an irregular breathing pattern during wakefulness and light sleep, which does not persist during

SWS. Such irregular breathing is not seen in nonmyotonic subjects with similar respiratory muscle weakness.

Myasthenia gravis

The majority of respiratory events in myasthenia gravis are central apneas. Sleep-disordered breathing in myasthenia gravis is associated particularly with diaphragmatic weakness. Sleep-disordered breathing may improve following treatment with thymectomy or prednisolone.

Treatment of sleep-disordered breathing in neuromuscular disease

Improved sleep architecture and daytime arterial blood gases, and increased ventilatory response to carbon dioxide, result from nocturnal ventilation in neuromuscular disease. Furthermore, non-invasive ventilation improved survival time and quality of life (QOL) in individuals with slowly and rapidly progressive neuromuscular disease when compared to historical controls. In a study of 14 children with neuromuscular disease, symptoms of daytime sleepiness and headache improved after initiation of non-invasive ventilation; sleep quality assessed by polysomnography also improved; hospitalization rates and healthcare costs decreased; QOL remained stable after non-invasive ventilation, despite disease progression. Despite the fact that randomized controlled trials are lacking, non-invasive ventilation is recommended in neuromuscular disease. Further studies are needed, however, to evaluate the optimum criteria for selection of subjects and timing of treatment initiation. Currently, there is no evidence that sleep studies improve the selection of subjects for non-invasive ventilation over and above evaluation of symptoms and daytime respiratory function.

Sleep and headache

Headache as a consequence of sleep disorders

Headache is not specific to any primary sleep disorder, and the relationship between sleep and headache has great individual variation. However, morning headache occurs up to three times more often among heavy snorers and people with obstructive sleep apnea than in the general population. Sleep apnea can trigger or cause sleep-related headaches. Those who complain of awakening with morning headaches of less than 30 minutes' duration are likely to suffer from OSA. In this group, morning headaches can be improved by treating the OSA with CPAP or uvulopalatopharyngoplasty. Interestingly, there is no evidence that the duration of nocturnal hypoxemia relates to headache complaints in individuals with OSA.

There is also a link between sleep and migraine. Migraine sufferers with poor sleep hygiene had a significant improvement in the frequency and duration of their symptoms when following instructions to improve sleep hygiene.

Cluster headaches may be triggered by hypoxemic events such as sleep apnea, the latter being more common during REM sleep. Sleep-disordered breathing occurs in the majority of people with cluster headache. OSA may even trigger cluster headache during susceptible periods.

Headache as a cause of sleep disorders

Migraine attacks may be precipitated by sleep deprivation or excessive sleep, and sleep may be associated with relief of migraine attacks. Waking with migraine often occurs out of REM sleep. Chronic paroxysmal hemicrania also seems to be related to REM sleep.

Hypnic headache syndrome is an unusual chronic headache that usually begins after age 60 years and occurs exclusively during sleep. Sleep in these individuals may be normal to markedly insufficient. The headache attacks, single or multiple in one night, occur exclusively during sleep and tend to present at a consistent time each night. The clinical spectrum of the disorder includes unilateral forms (about 40%), forms with a longer duration (up to 3 hours), and cases with onset in adolescence or young adulthood. To date the reported female/male ratio is 1.7/1. Pain is of severe intensity in less than one-third of cases and mild to moderate in about two-thirds. The location of pain is frontotemporal in over 40% of cases; headache is throbbing in 38% of cases, dull in 57%, and stabbing in less than 5%. Nausea is reported in 19% of cases; photophobia, phonophobia, or both are present in 6.8%. Mild autonomic signs (lacrimation, nasal congestion, ptosis) may rarely be present. Sufficient evidence, mainly from polysomnographic studies, indicates that hypnic headache is a primary REM sleep-related headache disorder of chronobiological origin. Lithium, melatonin, indomethacin, and caffeine at bedtime are among the most effective therapeutic options. Available data allow speculation that, in predisposed subjects, an age-related impairment of the suprachiasmatic nucleus could cyclically activate a mechanism leading to both a sudden awakening and headache. The mechanism may be precipitated by neurophysiologic events such as the strong reduction of firing occurring in the dorsal raphe nucleus during a REM sleep phase.

Sleep and multiple sclerosis

Sleep disorders are pervasive in people with multiple sclerosis (MS), although clinically underrecognized by most physicians. Increasing awareness in the medical community may contribute to early detection and treatment of sleep abnormalities in MS causing excessive daytime somnolence and fatigue.

Daytime fatigue in MS

At least three-quarters of MS individuals complain about fatigue, which is often difficult to treat. A relationship between fatigue and disrupted sleep or abnormal sleep cycles has been demonstrated in those with MS. MS causes sleep fragmentation in terms of both macro- and microstructure. Fatigue in MS can be partially explained by disruption of sleep structure, poor subjective sleep quality, pain, nocturia, and depression. Further studies have shown that the subjective complaint of fatigue is linked to destructive pathologic processes resulting in progressive brain atrophy in those with remitting–relapsing MS.

The treatment of choice for symptoms of severe daytime fatigue in MS is modafinil. For less severe symptoms of fatigue amantadin is suitable. However, the underlying cause of daytime somnolence in MS may be an associated sleep disorder. In the latter case, it makes sense to treat the sleep disorder before initiating symptomatic treatment for the fatigue with modafinil or amantadin.

Sleep disorders in MS

Sleep disturbance in MS is usually due to leg spasms, pain, immobility, nocturia, or medication. The most common sleep disorders seen in people with MS include circadian rhythm disorders, insomnia, nocturnal movement disorders, sleep-disordered breathing, narcolepsy, and RBD. More than one-third of those with MS suffer from RLS, suggesting that MS can cause RLS, or that MS and RLS may have common susceptibility factors. Most of these sleep disorders are due to specific CNS lesions. For example, damage of the biological clock, the circadian oscillator, which is situated in the suprachiasmatic nucleus (SCN), a small paired structure just above the optic chiasm, may cause circadian rhythm disorders. Disrupted sleep has the potential to cause daytime somnolence, increased fatigue, and unrefreshing sleep, and it may be associated with dangerous respiratory events with the risk of death during sleep, with demyelination in the medulla oblongata resulting in fatal sleep apnea. Awareness and treatment of these conditions is vital to improving health and QOL in people with MS.

It should be kept in mind that specific sleep disorders in MS may be due to specific demyelinating brain lesions, and therefore are potentially reversible. Similarly, drug treatment for sleep disorders in MS may not be a lifelong requirement.

Sleep and epilepsy

Sleep and epileptic seizures

About 20% of all seizures in people with epilepsy occur during sleep, usually out of non-rapid eye movement (NREM) sleep stage 2 and to a smaller extent out of slow-wave sleep (SWS). Epileptic seizures during REM sleep are an extremely rare phenomenon. Frontal lobe epilepsy seizures occur more often during sleep than temporal lobe epilepsy seizures. This fact is used for localizing the epileptogenic region. Seizures in temporal lobe epilepsy tend to generalize more often when occurring during sleep. This is not the case in frontal lobe epilepsy. Some epileptic syndromes, such as juvenile myoclonic epilepsy, are very sensitive to sleep deprivation, which can cause clusters of seizures. Sleep deprivation can result from most sleep disorders, or from lifestyle.

Seizures during the night disturb sleep architecture. Some studies have shown improved sleep with increased sleep efficiency, increased REM sleep, and decreased numbers of arousals following treatment of seizures. However, it is not quite clear if the improved sleep is based on the pharmacologic features of the antiepileptic medication or if it is due to reduced numbers of seizures. Epilepsy is associated with disturbed sleep architecture, and seizures seem to influence sleep architecture beyond the postictal phase. For example, seizures in temporal lobe epilepsy occurring during the day cause a significant decrease in REM sleep the following night.

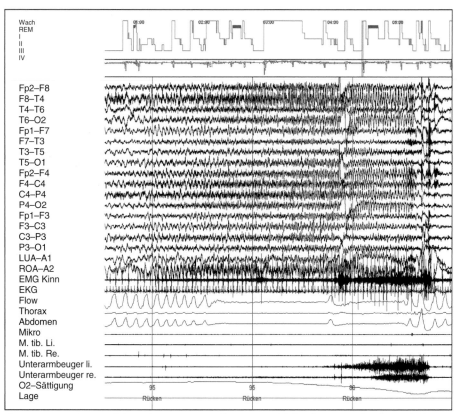

Fig. 9.6. Two minutes of the polysomnogram of a person with focal status epilepticus, which was based on an encephalitis with repeated EEG seizure patterns during sleep on the right central temporal region. These seizure patterns were associated solely with central sleep apneas.

Sleep apnea and epileptic seizures

Epileptic seizures may be associated with sleep apnea (Fig. 9.6). Single sleep apnea episodes, whether central or obstructive, may be seen with nocturnal epileptic seizures. An investigation of the incidence of sleep apnea in 39 individuals with epilepsy not responding to medical therapy revealed that 33% had obstructive sleep apnea (OSA). Seizure frequency, localization, type, numbers of antiepileptic drugs, and scores on the Epworth Sleepiness Scale were similar in individuals with and without OSA, but male gender and increased body mass index predisposed towards OSA.

One very small study investigating the effect of nasal continuous positive airway pressure (CPAP) ($n = 5$) or an intraoral snoring device ($n = 1$) in five adults and one child with epilepsy and OSA found a 45% reduction of the seizures in three and a 60% reduction of the seizures in one person. These reports support the hypothesis that adequate treatment of OSA improves seizure control in epilepsy.

Periodic limb movements during sleep and epilepsy

Twelve percent of those with epilepsy show increased numbers of periodic limb movements during sleep (PLMS). Since PLMS may result in fragmented sleep and thus increased risk for seizures, consideration should be given to treatment of the PLMS.

Conclusion

Thirty to forty percent of those with epilepsy do not achieve a seizure-free state with antiepileptic therapy. Good sleep quality and efficiency are important in epilepsy. Seizures, poor sleep hygiene, and primary sleep disorders may worsen sleep quality and therefore decrease seizure control. Sleep disorders should therefore be considered when evaluating and discussing treatment strategies for people with epilepsy.

FURTHER READING

Attarian HP, Brown KM, Duntley SP, Carter JD, Cross AH. The relationship of sleep disturbances and fatigue in multiple sclerosis. *Arch Neurol* 2004; **61**: 525–8.

Bourke SC, Gibson GJ. Sleep and breathing in neuromuscular disease. *Eur Resp J* 2002; **19**: 1194–201.

Clarenbach P, Wessendorf T. Sleep and stroke. *Rev Neurol* 2001; **157**: 46–52.

De Simone R, Marano E, Ranieri A, Bonavita V. Hypnic headache: an update. *Neurol Sci* 2006; **27** (Suppl 2): S144–8.

Eisensehr I, Noachtar S. Haematological aspects of obstructive sleep apnoea. *Sleep Med Rev* 2001; **5**: 207–21.

Eisensehr I, Schmidt D. Epilepsy and sleep disorders. *MMW Fortschr Med* 2005; **147**: 54–7.

Eisensehr I, Ehrenberg BL, Noachtar S, *et al.* Platelet activation, epinephrine, and blood pressure in obstructive sleep apnea syndrome. *Neurology* 1998; **51**: 188–95.

Eisensehr I, Linke R, Noachtar S, *et al.* Reduced striatal dopamine transporters in idiopathic rapid eye movement sleep behaviour disorder: comparison with Parkinson's disease and controls. *Brain* 2000; **123**: 1155–60.

Eisensehr I, Noachtar S, von Schlippenbach C, *et al.* Hypersomnia associated with bilateral posterior hypothalamic lesion: a polysomnographic case study. *Eur Neurol* 2003; **49**: 169–72.

Fleming WE, Pollak CP. Sleep disorders in multiple sclerosis. *Semin Neurol* 2005; **25**: 64–8.

Garcia-Borreguiro D, Larrosa O, Bravo M. Parkinson's disease and sleep. *Sleep Med Rev* 2003; **7**: 115–30.

Kaynak H, Altintas A, Kaynak D, *et al.* Fatigue and sleep disturbance in multiple sclerosis. *Eur J Neurol* 2006; **13**: 1333–9.

Malow BA, Bowes RJ, Ross D. Relationship of temporal lobe seizures to sleep and arousal: a combined scalp-intracranial electrode study. *Sleep* 2000; **23**: 231–4.

Marrie RA, Fisher E, Miller DM, Lee JC, Rudick RA. Association of fatigue and brain atrophy in multiple sclerosis. *J Neurol Sci* 2005; **228**: 161–6.

Moldofsky H. Sleep and pain. *Sleep Med Rev* 2001; **5**: 387–98.

Neau JP, Paquereau J, Meurice JC, Chavagnat JJ, Gil R. Stroke and sleep apnoea: cause or consequence? *Sleep Med Rev* 2002; **6**: 457–70.

Rains JC, Poceta JS. Headache and sleep disorders: review and clinical implications for headache management. *Headache* 2006; **46**: 1344–63.

Schenck CH, Callies AL, Mahowald MW. Increased percentage of slow-wave sleep in REM sleep behavior disorder (RBD): a reanalysis of previously published data from a controlled study of RBD reported in SLEEP. *Sleep* 2003; **26**: 1066–7.

10 Sleep and psychiatric disorders

Thomas C. Wetter, Elisabeth Zils, and Stephany Fulda

Introduction

Psychiatric disorders, in particular mood and anxiety disorders, are among the most common causes of sleep disturbances. According to previous studies, mental disorders have been reported in 35–53% of persons suffering from insomnia. In addition, longitudinal data show that insomnia sufferers are at increased risk for depression, anxiety disorders, and substance abuse. However, it is assumed that psychiatric disorders in those with sleep disturbances are often overlooked. Thus, exploring the individual's psychiatric history and obtaining current psychiatric findings is imperative for the diagnosis of sleep disturbances. Since, in general, the severity of sleep disturbances tends to correlate with the severity of the underlying psychiatric disorder, improved sleep is often indicative of an improvement in the psychiatric disorder. Sleep disturbances, especially insomnia, may be caused by a broad range of psychiatric disorders, in particular by mood and psychotic disorders, anxiety disorders, dementia, substance-related and personality disorders. However, there exist only a few systematic studies on the frequency of insomnia accompanying psychiatric diagnoses.

Mood disorders: depression and mania

Epidemiology and clinical features

The lifetime prevalence for mood disorders is estimated between 2% and 25% (major depressive disorder prevalence of 15% and up to 25% in women) and does not differ between ethnic groups. The 1-year incidence of depression is estimated between 10% and 15%. The etiology of mood disorders is not known, but a disturbed interplay between biological, genetic, and psychosocial factors plays an important role in the cause of mood disorders. Symptoms include changes in psychomotor activity, cognitive abilities, vegetative functions, and biological rhythms such as sleep, appetite, and libido. Individuals with depressed mood have a loss of energy, interest, and pleasure, states of anxiety, feelings of guilt, impairment of memory and concentration, and they may suffer from thoughts of suicide. The two major mood disorders are major depressive disorder and bipolar I disorder. The diagnostic criteria for major depressive disorder according to the fourth edition of the *Diagnostic and Statistical Manual of*

Sleep Medicine, ed. Harold R. Smith, Cynthia L. Comella, and Birgit Högl. Published by Cambridge University Press. © Cambridge University Press 2008.

Table 10.1. *DSM-IV criteria for major depressive episode.*

A. Five (or more) of the following symptoms have been present during the same 2-week period and represent a change from previous functioning; at least one of the symptoms is either (1) depressed mood or (2) loss of interest or pleasure.

1. Depressed mood most of the day, nearly every day, as indicated by either subjective report (e.g., feels sad or empty) or observation made by others (e.g., appears tearful). Note: In children and adolescents, can be irritable mood.

2. Markedly diminished interest or pleasure in all, or almost all, activities most of the day, nearly every day (as indicated by either subjective account or observation made by others).

3. Significant weight loss when not dieting or weight gain (e.g., a change of more than 5% of body weight in a month), or decrease or increase in appetite nearly every day. Note: In children, consider failure to make expected weight gains.

4. Insomnia or hypersomnia nearly every day.

5. Psychomotor agitation or retardation nearly every day (observable by other, not merely subjective feelings of restlessness or being slowed down).

6. Fatigue or loss of energy nearly every day.

7. Feelings of worthlessness or excessive or inappropriate guilt (which may be delusional) nearly every day (not merely self-reproach or guilt about being sick).

8. Diminished ability to think or concentrate, or indecisiveness, nearly every day (either by subjective account or as observed by others).

9. Recurrent thoughts of death (not just fear of dying), recurrent suicidal ideation without a specific plan, or a suicide attempt or a specific plan for committing suicide.

B. The symptoms do not meet criteria for a mixed episode.

C. The symptoms cause clinically significant distress or impairment in social, occupational, or other important areas of functioning.

D. The symptoms are not due to the direct physiological effects of a substance (e.g., a drug of abuse, a medication) or a general medical condition (e.g., hypothyroidism).

Mental Disorders (DSM-IV) specify a level of severity and duration of symptoms as minimum requirements to meet the diagnosis (Table 10.1). The hallmark of a manic episode (bipolar I disorder) is a euphoric mood with thoughts of high self-confidence, or irritable mood. Other signs are hyperactivity, disorganized behavior, emotional lability, and feelings of anger and hostility. Mood-congruent manic delusions include extraordinary abilities, but mood-incongruent delusions and hallucinations may also be present in mania. In addition, a person may show difficulties in concentrating, flight of ideas, or incoherent thinking.

Sleep features

Subjective complaints

About 80–90% of people with depression suffer from an impairment of sleep quality. Characteristic complaints are difficulties falling asleep and maintaining sleep with multiple awakenings at night, during which the individuals ruminate about their problems. A typical feature of severe depression is early morning awakening (at least

2 hours before the usual time of awakening) without falling asleep again (so called "terminal insomnia"). However, systematic studies could not confirm that waking up early in the morning is a specific symptom of a certain subtype of depressive disorders ("endogenous" vs. "neurotic" depression). As a consequence of disturbed nighttime sleep, a person may suffer from daytime sleepiness, which may mimic depressive features.

Depression is the most frequent cause of insomnia. Epidemiological studies have shown that the incidence of depressive disorders among people with severe sleep disturbances was increased compared to persons without sleep disturbances, confirming a high comorbidity of insomnia and depressive disorders. On the other hand, studies have also shown that insomnia is associated with an increased risk for the development of a depression.

Hypersomnia (and significant weight gain or increase in appetite) is a characteristic finding in depression with atypical features – these symptoms have been referred to as reversed vegetative symptoms. Hypersomnia has also been described in individuals with depressive episodes of bipolar depression. Up to 15% of those suffering from a major depression may show symptoms of hypersomnia, and it has been reported that hypersomnia is often observed during depressive episodes in bipolar disorders. Moreover, the increased need of sleep is one of the characteristic symptoms of the seasonal affective disorder. A thorough exploration will show whether the feeling of increased daytime fatigue and sleepiness could also be due to the lack of drive and listlessness. If a depressive person shows an increased tendency to fall asleep, other causes of hypersomnia (e.g., sleep-disordered breathing, periodic limb movement disorder, narcolepsy) should be considered for differential diagnosis. However, hypersomnia may also be a side effect of psychopharmacological medication comprising a strong sedative component. In a manic episode people typically perceive a decreased need for sleep and feel rested after only a few hours of sleep.

Polysomnographic findings

Systematic sleep studies using overnight polysomnography have shown that total sleep time, sleep efficiency, and slow-wave sleep (SWS) were reduced in people with depression, while the number of awakenings and waking periods at night were increased. In addition, changes were found in REM sleep, such as a shortened time period between sleep onset and the first REM episode (REM latency), a prolonged first REM period, and an increased number of eye movements during REM sleep (REM density) (Table 10.2). These findings suggest that REM sleep is disinhibited in depression.

The initial assumption that these changes are depression-specific could not be confirmed, in particular since REM sleep changes were also found in individuals with other psychiatric or sleep disorders. For example, symptoms of REM sleep disinhibition were also described in narcolepsy and schizophrenia. However, the full scope of polysomnographic REM sleep abnormalities, such as an increased REM density, an increased relative amount of REM sleep, and a shortened REM latency, has so far been reported only in depression. Pharmacological studies using

Table 10.2. *Sleep abnormalities in mood disorders.*

Mood disorder	Sleep EEG findings
Major depressive episode	↓sleep continuity (↑SL, ↓SE, ↓TST) ↓SWS ↓REML, ↑REMD; ↑REM% of TST
Manic episode	↓sleep continuity (↑SL, ↓SE, ↓TST) ↓SWS ↓REML, ↑REMD; ↑REM% of TST

SL, sleep latency; SE, sleep efficiency; TST, total sleep time; REML, REM sleep latency; REMD, REM density; SWS, slow-wave sleep.

cholinergic substances to investigate the phenomenon of REM sleep disinhibition suggest a supersensitivity of central cholinergic receptors in depressive individuals and support the hypothesis that there is an imbalance of central cholinergic and aminergic neurotransmission in favor of the cholinergic system.

Polysomnographic studies in depressive individuals suffering from hypersomnia showed basically normal sleep profiles. Hypersomnia could not be objectively verified as a symptom using the multiple sleep latency test. Seasonally depressed people also had substantially normal findings in polysomnographic studies. It appears that in depression the feeling of increased daytime fatigue or sleepiness is more of a subjective symptom. Regarding the sleep microstructure in people with depression, all-night spectral analysis showed a reduced power density, particularly in the low (0.25–3 Hz) frequency band. Sleep studies during manic episodes showed similar polysomnographic abnormalities as for depression, even with respect to REM sleep alterations (Table 10.2).

Effects of antidepressive treatment on sleep

To treat severe depression, a combination therapy of antidepressive drugs and psychotherapy is often necessary. Apart from their mood-improving properties, some of the currently available antidepressant substances exhibit a sedative effect that can be utilized for treating concurrent insomnia. In addition, specific antidepressants are effective drugs for the treatment of insomnia not due to a mental disorder. Almost all antidepressants have been shown to affect sleep continuity and sleep architecture. Typically, these medications are associated with a delayed onset of REM sleep, reduced amount of REM sleep, and increased SWS. The influence on REM sleep latency is the most consistent finding for tricyclic and tetracyclic antidepressants, selective serotonin (and noradrenaline) reuptake inhibitors (SSRIs or SNRIs), and monoamine oxidase inhibitors. This robust finding has generated the hypothesis that REM sleep suppression plays a pivotal role in the neurophysiological mechanisms underlying treatment response. However, trimipramine and trazodone do not exert an effect on REM sleep, indicating that no unambiguous relationship between clinical improvement and REM sleep suppression exists. Table 10.3 presents an overview of

Table 10.3. *Antidepressant drugs and their effects on sleep parameters.*

Antidepressant drug	Potentially affected sleep parameters			
	REM latency	REM sleep	Sleep continuity	Slow-wave sleep
Amitriptyline	↑↑↑	↓↓	↑↑↑	↔
Clomipramine	↑↑↑	↓↓↓	↑↑↑	↔
Desipramine	↑↑↑	↓↓	↑↑↑	↔
Maprotiline	↑↑↑	↓↓	↔	↔
Mianserin	↑	↓	↑↑↑	↔
Mirtazapine	↑	↔	↑↑↑	↔
Nefazodone	↔	↑↑↑	↑↑↑	↔
SSRIs	↑↑↑	↓	↓	↔
Trazodone	↑	↓	↑↑↑	↑
Trimipramine	↑	↔	↑↑↑	↔

↑↑↑, substantial increase (improvement); ↑, minor increase (improvement); ↓↓↓, major decrease; ↓↓, moderate decrease; ↓, minor decrease; ↔, no effect.

significant effects of antidepressants on sleep parameters. Regarding potential side effects on sleep quality, recent studies have shown that antidepressants may induce or aggravate restless legs syndrome (e.g., mirtazapine) or may increase the risk of periodic leg movements (e.g., venlafaxine and SSRIs).

Therapeutic use of sleep deprivation in depression

Total sleep deprivation for one whole night improves depressive symptoms in 40–60% of subjects. Most (50–80%) experience a relapse of depressive symptoms after recovery sleep, but in a few individuals improvements may last for weeks. In a small proportion of subjects (2–7%) sleep deprivation can lead to worsening of symptoms. Increased sleepiness and sometimes (hypo-) mania may also develop during sleep deprivation. About 10–15% of subjects experience an improvement only after the recovery night. The pattern of response to repeated sleep deprivation is highly variable, and each individual may respond at one time but not at another, or vice versa. An improved outcome for repeated as opposed to one-time sleep deprivation has not been clearly demonstrated. Partial sleep deprivation in the early part of the night (with sleep between 03:00 and 06:00 hours), or in the late part (i.e., remaining awake after 01:30 hours) is slightly less effective than total sleep deprivation. A selective deprivation of REM sleep is not associated with an increased response rate.

Newer studies suggest that the effect of sleep deprivation on depressive symptoms may be stabilized with antidepressant drugs, light therapy, or shifting of sleep times. However, the clinical feasibility of sleep deprivation therapy is considerably restricted by the fact that the majority of sleep deprivation responders experience a relapse of the depressive mood after the first night of sleep. There is evidence that, after a night of no sleep, shifting the sleep period to the late afternoon and early night may lower this risk, and avoiding sleep during this critical phase has an antidepressive effect.

The advantage of sleep deprivation consists in its more rapid efficacy as compared to antidepressants. Therefore, in some individuals, the time until the onset of the pharmacological effect can be therapeutically bridged by combining antidepressants and sleep deprivation therapy. However, the precise mechanisms underlying the effect of sleep deprivation in depression are still unknown.

Anxiety disorders: posttraumatic stress disorder, panic disorder, generalized anxiety disorder, obsessive–compulsive disorder

Epidemiology and clinical features

The group of anxiety disorders consists of phobic disorders, panic disorder, generalized anxiety disorder, and combined fear and depression. According to DSM-IV, obsessive–compulsive disorder and posttraumatic stress disorder also belong to this group.

People suffering from posttraumatic stress disorder (PTSD) have experienced a traumatic life event such as war, natural catastrophe, car accident, death of a very close person, or rape. The trauma is life-threatening or highly life-altering. People developing PTSD show a prolonged reaction to this traumatic event. They (1) re-experience the trauma, e.g., during situations similar to the traumatic event, suffering from "flashbacks" and nightmares, (2) avoid objects and situations reminding them of the trauma, (3) show signs of hyperarousal, e.g., sleep disturbances and hypervigilance, which did not exist before the trauma. Lifetime prevalence in the general population is about 1–9%, differing between studies. Women are more than twice as likely as men to develop PTSD after exposure to a psychological trauma.

People with panic disorder experience a discrete period of intense fear, accompanied by somatic and cognitive symptoms such as dyspnea, chest pain, tachycardia, palpitations, vertigo, dizziness, perspiration, nausea, sensory phenomena (paresthesia, hypesthesia, feelings of heat or cold), depersonalization, derealization, and losing control. These symptoms occur abruptly, unexpectedly, and without a special causative situation. The maximum of intensity is reached after about 10–20 minutes and symptoms usually decrease after 20–30 minutes but sometimes persist for hours. A concurrent agoraphobia often develops. Lifetime prevalence of this disorder is 3%, with women affected twice as often as men.

Phobic disorders include phobia, social phobia, and agoraphobia. Their common characteristic is an irrational fear of certain situations or objects that does not correspond to the actual danger. Fear and somatic symptoms are always evoked by the same situation or object. The trigger in agoraphobia is either a large place or a crowded situation. In social phobia, sufferers do not dare talk, eat, or even spend time together with other people. They are afraid of being judged by others and fear embarrassment. Specific phobia is characterized by an isolated triggering object or situation. Very common triggers in specific phobias are blood, spiders, exams, altitude, and closed, small rooms (claustrophobia). In all phobias the triggering factor is strictly avoided. Lifetime prevalence of phobic disorders ranges between 5% and 13%.

In generalized anxiety disorder (GAD) a person permanently worries about things of daily life. Contents of the fear are different and often change, e.g., their own or a relative's health, their children's achievement at school, their financial situation. Lifetime prevalence in men has been estimated at 6.6%, and in women 12.2%. Associated symptoms are restlessness, difficulty in concentration, being easily fatigued, irritability, elevated muscle tension, and sleep disturbances.

Obsessive–compulsive disorder (OCD) has a lifetime prevalence of 2–3%. A person with OCD suffers from obsessions or/and compulsions. Common contents of obsessions are aggression, sexuality, dirt, contamination, specific arrangements and orders, pathological doubts of correctly done actions. Sufferers recognize these thoughts or actions as being irrational.

Sleep features
Subjective complaints
The most frequent complaints in PTSD are difficulties falling asleep (sleep-onset insomnia), difficulties staying asleep (sleep-maintenance insomnia), and early morning awakening. Additionally, they often report nightmares. The content of these can be an exact replication of the trauma as well as other threatening and frightening themes. There are indications that in early stages the nightmares' contents mirror the trauma, but that they change over time to just threatening themes. Compared to individuals with insomnia without PTSD, those with PTSD have no difference in total sleep time, but complain about additional symptoms: fear of going to bed, waking up with the covers torn apart, fear of the dark, thinking of the trauma whilst lying in bed, talking and yelling during sleep, waking up confused or disorientated, waking up from a nightmare and finding it difficult to fall asleep again.

In panic disorder, complaints about insomnia, restless or disrupted sleep, as well as nocturnal panic attacks, are common: 44–71% of individuals with panic disorder have reported nocturnal panic attacks at least once in their life.

In social phobia, common complaints about sleep behavior are insomnia and nonrestorative sleep. It should be noted that sleep disturbances are not one of the most prominent symptoms in these individuals.

Sixty to seventy percent of people with GAD complain about insomnia. The severity of insomnia correlates positively with the severity of the anxiety disorder. This includes complaints of difficulty falling or staying asleep. There are also statements of restless or unsatisfying sleep in GAD.

People with OCD do not express characteristic sleep disturbances. Some report difficulties going to bed due to their compulsions, e.g., checking the front door or the stove. In other cases there may occur sleep complaints that can be attributed to a secondary depression.

Polysomnographic findings
PSG findings in anxiety disorders are inconsistent (Table 10.4). In PTSD, some studies showed a reduction of sleep efficiency, and elevated number of awakenings. Other investigators did not find any differences at all in sleep efficiency and number of

Table 10.4. *Sleep abnormalities in anxiety disorders.*

Anxiety disorder	Sleep EEG findings
Posttraumatic stress disorder	Normal or ↓sleep continuity
	Normal or↓REML; ↓ or ↑REM% of TST
	Flashback dreams usually arising from REM sleep
Panic disorder	Normal or ↓ sleep continuity
	Sleep panic attacks, usually arising at stage 2–SWS transition
Generalized anxiety disorder	↓sleep continuity
Obsessive–compulsive disorder	↓sleep continuity
	Normal or ↓REML

SWS, slow wave sleep; REML, REM sleep latency; TST, total sleep time.

awakenings. Surprisingly, there are higher awakening thresholds in SWS of people with PTSD in comparison to controls. The findings referring to REM sleep are very discordant. Congruent results were found only for REM density, which was higher in PTSD sufferers in four studies. Regarding these findings, the high comorbidity of depression in PTSD has to be taken into account, since an increased frequency of rapid eye movements is known for depression. One study reported a higher number of awakenings during REM sleep, which has not been replicated so far. Consistent results exist for an increased number of body movements in PTSD compared with healthy controls, although it has to be elucidated whether this is due to a medical or psychiatric cause.

The PSG findings in panic disorder show prolonged sleep latencies, a higher amount of wake time after sleep onset, and hence a decreased sleep efficiency compared to healthy controls. Regarding REM sleep measures in panic disorder, the findings are contradictory. Some studies found a reduction of REM latency and REM density whereas others did not. As mentioned above, nocturnal panic attacks occur in addition to daytime panic attacks. The symptoms are very similar, but dyspnea is reported more often nocturnally. Nocturnal panic attacks begin from late stage 2 or early stage 3 sleep and have to be distinguished from nightmares, other sleep-related events, and awakenings due to environmental factors.

The subjective reports on sleep disturbances in individuals with social phobia could not be confirmed using PSG studies. Sleep efficiency and REM sleep measures are not significantly different from those of healthy controls.

There are only a few studies investigating sleep in GAD. It is concluded that wake time after sleep onset and prolonged sleep latency are higher in GAD than in healthy controls. Moreover, total sleep time and sleep efficiency are reduced compared to controls. This mainly results in sleep-maintenance insomnia and – to a smaller extent – in sleep-onset insomnia.

The majority of sleep studies in OCD revealed normal REM latencies. It has been shown that sleep efficiency is significantly reduced, and the number of awakenings and early morning awakening tends to be higher than in controls. In addition, a negative correlation of the individuals' scores of the Y-BOCS, a rating inventory for obsession and compulsion, with total sleep time and sleep efficiency has been reported. Therefore, sleep efficiency seems to be reduced in people with OCD, either by a higher number of awakenings, by a reduction of total sleep time, or by a higher wake percentage after sleep onset.

Schizophrenia

Epidemiology and clinical features

The lifetime prevalence of schizophrenia has been reported as ranging from 1% to 2%, and about 0.025% to 0.05% of the total population is treated for schizophrenia in any single year. Schizophrenia is equally prevalent in men and women, but the onset and course of the disease differs. In general, the onset in women is later (25–35 years) and the outcome is better for women than for men with schizophrenia. The cause of schizophrenia is unknown, but a specific vulnerability for biological, psycho-social, and environmental factors seems to be crucial for the development of this disorder. Schizophrenia is often discussed as if it was a single disease, but the diagnostic category includes a group of disorders with heterogeneous presentations and probably heterogeneous causes. DSM-IV classifies the subtypes of schizophrenia based predominantly on clinical presentation (Table 10.5): paranoid (delusions or hallucinations), disorganized (disorganized behavior, inappropriate affect), catatonic (psychomotor disturbances including mutism, negativism, or excessive motor activity), undifferentiated (criteria of the paranoid, disorganized, or undifferentiated type are not met). Another classification is based on the presence or the absence of positive (productive) and negative symptoms. Positive symptoms are characterized by hallucinations, delusions, bizarre behavior, and formal thought disorders such as incoherence and illogicality. Typical negative symptoms are a flattened affect, a poverty of speech, anhedonia, social withdrawal, and cognitive impairment.

Sleep features
Subjective complaints
Although sleep disturbances are not included in the diagnostic criteria for schizophrenia, they may be a prominent complaint during the prodromal phase of the disease or during the exacerbation of schizophrenic symptoms. In addition, sleep problems may precede the onset of acute psychotic symptoms. Typically, individuals report sleep-onset and maintenance insomnia and frequent nocturnal awakenings. A strong correlation has been found between difficulty initiating sleep and positive symptoms, including delusions, hallucinations, and disorganization. Some people may suffer from disturbances of the circadian rhythm, including a complete reversal of the day/night pattern of sleep. Because of social withdrawal, substance abuse, excessive daytime napping, or effects of medication, sleep in schizophrenic individuals may also be severely impaired as a consequence of poor sleep hygiene. There are no systematic reports on excessive daytime sleepiness, but antipsychotic and

Table 10.5. *DSM-IV Diagnostic criteria for schizophrenia.*

A. Characteristic symptoms: two (or more) of the following, each present for a significant portion of time during a 1-month period (or less if successfully treated):
  1. Delusions.
  2. Hallucinations.
  3. Disorganized speech (e.g., frequent derailment or incoherence).
  4. Grossly disorganized or catatonic behaviour.
  5. Negative symptoms (i.e., affective flattening, alogia, or avolition).
     Note: Only one Criterion A symptom is required if delusions are bizarre or hallucinations consist of a voice keeping up a running commentary on the person's behavior or thoughts, or two or more voices conversing with each other.
B. Social/occupational dysfunction: for a significant portion of the time since the onset of the disturbance, one or more major areas of functioning such as work, interpersonal relations, or self-care are markedly below the level achieved prior to the onset (or when the onset is in childhood or adolescence, failure to achieve expected level of interpersonal, academic, or occupational achievement).
C. Duration: continuous signs of the disturbance persist for at least 6 months. This 6-month period must include at least 1 month of symptoms (or less if successfully treated) that meet Criterion A (i.e., active-phase symptoms) and may include periods of prodromal or residual symptoms. During these prodromal or residual periods, the signs of the disturbance may be manifested by only negative symptoms or two or more symptoms listed in Criterion A presented in an attenuated form (e.g., odd beliefs, unusual perceptual experiences).
D. Schizoaffective and mood disorder exclusion: schizoaffective disorder and mood disorder with psychotic features have been ruled out because either (1) no major depressive, manic, or mixed episodes have occurred concurrently with the active-phase symptoms; or (2) if mood episodes have occurred during active-phase symptoms, their total duration has been brief relative to the duration of the active and residual periods.

sedative medication may result in sleepiness. Importantly, sleep-disordered breathing may show a higher prevalence in people with schizophrenia.

Polysomnographic findings

The results of all-night polysomnographic studies have to be interpreted in the context of individual characteristics (i.e., the subtype of schizophrenia, phases of the illness, age), the status of medication, and specific comorbid sleep disorders (such as sleep apnea syndrome, periodic limb movement disorder). In addition, other coexistent psychiatric (e.g., substance abuse) or somatic disorders may influence sleep. Therefore, controversy exists about the significance of sleep EEG findings in those with schizophrenia (Table 10.6). Compared with healthy controls of a similar age, never-medicated schizophrenic patients show an increase in sleep latency, in wake time after sleep onset, and in the number of nocturnal awakenings. Regarding sleep architecture, there is a reduction in the relative amount of sleep stage 2 and only a moderate reduction in SWS. REM sleep latency is shortened and the absolute

Table 10.6. *Sleep abnormalities in schizophrenia, eating disorders, and alcohol abuse.*

Disorder	Sleep EEG findings
Schizophrenia	↓sleep continuity
	Normal or↓SWS
	Normal or↓REML
Alcohol abuse	↓sleep continuity
	↓SWS
	Normal or↓REML
	Normal or ↑REM% of TST
	↑REMD
Eating disorders	Normal or↓sleep continuity
	Normal or↓SWS
	Normal or↓REML
	Normal or↓or ↑REMD

SWS, slow-wave sleep; REML, REM sleep latency; REMD, REM density; TST, total sleep time.

amount of REM sleep is decreased. Disturbed sleep continuity, reduced deep sleep, and shortened REM latency were also described in polysomnographic studies with depressed individuals. However, those with schizophrenia do not show increased first REM period duration or density. Interestingly, the sleep profile in schizophrenia parallels the one observed in delusional depression, suggesting that similar pathophysiologic mechanisms may underlie both psychotic disorders. This concept is supported by similar patterns of clinical responses.

Quantitative sleep EEG analyses revealed reductions in delta and theta power in schizophrenia compared with matched controls. Delta deficits were more pronounced in the 1–2 Hz delta frequency range, possibly reflecting thalamocortical dysfunction in schizophrenia. This view is supported by observations of reduced thalamic volume, synaptic density, and metabolism in schizophrenia.

Effects of antipsychotic medication

A reduction of SWS has not been confirmed in polysomnographic studies on drug-naive subjects, indicating that SWS changes may reflect the remnant of prior neuroleptic treatment rather than the pathophysiology of the disorder itself. In addition, these studies indicate that withdrawal of drug therapy influences sleep findings. These factors may partly explain the discrepancies in the literature regarding sleep findings in schizophrenia. However, a meta-analysis of sleep in people with schizophrenia without neuroleptic treatment at the time of sleep recording showed that they have sleep disorders that are not necessarily a consequence of neuroleptic treatments. Many of the antipsychotically active substances have a sedative effect. Examples are levomepromazine, thioridazine, perazine, zuclopenthixole, and the atypical neuroleptics clozapine, olanzapine, and quetiapine. Although the typical neuroleptics melperone and pipamperone have only a weak antipsychotic effect, they are sedative and sleep-promoting and thus suitable as an additional treatment for psychotic individuals with sleep disturbances rather than as a sole therapy of psychosis. Haloperidol, benperidol and flupentixol have a strong antipsychotic effect but may also decrease sleep latency, although this has been challenged recently.

In summary, typical and atypical antipsychotics tend to improve sleep induction and/or sleep maintenance. However, these drugs may also show several differential effects on sleep architecture and REM sleep parameters that may be attributed to their selectivity for receptor types and transmitter systems, because dopaminergic, serotoninergic, and cholinergic neurotransmission all modulate sleep in a complex way.

Dementia

The majority of people with dementia suffer from sleep disturbances. Although, with respect to their nature, these are similar to the typical sleep changes occurring during the normal process of aging, they are much more serious. Characteristically, there is an increased number of waking periods at night, increased periods of reduced vigilance, and increased daytime sleepiness. The phenomenon of nighttime insomnia combined with a state of anxiety and confusion is referred to as "sundowning" syndrome. Nocturnal sleep disruption in these individuals, and consequently in the spouse or caregiver, represents a major cause of institutionalization.

Polysomnographic studies including subjects with dementia report disturbed sleep continuity including delayed sleep-onset latency, frequent waking periods at night, a reduced deep sleep percentage, and an increased number of light sleep phases. In contrast to depression, dementia tends to result in decreased REM sleep in the sense of a reduced REM sleep rate and a delayed REM latency. In addition, fewer sleep spindles and K complexes were reported.

Sedating neuroleptics (such as melperone or pipamperone) may be suitable for treatment of sleep disturbances because these substances are well tolerated (e.g., no muscle relaxation and breathing depression) and may positively influence both insomnia and anxiety/confusion with only minor hangover effects. However, systematic polysomnographic studies of these drugs in dementia are lacking. Benzodiazepines are often used to ameliorate sleep disturbances, but may induce paradoxical reactions (increased anxiety and confusion) and an exacerbation of respiratory dysfunction. The administration of benzodiazepines with long half-lives such as diazepam should be avoided because of daytime sedation and unfavorable influence on the structure of the sleep/wake rhythm.

Substance abuse: alcohol, hypnotics, stimulants

Alcohol

Although alcohol is often sedating and commonly used as a self-administered sleeping substance, its usefulness is limited by arousing effects, sleep fragmentation, and hangover effects. In addition, alcohol use may induce apneas in those at risk of sleep-disordered breathing and may increase the number of periodic leg movements during sleep. Both acute and chronic consumption of alcohol result in considerable sleep changes. In healthy persons, acute doses lead to reduced sleep latency, increases in SWS and delta EEG power, and increased wake or light (stage 1) sleep in the second half of the sleep period. In addition, a dose-dependent suppression of REM sleep and a REM "rebound" in the second half is reported. However, a tolerance to sedative and sleep-stage effects develops within repeated nights of administration.

In individuals with alcohol abuse or dependence, many types of sleep disturbances have been attributed to the effects of alcohol or alcohol withdrawal. Chronic alcohol addicts very often suffer from substantial insomnia, which frequently persists even after long alcohol-free periods. Polysomnographic studies with alcohol-dependent subjects that were performed during an alcohol-free period revealed impaired sleep continuity, a reduced deep sleep rate, and signs of REM sleep disinhibition in the sense of increased REM sleep and increased REM density (Table 10.6).

If symptoms of insomnia persist despite long-term withdrawal, sedative antidepressants may be helpful. Acamprosate, a drug successfully used in maintaining abstinence following alcohol withdrawal, may also ameliorate both sleep continuity and sleep architecture.

Hypnotics

Paradoxically, hypnotics may contribute to chronic sleep disturbances when administered over longer periods by developing both addiction and withdrawal symptoms, in particular a "rebound insomnia." This applies in particular to benzodiazepine hypnotics. Rebound insomnia may be observed after only a few weeks of administration, and it is assumed that it may trigger the long-term consumption of hypnotics. Rapid development of tolerance is especially true for benzodiazepines with a short half-life (e.g., triazolam) and seems to be less common in newer hypnotics such as zolpidem or zaleplon. Persons taking benzodiazepines over a prolonged time without increasing the dosage ("low dose dependency") and suffering from insomnia should slowly reduce the dosage and take sedative antidepressants, which may be helpful for treating rebound insomnia. Importantly, side effects of hypnotics include exacerbation of sleep-disordered breathing and drug-induced sleepwalking.

Stimulants

The use of stimulants results in an increased vigilance, which is utilized therapeutically for the treatment of hypersomnias such as narcolepsy. Stimulant drug abuse may lead to markedly disturbed sleep continuity. Polysomnographic studies found prolonged sleep onset time, shortened total sleep time, and REM sleep suppression in the sense of a reduced REM sleep rate and a delayed REM latency after administration of amphetamines. Withdrawal of amphetamines is followed not only by a depressive and dysphoric mood, but also by symptoms of hypersomnia and, polysomnographically, a REM sleep rebound.

Eating disorders

Anorexia nervosa and bulimia nervosa are classified as eating disorders characterized by abnormal patterns of eating behavior as a consequence of fear of losing control and becoming overweight. The core features of anorexia nervosa according to DSM-IV are a refusal to maintain body weight at or above a minimally normal weight for age and height, an intensive fear of gaining weight, even though underweight, a disturbance in the way in which one's body weight is experienced. Diagnostic criteria for bulimia nervosa include recurrent episodes of binge eating and recurrent inappropriate compensatory behavior in order to prevent weight gain, such as self-induced vomiting.

Both anorexia nervosa and bulimia nervosa are often accompanied by additional psychiatric disorders, the most common being a major depressive episode. However, complaints about disturbed sleep are rare. Sleep studies in anorexia and bulimia showed a disturbed sleep maintenance comprising reduced sleep efficiency, increased intermittent wake time, and an increased amount of sleep stage 1. Mixed results are found regarding the amount of SWS and slow-wave activity (Table 10.6). Conflicting observations are also related to REM sleep parameters: REM latencies are shortened or prolonged, REM densities are increased, normal, or decreased, and no systematic associations between REM latency and REM density (as typical for major depression) are present. In people with bulimia nervosa, however, a limited number of studies report that SWS, REM latencies, and REM density are the same as in healthy persons.

Personality disorders

The term "personality disorder" describes enduring patterns of inner experiences and behavior that deviate markedly from the culturally expected and accepted standards. These patterns have an onset in adolescence or early adulthood, are stable over time, and cause a behavior that is inflexible, maladaptive, or otherwise dysfunctional across a broad range of personal and social situations, leading to personal distress or adverse impact on the social environment. Personality disorders are grouped into three clusters in DSM-IV. Cluster A includes the paranoid, schizoid, and schizotypal personality disorders; cluster B covers the antisocial, histrionic, borderline, and narcissistic type; and cluster C contains the avoidant, the dependent, and the obsessive–compulsive personality disorders. The prevalence of personality disorders is estimated between 2% and 40% in the clinical and around 10% in the general population, depending on the subtype of these disorders.

Up to now there are no studies systematically examining subjective complaints due to sleep disturbances in people with personality disorders, but clinical observations show that many of them also report chronic sleep disturbances. With respect to the development of insomnia, the high comorbidity of a personality disorder with other psychiatric disorders such as depression and addiction disorders has to be taken into account. Polysomnographic studies with individuals suffering from a personality disorder, which included almost exclusively those with a borderline personality disorder, found an increased sleep-onset latency, a higher number of waking periods at night, and a reduced sleep efficiency. In some non-depressed borderline individuals, signs of REM sleep disinhibition in the sense of a shortened REM latency were reported.

FURTHER READING

Adrien J. Neurobiological bases for the relation between sleep and depression. *Sleep Med Rev* 2002; **6**: 341–51.

American Academy of Sleep Medicine. *The International Classification of Sleep Disorders: Diagnostic and Coding Manual*, 2nd edn (ICSD-2). Westchester, IL: American Academy of Sleep Medicine, 2005.

American Psychiatric Association. *Diagnostic and Statistical Manual of Mental Disorders*, 4th edn (DSM-IV). Arlington, VA: American Psychiatric Association, 1994.

Benson KL, King R, Gordon D, Silva JA, Zarcone VP Jr. Sleep patterns in borderline personality disorder. *J Affect Disord* 1990; **18**: 267–73.

Bliwise DL. Sleep disorders in Alzheimer's disease and other dementias. *Clin Cornerstone* 2004; **6** (Suppl. 1A): S16–28.

Buysse DJ, Hall M, Begley A, *et al.* Sleep and treatment response in depression: new findings using power spectral analysis. *Psychiatry Res* 2001; **103**: 51–67.

Charon F, Dramaix M, Mendlewicz J. Epidemiological survey of insomniac subjects in a sample of 1,761 outpatients. *Neuropsychobiology* 1989; **21**: 109–10.

Chouinard S, Poulin J, Stip E, Godbout R. Sleep in untreated patients with schizophrenia: a meta-analysis. *Schizophrenia Bull* 2004; **30**: 957–67.

Coleman RM. Sleep–wake disorders based on a polysomnographic diagnosis. *JAMA* 1982; **247**: 997–1003.

Craske MG, Tsao JC. Assessment and treatment of nocturnal panic attacks. *Sleep Med Rev* 2005; **9**: 173–84.

Giedke H, Schwärzler F. Therapeutic use of sleep deprivation in depression. *Sleep Med Rev* 2002; **6**: 361–77.

Harvey AG, Jones C, Schmidt DA. Sleep and posttraumatic stress disorder: a review. *Clin Psychol Rev* 2003; **23**: 377–407.

Kaplan HI, Sadock BJ. *Synopsis of Psychiatry*, 8th edn. Baltimore: Williams & Wilkins, 1998.

Lauer CJ, Krieg JC. Sleep in eating disorders. *Sleep Med Rev* 2004; **8**: 109–18.

Lauer CJ, Schreiber W, Pollmächer T, Holsboer F, Krieg JC. Sleep in schizophrenia: a polysomnographic study on drug-naive patients. *Neuropsychopharmacology* 1997; **16**: 51–60.

Monti JM, Monti D. Sleep disturbances in generalized anxiety disorder and its treatment. *Sleep Med Rev* 2000; **4**: 263–76.

Monti JM, Monti D. Sleep in schizophrenia patients and the effects of antipsychotic drugs. *Sleep Med Rev* 2004; **8**: 133–48.

Papadimitriou GN, Linkowski P. Sleep disturbance in anxiety disorders. *Int Rev Psychiatry* 2005; **17**: 229–36.

Riemann D, Berger M, Voderholzer U. Sleep and depression – results from psychobiological studies: an overview. *Biol Psychol* 2001; **57**: 67–103.

Robinson D, Walsleben J, Pollack S, Lerner G. Nocturnal polysomnography in obsessive–compulsive disorder. *Psychiatry Res* 1998; **80**: 257–63.

Roehrs T, Roth T. Sleep, sleepiness, sleep disorders and alcohol use and abuse. *Sleep Med Rev* 2001; **5**: 287–97.

Tandon R, Shipley JE, Taylor S, *et al.* Electroencephalographic sleep abnormalities in schizophrenia. *Arch Gen Psychiatry* 1992; **49**: 185–94.

Tsuno N, Besset A, Ritchie K. Sleep and depression. *J Clin Psychiatry* 2005; **66**: 1254–69.

Wetter TC, Lauer CJ, Gillich G, Pollmächer T. The electroencephalographic sleep pattern in schizophrenic patients treated with clozapine or classical antipsychotic drugs. *J Psychiatr Res* 1996; **30**: 411–19.

Wilson S, Argyropoulos S. Antidepressants and sleep: a qualitative review of the literature. *Drugs* 2005; **65**: 927–47.

11 Sleep and medical disorders

Andrea Iaboni and Harvey Moldofsky

Introduction

Addressing sleep disturbance in those who are medically ill should be a high priority. Primary sleep disorders, nocturnal disease symptoms, pain, medications, unhealthy lifestyle factors, depression, anxiety, and stress can all contribute to poor-quality sleep. The resulting sleep disturbance can aggravate the underlying disease process and impair daytime functioning.

In this chapter, we describe both the impact of medical diseases and their treatments on sleep, and how disordered sleep can contribute to medical illnesses. Assessment of sleep disturbance is essential to a 24-hour approach to managing medical illness.

Cardiovascular disease and sleep

Cardiovascular parameters such as blood pressure and heart rate, and cardiovascular events such as myocardial infarction and sudden cardiac death, all show circadian rhythms. Awakening in the morning hours is a stress on the cardiovascular system. The sympathetic nervous system is stimulated, catecholamines are released, and blood pressure surges. These changes are believed to cause an excess incidence of morning myocardial infarctions and sudden cardiac death (Fig. 11.1).

Loss of normal circadian rhythms is also associated with disease. The best example is the case of nocturnal hypertension. Blood pressure normally falls 10–20% at night, commonly termed a "dipper" pattern (Fig. 11.2). "Non-dippers" are usually people with secondary hypertension who have lost their drop in blood pressure during sleep. However, non-dipping also occurs in up to 30% of individuals with essential hypertension. The non-dipper pattern is associated with increased risk of hypertensive end-organ damage – i.e., left ventricular hypertrophy, myocardial infarction, albuminuria, and stroke. In fact, nighttime blood pressure is a better prognostic marker for cardiovascular mortality than daytime blood pressure. Measurement of the 24-hour ambulatory blood pressure pattern provides important prognostic information, and is useful for identifying potentially dangerous morning surges. Research

Sleep Medicine, ed. Harold R. Smith, Cynthia L. Comella, and Birgit Högl. Published by Cambridge University Press. © Cambridge University Press 2008.

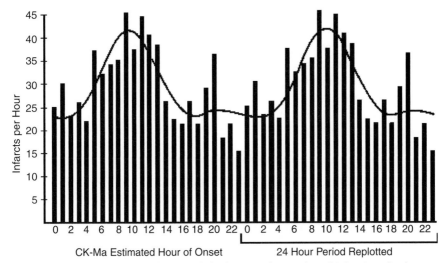

Fig. 11.1. Circadian distribution of myocardial infarction: the number of infarctions (in the MILIS database) beginning during each hour of the day. Reprinted with permission from Muller JE. Circadian variation in cardiovascular events. *Am J Hypertens* 1999; **12**: 35S–42S.

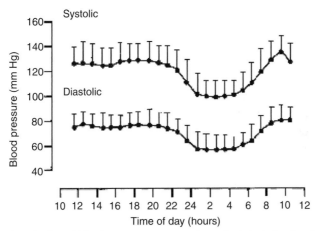

Fig. 11.2. Circadian rhythm of blood pressure: mean and standard deviation hourly values (*n* = 50). Reprinted with permission from Broadhurst P, Brigden G, Dasgupta P, Lahiri A, Raftery EB. Ambulatory intra-arterial blood pressure in normal subjects. *Am Heart J* 1990; **120**: 160–6.

into the benefits of pharmacological restoration of the nocturnal dip and control of morning surges is ongoing (see Drugs and sleep, later in this chapter).

Obstructive sleep apnea and cardiovascular disease

Obstructive sleep apnea (OSA), along with smoking, diabetes, dyslipidemia, and hypertension, is an important risk factor for coronary artery disease. In large epidemiological studies, the association between heart disease and OSA is independent of such confounders as obesity and age.

The acute pathophysiological effects of the apnea–arousal cycle include:
- hypoxemia
- increased negative intrathoracic pressure
- decreases in cardiac output
- activation of the sympathetic nervous system
- acute hypertension.

Chronic pathophysiological changes associated with this process include the following persistent elevations:
- sympathetic tone
- platelet activation
- inflammatory mediators
- C-reactive protein
- vascular endothelial dysfunction.

All of these effects have been suggested to promote artherogenesis in OSA.

Other important cardiovascular effects of OSA include:
- *Essential hypertension.* 40% of hypertensive adults have some degree of sleep-disordered breathing, which increases to 80% in treatment-refractory hypertension.
- *Cardiac arrhythmias.* Bradyarrhythmias, prolonged sinus pauses, and increased ventricular ectopy are common; atrial fibrillation is also markedly increased in people with OSA.
- *Pulmonary hypertension.* In most cases the elevations are modest with the exception of the overlap of OSA and chronic obstructive pulmonary disease, where pulmonary hypertension and cor pulmonale are common (see Respiratory disease and sleep, below).
- *Insulin resistance* (see Other medical illness and sleep, below).

Untreated OSA is associated with an increased risk of mortality in people with coronary artery disease. This underlines the importance of investigating suspected sleep-related respiratory disturbances in individuals with significant cardiovascular risk factors, and in those with hypertension refractory to treatment. With good compliance, therapeutically titrated nasal continuous positive airway pressure (CPAP) is effective at lowering OSA-associated hypertension and reducing the occurrence of arrhythmias.

Congestive heart failure

Several cardinal symptoms of congestive heart failure (CHF), i.e., orthopnea and paroxysmal nocturnal dyspnea, involve disruption of sleep. Sleep-disordered breathing is common in CHF, with 15–30% of individuals with CHF diagnosed with OSA, and 30–40% diagnosed with central sleep apnea (CSA). OSA is believed to exacerbate CHF through its effect on blood pressure, cardiac output, and ventricular function.

Cheyne–Stokes respiration with central sleep apnea (CSR-CSA) is common in heart failure. CSR refers to a crescendo–decrescendo pattern of respiration with periods of central apnea at the nadir and momentary arousals at the peak of the ventilatory effort. The resulting apnea–arousal cycles cause fragmented sleep and daytime sleepiness. CSR-CSA is also associated with increased mortality. Key risk factors for CSR-CSA in CHF are:

- male gender
- awake hypocapnia ($PaCO_2 < 38$ mm Hg)
- older age
- atrial fibrillation.

Unlike OSA, obesity is not a risk factor.

Management of sleep-disordered breathing in CHF includes:

(1) Optimal medical management of CHF.
(2) Nasal CPAP in OSA and CSR-CSA reduces the number of apneic events, improves nocturnal oxygenation and left ventricular ejection fraction (LVEF), but does not improve survival.
(3) Nocturnal oxygen reduces CSA frequency if individual is hypoxemic.
(4) Adaptive servo-ventilation (ASV), a new and promising device, decreases CSA frequency, improves LVEF, reduces arousals from sleep, and increases slow-wave sleep.
(5) Medications (more study required): oral theophylline reduced the number of apnea events and the duration of oxygen desaturations during sleep temazepam decreases arousals from sleep in CSR-CSA, but does not improve the underlying sleep-respiratory disturbance.

Nocturnal angina

Nocturnal angina may herald an acute coronary event. Several sleep-related factors predispose to coronary artery ischemia at night:

- nocturnal hypoxemia secondary to OSA
- nocturnal autonomic surges associated with REM sleep
- nocturnal hypotension and bradycardia associated with NREM sleep
- vasospasm associated with Prinzmetal's variant angina (most commonly occurs between midnight and 07:00 during REM sleep).

Individuals at risk are those who have the following:

- known coronary artery disease with significant stenosis
- untreated OSA with oxygen desaturations
- valvular disease such as aortic stenosis or regurgitation
- vasospasm associated with Prinzmetal's variant angina
- excessive antihypertensive use or excessive beta-adrenergic blockade.

An urgent cardiac workup is indicated. Useful diagnostic tests for identifying sleep-related factors include overnight oximetry, 24-hour blood pressure and electrocardiogram monitoring, and polysomnography to assess for OSA.

Management includes appropriate interventions for critical stenosis or valvular disease, nasal CPAP for OSA, and nitrates and calcium-channel blockers for variant angina.

Nocturnal arrhythmia and sudden death

Common and normal rhythm changes seen in sleep include:

- sinus pauses
- sinus bradycardia
- first-degree AV block.

While most cardiac events occur during waking hours, 15–20% of automatic implantable defibrillator discharges take place during sleep. REM sleep in particular is a period of arrhythmogenesis associated with bursts of sympathetic activity. Paroxysmal atrial fibrillation peaks in the early morning between 02:00 and 05:00.

Cyclic heart rate fluctuations often occur with OSA. Sinus bradycardia occurs during the apneic phase and the heart rate rises sharply at the termination of the apnea. Nocturnal brady-tachycardia in 24-hour ambulatory electrocardiograms provides an important clue to identify people with OSA.

The Brugada syndrome and sudden unexplained nocturnal death syndrome (SUNDS) are two related rare phenomena. Both are causes of sudden cardiac death due to ventricular fibrillation, predominantly between 20:00 and 08:00, affecting young, healthy men without structural heart disease, with a higher incidence in Asian countries. The Brugada syndrome is characterized by distinct ST segment elevations in the right precordial ECG leads and is associated with a mutation in a gene encoding a cardiac sodium channel. A family history of sudden death is common. "Kiroshi," a Japanese term, is used to describe sudden death in otherwise healthy young people following prolonged episodes of overwork and sleep deprivation.

Respiratory disease and sleep

Asthma

Airway function has a normal circadian variation, with peak airflow in the afternoon and the lowest in the early morning at about 04:00. In people with asthma, this morning trough is associated with worsening of asthma symptoms and sleep disturbance. Early-morning forced expiratory volumes can drop as much as 20–40% in those with asthma (Fig. 11.3). Sleep disruption affects up to 40% of asthmatics, and causes significant daytime impairment, noted in particular in school performance and attendance by children with asthma. An excess of asthma attacks and of asthma-related deaths occurs at night.

Sleep-related pathophysiological factors involved in nocturnal asthma include:

- Airway inflammation increases at night, with higher numbers of airway eosinophils and leukocytes.
- Circadian changes in circulating catecholamines, with an early-morning trough in epinephrine and increased vagal parasympathetic tone at night can worsen airway resistance.
- Snoring and OSA in people with asthma worsens nocturnal symptoms.
- Allergens such as dust mites and pet dander are often concentrated in the bedroom.
- Allergic rhinitis is common in asthma and postnasal drip can lead to airway irritation and reflex bronchoconstriction.
- Cool, dry air at night contributes to bronchospasm.
- Gastroesophageal reflux has been shown to worsen bronchoconstriction.

Nocturnal asthma is a marker for poor asthma control. The management includes optimizing medical treatment, identifying contributing medical and environmental conditions:

A

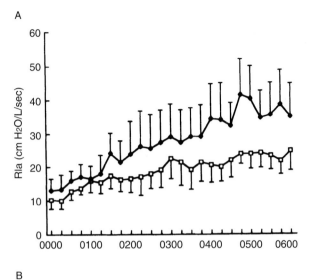

B

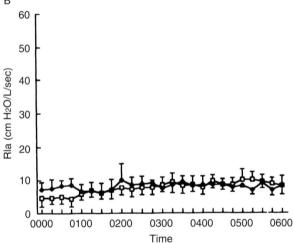

Fig. 11.3. Nocturnal changes in lower airway resistance (Rla) during sleep (◆) and with prevention of sleep (□) in six individuals with asthma (A) and four normal controls (B). Bars, SE. Reprinted with permission from Soutar CA, Costello J, Ijaduola O, Turner-Warwick M. Nocturnal and morning asthma: relationship to plasma corticosteroids and response to cortisol infusion. *Thorax* 1975; **30**: 436–40.

(1) Step-up asthma management until control has been achieved. This includes inhaled corticosteroids and, in many cases, the addition of a long-acting beta-adrenergic agent or leukotriene modifier.

(2) Adjust the timing and dosing of medications to give a maximal level in the early morning hours (see Drugs and sleep, below).

(3) Sleep environmental control includes replacement of pillows and bedding with non-allergenic materials, removing pets from the bedroom, frequent cleaning of bedroom and mattress, and warming and humidifying the air.

(4) In those with allergic rhinitis, nasal anti-inflammatory therapy with topical steroids and nasal saline rinses improves postnasal drip and minimizes nocturnal symptoms.

(5) Assess for gastroesophageal reflux disease (GERD), and manage with lifestyle changes and pharmacologic therapies if necessary (see Gastroesophageal reflux and sleep, below).

(6) Assess for OSA in individuals with a suggestive history. Nasal CPAP improves nocturnal asthma in those with concomitant OSA.

Chronic obstructive pulmonary disease

Chronic obstructive pulmonary disease (COPD) is characterized by cough and dyspnea associated with irreversible airflow obstruction, with a progression to respiratory failure. Poor sleep quality is common in people with COPD, with 50% describing subjective disturbed sleep (Table 11.1).

Sleep-related changes in respiratory physiology can result in nocturnal oxygen desaturation and respiratory compromise in people with diseased lungs (Fig. 11.4). Examples include:

- decreased ventilatory drive
- decreased lung volume
- increased upper airway resistance
- decreased ventilatory responsiveness to hypercapnia and hypoxemia
- low muscle tone in REM sleep, impairing ribcage movement and airway patency.

Although OSA is found in COPD at about the same rate as in the general population, those with both COPD and OSA are at particular risk because:

- In hypoventilating hypoxemic individuals with COPD the SaO_2 is on the steep portion of the oxyhemoglobin dissociation curve, leading to severe desaturations with relatively small changes in partial pressure of oxygen during apneic events.
- Severe nocturnal oxygen desaturations predispose to pulmonary hypertension, cor pulmonale, polycythaemia, and cardiac dysrhythmias.

Table 11.1. *Sleep changes in chronic obstructive pulmonary disease (COPD).*

Sleep changes
Sleep architecture changes: increased frequency of arousals, increased frequency of sleep stage changes, decreased total sleep time, poor sleep efficiency
OSA
Nightmares
Insomnia
Daytime sleepiness
Factors
Nocturnal cough, sputum, wheeze, dyspnea
Orthopnea
Smoking
Nocturnal hypoxemia and hypercapnia
Depression

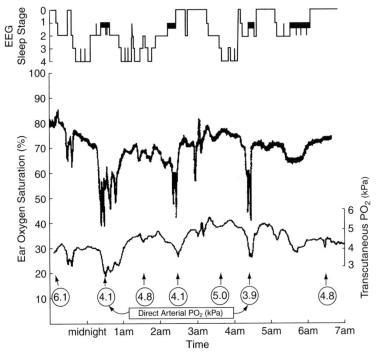

Fig. 11.4. Overnight changes in sleep stage, oxygen saturation, and transcutaneous PO_2, with intermittent measurement of PaO_2, in COPD with nocturnal hypoxemia. Reprinted with permission from Douglas NJ. Sleep in patients with chronic obstructive pulmonary disease. *Clin Chest Med* 1998; **19**: 115–25.

The management of COPD should take account of a number of sleep-related issues:

(1) Ask about symptoms consistent with OSA such as snoring, witnessed apneas during sleep, and excessive daytime sleepiness.

(2) Optimize COPD management to improve nocturnal symptoms such as cough and dyspnea. Pharmaceutical agents that benefit nocturnal SaO_2 and improve sleep quality include anticholinergic agents and sustained-release theophylline.

(3) Awake arterial blood gas levels are the best prognostic indicators, and in most cases polysomnography is not necessary.

(4) Overnight sleep studies are indicated where there is the suspicion of OSA or the person develops complications such as polycythemia or cor pulmonale, which are not fully explained by the awake oxygen levels.

(5) CPAP, in those with COPD and OSA, improves nocturnal gas exchange, reduces respiratory muscle fatigue, and improves functional status.

(6) Long-term oxygen (> 15 hours/day) reduces mortality in COPD, and consensus guidelines have been developed. In general, oxygen therapy is indicated when $PaO_2 < 55$ mm Hg ($SaO_2 < 88\%$) or when $PaO_2 = 55$–59 mm Hg in those with pulmonary hypertension, peripheral edema, or polycythemia.

(7) Oxygen does not benefit individuals with isolated nocturnal desaturations, except if there is cor pulmonale.

(8) Hypercapnic individuals may benefit from nocturnal bilevel positive pressure ventilation, but the evidence for its long-term use in COPD is limited.

(9) Avoid sedative medications, particularly benzodiazepines, for the treatment of insomnia because of the risk for respiratory depression.

Gastroesophageal reflux and sleep

About 7% of the population experience heartburn on a daily basis and 15% have weekly symptoms. In individuals with heartburn at least once weekly, three-quarters complain of heartburn affecting their sleep. Gastroesophageal reflux (GER) is caused by loss of the pressure gradient between the lower esophageal sphincter and stomach, most commonly by transient relaxations of the lower esophageal sphincter, resulting in reflux of gastric contents into the esophagus.

Reflux that occurs at night during sleep results in prolonged acid contact with the esophageal mucosa and an increased risk of proximal migration of acidic contents. Nighttime reflux may predispose to serious complications such as erosive esophagitis and epithelial reactive changes that may contribute to the development of Barrett's esophagus. Other important clinical problems that are associated with proximal acid migration include exacerbation of bronchial asthma, chronic cough, hoarseness, and laryngitis.

Contrary to popular belief, the recumbent sleep posture is not the main problem – awake supine persons clear acid in much the same way as upright individuals – but rather changes in GER defence mechanisms that are associated with sleep:

- a dramatic decrease in the production of saliva during sleep, important for neutralizing acid reflux
- a decreased frequency of swallowing, with a near absence of swallowing in slow-wave sleep
- delayed gastric emptying during sleep
- impaired perception of heartburn.

Esophageal acid contact triggers protective awakenings, resulting in fragmented, poor-quality sleep and impairing daytime functioning. GER disease (GERD) is frequently comorbid with OSA, with one study finding > 100 reflux episodes per night in individuals with OSA. The nature of this link is still uncertain, but interestingly, treatment of OSA by CPAP improves nocturnal GER symptoms. OSA and GER also share a central risk factor: obesity. Obesity contributes to GER through increased intra-abdominal pressure and slower gastrointestinal transit times, and weight loss has been shown to improve GER.

The ICSD-2 criteria for the diagnosis of sleep-related GERD include recurrent awakenings from sleep with shortness of breath or heartburn and one of:

(i) a sour bitter taste in the mouth upon awakening from sleep

(ii) sleep-related coughing or choking

(iii) awakening from sleep with heartburn.

The gold standard for diagnosis of sleep-related GERD is polysomnography with continuous esophageal pH monitoring, although this test is not commonly available.

Table 11.2. *Management of nocturnal gastroesophageal reflux disease (GERD).*

Lifestyle modifications
    No food in the 3 hours before bedtime and avoidance of large meals
    Avoidance of caffeine, alcohol, mint, tomato-based foods, spicy foods, citrus, soft drinks
    Smoking cessation
    Weight reduction
    Avoidance of medications that promote GER (Ca channel blockers, anticholinergic
       medications, theophylline, prostaglandins, bisphosphonates)
    Elevate head of bed by 150 mm using blocks or wedges

Medical therapy
    Proton pump inhibitors
       Given before breakfast and supper to suppress gastric acid production
       Nocturnal acid breakthrough can occur
    H2 receptor antagonists
       Can be used at bedtime to control nocturnal acid secretion
    Promotility agents
       High side-effect profile

Surgical therapy
    Antireflux surgery in individuals with disease complications

Twenty-four-hour ambulatory esophageal pH measurement is useful when the diagnosis is in question. In individuals with dysphagia, odynophagia, severe and/or chronic heartburn, and poor response to treatment, endoscopic examination is warranted. The differential diagnosis of nocturnal chest pain includes angina, which may require cardiac investigations.

Management strategies are outlined in Table 11.2.

End-stage renal disease and sleep

People with end-stage renal disease (ESRD) on hemodialysis or peritoneal dialysis sleep very poorly. Subjectively, a high proportion complain of shortened and fragmented sleep, daytime sleepiness, and restless legs. Polysomnography shows that the total sleep times and sleep efficiencies are low; the number of arousals and wake time are both high. Daytime sleepiness is also common, with most dialysis patients taking daytime naps and many – about 50% in one study – reporting unintentional naps. Overall, sleep disturbance in those receiving dialysis is associated with considerable functional impairment, poor health and wellbeing.

Primary sleep disorders are common. They include the following:

- OSA frequency is 30–80% in ESRD versus 2–4% in the general population. This association may be explained in part by significant overlap in common comorbid conditions for OSA and renal disease, including cardiovascular disease, diabetes, and obesity, as well as by demographic factors such as age and male gender. The cardiovascular impact of OSA (see above) is of particular concern in people with renal disease, in whom mortality from cardiovascular causes is high.

- Restless legs syndrome (RLS) and periodic limb movement disorder (PLMD) occur in about 80% of people receiving dialysis. Waking restlessness and unpleasant sensations in the lower limbs with sleep fragmentation are associated with difficulties in initiating and maintaining sleep.

Various contributing risk factors for these sleep disturbances include disease, treatment, and lifestyle factors (Table 11.3).

The clinical presentation of people with ESRD and sleep apnea is often atypical – they are not necessarily obese and less commonly have a history of snoring. Daytime sleepiness is common in many of those on dialysis and is thus not specific for

Table 11.3. *Factors contributing to poor sleep in people receiving dialysis.*

Disease factors
 Uremia, subclinical uremic encephalopathy
 Pruritis
 Edema
 Anemia
 Comorbid illnesses
 Peripheral neuropathy
 Secondary hyperparathyroidism
 Renal bone disease, bone pain
 Acid–base and electrolyte abnormalities
 Vitamin deficiencies

Treatment factors
 Early-morning dialysis scheduling
 Release of sleep-promoting inflammatory cytokines during dialysis
 Alteration in body temperature rhythms by dialysis
 Abnormal retention of melatonin altering circadian melatonin rhythm
 Tyrosine deficiency leading to neurotransmitter production changes
 Medications

Psychological factors
 Mood disorder
 Anxiety
 Psychosocial strain (finances, grief, loneliness)

Lifestyle factors
 Alcohol
 Caffeine
 Smoking
 Sedentary lifestyle
 Poor sleep hygiene

Adapted from Parker KP. Sleep disturbances in dialysis patients. *Sleep Med Rev* 2003; **7**: 131–43.

sleep apnea. Because restless and disturbed sleep is common there should be a high index of suspicion for a complicating primary sleep disorder. Polysomnography helps to clarify the nature and severity of the primary sleep disorder and aid in the management of ESRD.

Treatment considerations include the following:

(1) Optimized uremia control improves sleep and sleepiness.
(2) Renal transplantation alleviates both RLS and sleep apnea.
(3) Lifestyle modifications such as avoiding caffeine, nicotine, and evening alcohol, and basic sleep hygiene practices.
(4) If possible, adjust dialysis timing, frequency, or modality to better suit the individual's sleep schedule and lifestyle. In particular, nocturnal frequent home hemodialysis reduces RLS and sleep apnea, and improves sleep quality and social functioning.
(5) Nasal CPAP for OSA.
(6) Treat anemia with iron and recombinant erythropoeitin to improve RLS/PLMD.
(7) Review medications with special consideration given to the use of drugs known to worsen RLS (e.g., SSRI antidepressant and dopamine antagonists).
(8) Dopamine agonists (e.g., primipexole and ropinorole) are effective for RLS in those on dialysis.
(9) Clonazepam and gabapentin may reduce restlessness and nocturnal arousals.

Chronic pain and rheumatological disorders

Disruption of sleep is common in people with arthritic or muscular pain. Pain is a significant risk factor for insomnia, and the majority of people with pain suffer from difficulties initiating and maintaining sleep. Pain, sleep disturbance, and low mood are all believed to contribute to fatigue, a common complaint of those with rheumatic disorders.

Painful stimuli administered during the night disrupt sleep, resulting in decreased slow-wave sleep, increased light sleep, and increased sleep fragmentation. Not only does pain interfere with sleep, but disturbances of sleep also contribute to musculoskeletal pain and fatigue. Using noises to interrupt stage 4 slow-wave sleep in healthy sedentary controls results in complaints of unrefreshing sleep, aching, and fatigue, which are features of fibromyalgia and chronic fatigue syndrome. The disruption of slow-wave sleep produces a generalized hyperalgesic state, while a recovery night of slow-wave sleep raises pain tolerance thresholds. Interestingly, pain symptoms were not induced by the disruption of slow-wave sleep in a small group of physically fit long-distance runners, suggesting that physical fitness plays a significant preventive role in fibromyalgia. Indeed, cardiovascular fitness treatment programs improve tenderness, fatigue, and wellbeing.

In summary, there is an interrelationship of pain and sleep problems in rheumatic disorders. Therefore, sleep physiological disturbances should be considered in the assessment and management of these chronic painful illnesses.

Nonarticular musculoskeletal pain and sleep

Fibromyalgia syndrome

Fibromyalgia syndrome (FMS) affects 2% of the population, about 80% of whom are women. More than 90% of people with fibromyalgia describe disturbed sleep. Unrefreshing sleep is associated with the characteristic diffuse myalgia, multiple tender points in specific anatomic regions, and pervasive fatigue. The poorer the sleep, the greater the number of tender points. The FMS symptoms of myalgia, fatigue, unrefreshing sleep, and psychological distress are also found in individuals with other illness without defined disease pathology, such as chronic fatigue syndrome, irritable bowel syndrome, and temporomandibular joint disorder. Moreover, the symptoms and sleep disturbances that are features of FMS also occur in those with defined rheumatic disease pathology, such as osteoarthritis, rheumatoid arthritis, primary Sjögren's syndrome and systemic lupus erythematosis (SLE).

Sleep in FMS is light and unrefreshing with frequent arousals. Restless legs syndrome affects 20% of individuals. Sleep apnea may be the underlying problem in obese men and women diagnosed with FMS. The most common finding in FMS is the intrusion of an arousal pattern (alpha waves) in the EEG NREM sleep, termed the alpha-EEG sleep disorder. This sleep physiological disturbance and the ensuing unrefreshing sleep are associated with a daytime hyperalgesic state and pervasive fatigue.

The etiology of unrefreshing sleep, chronic pain, and fatigue in FMS is unknown. Various hypotheses have been proposed, including:

- Triggering noxious events such as psychological trauma, injuries, and febrile illnesses. Some people with FMS report no specific event that heralds the onset of symptoms.
- Alterations in the function of the sleeping/waking brain, such as increased nocturnal sympathetic activity and disturbances in the hypothalamic–cortical adrenal axis.
- A combination of environmental factors and genetic predisposition.

Treatment goals in FMS include the improvement of both pain and sleep, and the implementation of healthy behavioral changes with the aim of improving function and wellbeing. To date no specific treatment has been shown to have long-lasting remedial benefits. Most studies are for short-term periods and are beneficial for the self-ratings of sleep and pain symptoms in a small proportion of the individuals who complete the studies and who can tolerate the treatments. Various treatment options are outlined in Table 11.4, including behavioral, medical, and alternative therapies. The best evidence for the management of FMS supports aerobic exercise, cognitive behavioral therapy, and low-dose tricyclic (e.g., amitriptyline, cyclobenzaprine) or SNRI (e.g., duloxetine, milnacipran) medications.

Back pain

Acute low back pain is the most common of all musculoskeletal disorders in adults. Most back injuries resolve within 3 months. There is a direct relationship between the intensity of pain and the degree of sleep disturbance. For those with chronic pain, their pain symptoms may generalize, taking on the features of FMS with

Table 11.4. *Treatment strategies in fibromyalgia.*

Medications

  Good evidence for efficacy (> 1 RCT)

    Amitriptyline, 25–50 mg at bedtime (may lose effectiveness with time)

    Cyclobenzaprine, 10–30 mg at bedtime

    Tramadol or tramadol/acetominophen, 200–300 mg daily

  Modest evidence for efficacy (1 RCT)

    Dual-reuptake inhibitors (milnacipran, duloxetine)

    Serotonin reuptake inhibitors (fluoxetine, sertraline)

    Pregabalin

    Sodium oxybate

    Growth hormone (in GH-deficient individuals)

  No evidence for efficacy

    Opioids, nonsteroidal anti-inflammatory drugs, corticosteroids, benzodiazepenes and nonbenzodiazepene hypnotics, thyroid hormone, dehydroepiandrosterone, valacyclovir, melatonin

Nonmedicinal therapies

  Good evidence for efficacy (> 1 controlled trial)

    Cardiovascular exercise

    Cognitive behavioral therapy

    Patient education groups

  Modest evidence for efficacy

    Strength training

    Acupuncture

    Hypnotherapy

    Biofeedback

    Balneotherapy

    Massage therapy

  Weak or no evidence for efficacy

    Chiropractic therapy, ultrasound, electrotherapy, tender point injections, flexibility exercise

Adapted from Goldenberg DL, Burckhardt C, Crofford L. Management of fibromyalgia syndrome. *JAMA* 2004; **292**: 2388–95.

unrefreshing sleep, psychological distress, and functional disability. In such people, polysomnography shows high amounts of alpha-EEG NREM sleep.

See FMS for management strategies for improving chronic pain and nonrestorative sleep.

Articular rheumatological and connective tissue diseases and sleep

Osteoarthritis

Osteoarthritis (OA) is the most common arthritic disease affecting the older population. Pain in OA is associated with light and restless sleep. This poor-quality sleep is linked to depression and impaired physical functioning. Sleep disturbance can also aggravate pain: in one study of people with osteoarthritis of the fingers, disrupted sleep due to periodic limb movements predicted the presence of generalized morning pain and stiffness. The prevalence of sleep apnea in OA is unknown, but both are common conditions in obese individuals and thus considerable overlap can be expected. Because disordered sleep is known to promote pain, the presence of a primary sleep disorder should be considered in the assessment and management of people with OA who complain of generalized musculoskeletal pain and morning stiffness.

Management includes the following:

(1) Medications to control night pain:
   - Anti-inflammatory drugs improve both the quality of sleep and morning stiffness.
   - Narcotic pain medications improve hip and knee osteoarthritic pain and sleep problems. However, beware of the respiratory depressant effect of narcotics on sleep.
(2) Joint replacement surgery improves night pain, sleep, and quality of life.
(3) Treatment of comorbid primary sleep disorder, e.g., OSA, RLS.

Ankylosing spondylitis

People with ankylosing spondylitis (AS) commonly experience fatigue, which has been linked to pain, stiffness, sleep disturbance, and functional disability. More than 60% of those with AS complain of too little sleep as a result of night pain. In a small study, two out of seventeen fatigued individuals with AS had OSA diagnosed by night oximetry. Treatment with nasal CPAP improved their fatigue and daytime sleepiness.

Rheumatoid arthritis

Fatigue and poor-quality, nonrestorative sleep are significant sources of distress for people with rheumatoid arthritis (RA). Subjective disturbed sleep in RA is common and has been linked to pain, mood, and disease activity.

Polysomnography in RA shows high levels of alpha-EEG NREM sleep. Alpha-EEG sleep in RA has been associated with the severity of morning joint pain and stiffness and with the number of fibromyalgia tender points. Periodic limb movements with arousals are also frequently seen, both in adult and in juvenile RA.

Case reports and small studies have identified OSA in fatigued individuals with RA. In one small study, six out of ten non-obese people with RA and retrognathia were found to have OSA, and all were effectively treated with CPAP.

Risk factors for central and mixed sleep apnea in RA include:

- retrognathia secondary to temporomandibular joint destruction
- cervical spine disease leading to narrowing of upper airway
- cervical spine disease causing compression of the respiratory centers in the brainstem
- weight gain
- atrophy of pharyngeal muscles due to steroid medications.

Management of sleep disturbance in RA requires:

(1) Identifying and addressing underlying primary sleep disorders. Hypnotics improve subjective sleep quality but do not benefit disease activity, sleep architecture, or symptoms such as pain, fatigue, daytime function, or sleepiness.

(2) Treating the pain.

(3) Treating the disease.

(4) Anti-TNF biologic agents used to suppress RA disease activity improve sleep, possibly by suppression of the adverse effects on CNS functions of inflammatory-derived TNF-α. In individuals receiving their first infusion of infliximab, a drug that neutralizes TNF-α, there were no immediate changes in disease activity, but there was an improvement in overnight sleep physiology and daytime alertness.

Systemic lupus erythematosis

About 80% of people with systemic lupus erythematosis (SLE) experience fatigue during the course of their disease. Fatigue is a disabling symptom that is associated with significantly impaired function, psychological distress, and impaired quality of life, and is unresponsive to current treatments for SLE. Fibromyalgia is a common comorbidity, seen in up to 47% of individuals with SLE.

Fatigue in SLE has been most consistently associated with subjective poor-quality sleep and depressed mood. Two polysomnographic studies have identified that primary sleep disorders occur frequently in those with SLE: OSA occurs in 20–25%, PLMS in 25–35%, and there is a high prevalence of excessive daytime sleepiness. As in RA and FMS, alpha-EEG NREM sleep disturbance is common in fatigued individuals with SLE.

Management of fatigue in SLE includes identifying and treating underlying sleep disorders or mood disorders. As in fibromylagia, exercise programs have been shown to be effective in improving wellbeing.

Other medical illness and sleep

Circadian sleep/wakefulness is intricately linked to neuroendocrine and neuroimmune functions. Sleep deprivation or disturbance can cause significant perturbation of the endocrine and immune systems.

Insulin resistance

Disordered sleep and impaired glucose tolerance is of enormous public health concern because of its prevalence and association with cardiovascular disease. Experimental sleep restriction increases appetite and impairs glucose metabolism. Epidemiological studies have found an association between chronic sleep loss and both obesity and type 2 diabetes. Insulin resistance and OSA have also been linked, independent of body mass or waist circumference, although the direction of the association is uncertain. One hypothesis is that hypoxemia and sleep fragmentation may lead to altered glucose metabolism through changes in the HPA axis, autonomic nervous system, and increases in proinflammatory cytokines. There is conflicting evidence about whether CPAP can improve insulin sensitivity in these individuals, with the biggest improvements seen in non-obese people with sleep apnea.

Infectious disease

The immune system interacts with and is influenced by the sleep/wake system. Most people will have experienced an increase in sleepiness when ill with an infection.

Proinflammatory cytokines such as IL-1 and TNF-α are often somnogenic and can also alter the structure of sleep. Sleep deprivation weakens the immune system: for example, sleep deprived subjects have a blunted immune response to vaccination.

Table 11.5 summarizes some of the limited information available about a variety of endocrine, infectious, and other diseases that interact with sleep.

Drugs and sleep

People with chronic medical illness take multiple medications. Many medications disrupt sleep, increase daytime sleepiness, or exacerbate an underlying sleep disorder. A list of various medications and their effects on sleep is given in Table 11.6.

Circadian rhythms in human physiology should be considered when deciding about the timing and route of administration of medications. As already discussed, many disease symptoms and exacerbations follow a circadian pattern, e.g., asthma attacks in the early morning. The field of chronopharmacology assesses the timing, dosing, and delivery of medications to match the circadian rhythms of the target. This is complicated by circadian variations in pharmacokinetic parameters such as drug absorption and metabolism due to daily rhythms in gastric pH, gastro-intestinal motility, blood flow to the kidney, and biliary and liver function. The result is that a given dose of a given medication will have different kinetics if given in the evening instead of the morning. Circadian time must be considered as an important variable influencing a drug's pharmacokinetics and/or its beneficial or untoward effects.

"Chronokinetics" is especially important in oncology, where the aim is to limit side effects while enhancing the desired effects of a variety of toxic chemotherapeutic agents. Other examples include chronotherapeutics of asthma, hypertension, and dyslipidemia.

Conclusion

(1) When someone complains of sleep problems in association with a medical illness, it is important to make detailed clinical inquiries, including discussion with a bed partner, in order to determine whether a primary sleep disorder is complicating the diagnosis and management.

(2) Pay particular attention to loud snoring, apneas during sleep, nocturnal choking or gasping, restlessness, unexplained fatigue, and excessive daytime sleepiness.

(3) Nocturnal pain can be a significant source of sleep disruption and should be optimally managed.

(4) When a sleep disorder is suspected, overnight polysomnography is crucial to clarify the diagnosis and severity, and to facilitate management (Table 11.7).

(5) Chronotherapeutics is important for the proper determination of the timing and dose of administration of medications to optimize their benefit and minimize adverse effects.

Table 11.5. *Other medical illnesses and sleep.*

Disease	Sleep changes	Factors involved
HIV/AIDS	Insomnia	Psychosocial stressors
	Fragmented sleep	Depression and anxiety
	Daytime sleepiness	Pain
	Slow-wave sleep shifted to later	HIV or AIDS-related symptoms
	half of night in early disease stages	OSA secondary to lipodystrophy and
		lymphadenopathy
		Drugs (AZT and insomnia; Nevirapine/Efaviranez and vivid dreams)
Lyme disease	Fragmented sleep	Depression
	Unrefreshing sleep	Pain
		Fibromyalgia/chronic fatigue
		Lyme encephalopathy
Viral hepatitis	Fatigue	Pruritis
	Subjective poor-quality sleep	IFNα-related neuropsychiatric symptoms
		Psychosocial stressors
Cirrhosis	Daytime sleepiness	Subclinical hepatic encephalopathy
	OSA	Ascites
		Pruritis
Functional bowel syndromes	Subjective poor sleep quality	Depression
		Pain
		Autonomic dysregulation
Hypothyroidism	Unrefreshing sleep	Obesity
	OSA	Euthyroid sick syndrome can be secondary to OSA
	Daytime sleepiness	Thyroid hormone replacement improves OSA
	Fatigue	
Acromegaly	OSA	Macroglossia, increased pharyngeal soft tissue
	CSA	Craniofacial abnormalities
	Daytime sleepiness	

Table 11.5. (cont.)

Disease	Sleep changes	Factors involved
Cushing's disease	OSA	Growth hormone excess
	Daytime sleepiness	Visceral obesity
Polycystic ovary syndrome	OSA	Obesity
	Daytime sleepiness	Insulin resistance associated with OSA
		Increased androgens
Hypogonadism (male)	OSA	Testosterone replacement worsens OSA
		Treatment of OSA increases testosterone and improves libido
Menopause	Insomnia	Depression
	OSA	Vasomotor symptoms (hot flushes, sweats)
		Age, hormonal changes
		Weight gain
		HRT has been shown to improve subjective sleep quality and OSA
Cancer	Insomnia	Pain
	Restless legs	Depression, anxiety
	Daytime sleepiness	Chemotherapy
	OSA in head/neck cancer	Medications (steroids)
		Hormonal therapies (tamoxifen, androgen ablation) precipitate menopausal symptoms
Sickle cell disease	Fragmented sleep	Pain
	OSA	Obstructive adenotonsillar hypertrophy
		Nocturnal oxygen desaturations, risk for inducing sickle crisis or stroke

Table 11.6. *Medications and their effects on sleep.*

Drug class	Effect on sleep	Chronopharmacological considerations
Cardiovascular drugs		
Beta-blockers	Increased awakenings and wakefulness	Lipophilic drugs (i.e., propranolol) have higher rates of sleep disturbance, hydrophilic (i.e., atenolol) have lowest
	Daytime sleepiness due to disrupted sleep	Lowers diurnal blood pressure with less effect on nocturnal blood pressure
Calcium channel blockers	Abnormal dreams	Fewer side effects when dosed at bedtime
	Abnormal dreams	Better efficacy, circadian profile, and control of morning surge when chronotherapeutic preparations dosed at night
	Can worsen reflux	
ACE inhibitors	Risk of nocturnal hypotension in elderly	Ramipril dosed at bedtime in landmark HOPE trial
		ACE-I dosed at night can cause nocturnal hypotension
		Fewer side effects when dosed at bedtime
Angiotensin II receptor blockers	Unknown	Long-acting ARB can reduce morning surge
Statins	Well tolerated	Better lipid control when given at night
Amiodarone	Insomnia, abnormal dreams	Use minimum effective dose, give once daily in morning
Diuretics	Sleep disruption due to nocturia	Better tolerated when dosed early in day
Respiratory drugs		
Theophylline	Insomnia and sleep disruption	Structurally related to caffeine
	Can worsen reflux	SR theophylline dosed at 18:00 effective at treating nocturnal asthma
Corticosteroids (inhaled)	Well tolerated	Can increase evening dose to target nocturnal asthma
Corticosteroids (oral)	Insomnia, abnormal dreams	Single dose at 15:00 more effective than doses at 08:00 or 20:00 at improving nocturnal asthma with minimal adrenal suppression
Beta-agonists	Insomnia (oral formulations only)	Inhaled long-acting beta-agonists dosed at bedtime as effective as SR theophylline with less sleep disturbance

Table 11.6. (cont.)

Drug class	Effect on sleep	Chronopharmacological considerations
Leukotriene modifiers	Inhaled forms well tolerated	Improves subjective sleep in individuals with combination allergic rhinitis and asthma
Anticholinergics (inhaled)	Unknown	Tiotropium equally effective at improving nocturnal oxygen saturation when taken in the morning and the evening
	Well tolerated	Ipatropium at bedtime improves sleep in COPD
		Can be used as a bedtime medication in nocturnal asthma
Other drugs		
Fluoroquinolones	Insomnia	Ofloxacin has highest reported incidence of insomnia
Amantadine	Insomnia, abnormal dreams	
Bisphosphonates	Worsen reflux	Dose in AM, avoid recumbance
Thyroid hormone	Insomnia	Monitor for exogenous subclinical hyperthyroidism
Androgen hormone replacement	Worsens OSA	Bedtime testosterone patch application replicates normal circadian hormone rhythm
Estrogen hormone replacement	Improves OSA	
	Improves subjective sleep quality	
TCA, SSRI, lithium, neuroleptics	Sedation, daytime sleepiness	
	Worsen RLS	
Transdermal nicotine	Insomnia	
Caffeine-containing drugs	Insomnia	
Benzodiazepenes, barbiturates, narcotics	Sedation, daytime sleepiness	
	Insomnia in withdrawal	
	Depress respiratory drive	
	Exacerbate respiratory failure in COPD	
	Worsen OSA	

Table 11.7. *Indications for polysomnography in medical disorders.*

- Patients with congestive heart failure if they have nocturnal symptoms suggestive of sleep-disordered breathing (disturbed sleep, nocturnal dyspnea, snoring) or if they remain symptomatic despite optimal medical management (*standard*)
- Patients with coronary artery disease where there is suspicion of sleep apnea (*guideline*)
- Patients with history of stroke or transient ischemic attacks where there is suspicion of sleep apnea (*option*)
- Patients being evaluated for significant tachyarrhythmias or bradyarrhythmias where there is a suspicion that OSA or CSA is present (*guideline*)
- Patients with neuromuscular disorders and sleep related symptoms (*standard*)
- Patients with chronic lung disease if symptoms suggest a diagnosis of OSA or periodic limb movement sleep disorder (*standard*)
- In any patient when a diagnosis of OSA or periodic limb movement disorder is suspected (*standard*)

standard, high degree of clinical certainty; *guideline,* moderate degree of clinical certainty; *option,* uncertain clinical use. Based on : American Academy of Sleep Medicine. Practice parameters for the indications for polysomnography and related procedures. *Sleep* 2005; **28**: 499–521.

FURTHER READING

Celli BR, MacNee W, ATS/ERS Task Force. Standards for the diagnosis and treatment of patients with COPD: a summary of the ATS/ERS position paper. *Eur Respir J* 2004; **23**: 932–46.

DeVault KR, Castell DO. Updated guidelines for the diagnosis and treatment of gastroesophageal reflux disease. *Am J Gastroenterol* 2005; **100**: 190–200.

Goldenberg DL, Burckhardt C, Crofford L. Management of fibromyalgia syndrome. *JAMA* 2004; **292**: 2388–95.

Gula LJ, Krahn AD, Skanes AC, Yee R, Klein GJ. Clinical relevance of arrhythmias during sleep: guidance for clinicians. *Heart* 2004; **90**: 347–52.

Kryger MH, Roth T, Dement WC, eds. *Principles and Practice of Sleep Medicine,* 4th edn. Philadelphia, PA: Saunders, 2005.

Lemmer B. Relevance for chronopharmacology in practical medicine. *Semin Perinatol* 2000; **24**: 280–90.

Martin RJ, Banks-Schlegel S. Chronobiology of asthma. *Am J Respir Crit Care Med* 1998; **158**: 1002–7.

Parker KP. Sleep disturbances in dialysis patients. *Sleep Med Rev* 2003; **7**: 131–43.

12   Sleep and pediatrics

Roberta M. Leu and Carol L. Rosen

Introduction

Sleep disorders are common health issues in childhood that are serious and treatable, but that often go undetected. The National Sleep Foundation's *Sleep in America* poll in 2004 found that as many as 69% of parents believe their child has a sleep problem, but over half of doctors do not ask parents about their child's sleep, and only 10–14% of parents raise the issue with their child's doctor. Chronic sleep problems constitute one of the most common sources of parent concerns and have a major negative impact on child and family functioning. Sleep affects every aspect of a child's physical, emotional, cognitive, and social development. Sleep problems exacerbate nearly any medical, psychiatric, developmental, or psychosocial problem in childhood. The aims of this chapter are to help clinicians understand developmental changes in sleep patterns, screen for and identify common pediatric sleep disorders, know what tests and treatments to consider, and decide when to refer to a specialist.

Prevalence

Insufficient sleep is the most common sleep disorder in both adults and children, affecting 10% of children and 33% of teenagers, with excessive television viewing, 24/7 lifestyles and bedroom electronics contributing to its high prevalence. Insufficient sleep has also been shown to be a risk factor for obesity in multiple epidemiological studies of children and adults. Table 12.1 summarizes the prevalence of common sleep disorders in children.

Normal sleep in children

What is "enough" sleep?

While there are individual variations in both sleep needs and tolerance of sleep loss, the simple answer is "the amount of sleep that a child (or anyone) needs to feel well rested." Parents are good at recognizing when their child is "overtired"

Sleep Medicine, ed. Harold R. Smith, Cynthia L. Comella, and Birgit Högl. Published by Cambridge University Press. © Cambridge University Press 2008.

Table 12.1. *Prevalence of common sleep disorders in children.*

Insomnia: 10% teens (1/2 associated with a psychiatric diagnosis)
   Behaviorally based "insomnia" in younger children: 25%
Circadian sleep disorders (e.g., delayed sleep phase type): 7% of teens
Partial night wakings (parasomnias)
   Night terrors: 2–3%
   Sleepwalking: 5%
Rhythmic movement disorders (e.g., head banging, body rocking): 3–15%
   Bruxism: 14%
Restless legs syndrome: mild symptoms, 2%; moderate or severe symptoms, 0.5%
Obstructive sleep apnea: 2%
Narcolepsy: 0.5%

Table 12.2. *Reference values for sleep duration from infancy to adolescence.*

Age group	Hours of sleep
Newborn (0 to 2 mo)	16 to 20[a]
Infant (2 to 12 mo)	9 to 13 nighttime, 0.5 to 6 daytime
Toddler (12 mo to 3 yr)	10 to 13 nighttime, 0.5 to 4 daytime
Pre-school (3 to 5 yr)	10 to 13 nighttime, 0.7 to 3 daytime; daytime napping less common after age 5 yrs
School age (6 to 12 yr)[b]	8 to 11 nighttime; napping suggests insufficient sleep, a primary sleep disorder, or medication effect
Adolescent (13 to 18 yr)[c]	7 to 10 nighttime; napping may reappear, associated with insufficient sleep, a primary sleep disorder, or medication effect

Note:
[a]Total duration in 24 hours, includes daytime sleep
[b]At least 9 hours sleep is recommended by sleep professionals
[c]At least 8 hours sleep is recommended, 9 may be optimal

(whiny, cranky, moody, "hyper") in association with an acute sleep loss like a missed nap or late bedtime, but do not always associate these daytime symptoms with more chronic sleep loss. Total sleep duration decreases from an average of 14 ± 2 hours at 6 months of age to an average of 8 ± 1 hours at 16 years of age, with the greatest variability in infants and toddlers. Consolidation of nocturnal sleep occurs during the first 12 months after birth, with a decreasing trend of daytime sleep. Daytime napping typically disappears after age 5 years in monophasic sleep cultures. Table 12.2 summarizes normative data for sleep at different ages from a large population-based study. The sleep duration at the lowest percentile values begins to deviate from the recommendations of sleep professionals and sleep advocacy groups.

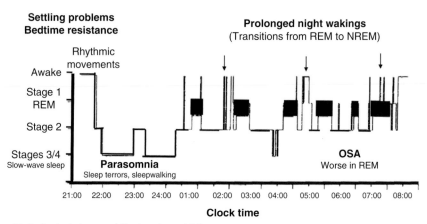

Fig. 12.1. Typical sleep architecture in a child.

Sleep architecture and clinical sleep disorders

The distribution of various sleep stages in a child across the night is shown in Fig. 12.1. A basic knowledge of sleep architecture and its developmental changes help to explain the etiology for many of the pediatric sleep disorders. Night wakings are most commonly experienced by infants and toddlers as prolongations of the normal nighttime arousals that occur at the end of each ultradian sleep cycle. The partial-arousal parasomnias (sleepwalking and sleep terrors) usually occur within 1–2 hours after sleep onset because that time period is when deep (stages 3 and 4), non-rapid eye movement (NREM), slow-wave sleep predominates. The increased prevalence of sleepwalking and sleep terrors in preschool-aged children is related to the relative increased proportion of slow-wave sleep in this age group. Factors that create rebound conditions for slow-wave sleep (sleep deprivation, withdrawal of medication that had suppressed slow-wave sleep) increase the likelihood of partial-arousal para-somnias. Conversely, nightmares are associated with rapid eye movement (REM) sleep. Obstructive sleep apnea (OSA) is most prominent in REM sleep, where the normal REM-related atonia exacerbates upper airway collapse in vulnerable airways.

Screening for sleep disorders

Pediatric sleep expert Dr. Judith Owens designed a simple five-item screening in-strument that uses the mnemonic "BEARS" to obtain sleep-related information and identify sleep problems in children aged 2–18 years in the primary care setting (Table 12.3). Tapping into multiple symptom domains of Bedtime and sleep-onset difficulties, Excessive sleepiness, Awakenings, Regular sleep/wake schedule, and Snoring/sleep-disordered breathing, this tool provides significantly more information about children's sleep than the use of a standard single question like "Does your child have any sleep problems?" Clinical problems such as excessive daytime sleepiness or suspected sleep apnea are likely to require additional diagnostic testing with poly-somnography, while atypical night wakings may require clinical or video EEG when paroxysmal disorders are suspected.

Table 12.3. *The "BEARS" algorithm for screening for sleep disorders in children.*

Symptom domain	Sleep or other primary disorders with sleep-related symptoms
Bedtime problems	Inadequate sleep hygiene, insomnia, restless legs syndrome, anxiety disorder
Excessive daytime sleepiness[a]	Hypersomnolence disorders (narcolepsy, idiopathic hypersomnia)
Awakenings during the night[b]	Parasomnia (sleep terrors, sleepwalking), nightmares, REM sleep behavior disorder, sleep-related epilepsy, insomnia, rhythmic movement disturbance, bruxism, anxiety or mood disorder
Regularity and duration of sleep	Circadian rhythm disorders, inadequate sleep hygiene, insufficient sleep
Snoring/Sleep apnea[c]	Obstructive sleep apnea, sleep-disordered breathing

Note:
[a]Nocturnal polysomnography is important to determine that no other sleep disorder is causing sleep fragmentation; daytime multiple sleep latency testing (MSLT) is important to document presence and severity of hypersomnolence and whether sleep-onset REM periods are associated with the daytime sleep episodes when hypersomnolence disorders such as narcolepsy and idiopathic hypersomnia are being considered
[b]Polysomnography with extended EEG montage and/or video EEG are likely to be needed to differentiate nocturnal epilepsy vs. parasomnia disorder vs. waking behaviors if clinical evaluation and EEG are insufficient to make a diagnosis
[c]Polysomnography used in confirming the presence and determining severity of the disorder

Healthy sleep habits

Sleep/wake schedules that give children the opportunity for sufficient sleep, positive bedtime routines at night, dark quiet sleep environments, and avoidance of "sleep stealers" like caffeinated beverages during the day are the lifestyle choices that help children develop healthy sleep habits. Parents should also be role models for their children, endorsing the importance of sleep. In contrast, inadequate sleep hygiene characterized by irregular sleep/wake schedules, irregular sleep locations (living room couch, parent's bed), family shift-work schedules or erratic parental sleep schedules, bedroom electronics (TVs, gaming devices) can be a pervasive way of life in some families. These lifestyle issues can be a major contributor to a child's trouble falling asleep, and to problematic night waking activities, and can result in chronic insufficient sleep with daytime dysfunction.

In trying to understand a child's sleeplessness or sleepiness, it is important to identify the child's usual bedtime, actual sleep onset time, wake time, and daytime napping for both weekdays and weekends. Having the parent describe a typical day in terms of the child's day care or school, meal times, and the details and locations of bedtime routines helps to put the child's sleep problems in a family context. Sleep deprivation in infants and toddlers may be the result of chronic early-morning awakenings by parents secondary to an early work start time. The lure of multimedia and the pressures of increased school work and extracurricular activities may place demands on a child's and teenager's time, preventing them from having adequate time to sleep at night. Regularizing the sleep/wake schedule to ensure adequate sleep time and optimizing the sleep environment to facilitate sleep can go a long way in solving insomnia-like sleep problems in children and teens.

Common sleep disorders in children

Figure 12.2 shows the most common sleep disorders in children and the age group(s) in which these disorders commonly present. The *International Classification of Sleep Disorders* (ICSD-2) has organized sleep disorders into six broad clinical categories: insomnia, sleep-disordered breathing, hypersomnia, circadian rhythm sleep disorders, parasomnias, and sleep-related movement disorders. In the remainder of this chapter, we describe the clinical presentation, basic evaluation, and management strategies for the most common sleep disorders in children in these categories.

- Insomnia: behavioral insomnia of childhood
- Sleep-disordered breathing: obstructive sleep apnea
- Hypersomnias: narcolepsy
- Circadian rhythm sleep disorders: delayed sleep phase type
- Parasomnias: sleep terrors, confusional arousals, sleepwalking
- Sleep-related movement disorders: restless legs syndrome/periodic limb movement disorder, rhythmic movement disorder

Insomnia

Behavioral insomnia of childhood

As the name suggests, children with this type of insomnia have difficulty falling asleep or maintaining sleep for behavioral reasons. Behavioral insomnia of childhood is

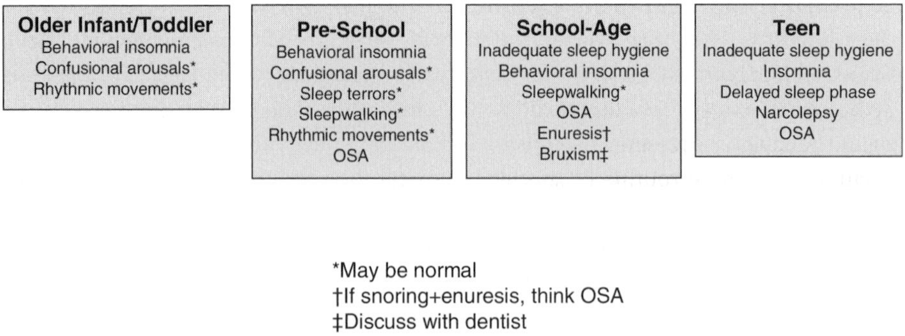

Older Infant/Toddler	Pre-School	School-Age	Teen
Behavioral insomnia	Behavioral insomnia	Inadequate sleep hygiene	Inadequate sleep hygiene
Confusional arousals*	Confusional arousals*	Behavioral insomnia	Insomnia
Rhythmic movements*	Sleep terrors*	Sleepwalking*	Delayed sleep phase
	Sleepwalking*	OSA	Narcolepsy
	Rhythmic movements*	Enuresis†	OSA
	OSA	Bruxism‡	

*May be normal
†If snoring+enuresis, think OSA
‡Discuss with dentist

Fig. 12.2. Developmental overview of common sleep problems by age group.

estimated to have a prevalence of 10–30% as it occurs in multiple age groups from infants to pre-school-aged children, while "special needs" children with complex medical or neurodevelopmental comorbidities experience even higher rates. Longitudinal data suggest that sleeping problems may persist over time, especially in young children.

This diagnosis has been divided into two subtypes: sleep-onset association type and limit-setting type. Although the sleep-onset association type predominates in infants and the limit-setting disorder type is more prevalent in toddlers and pre-school-aged children, many children have features of both subtypes. Behavioral insomnia of childhood is diagnosed by clinical history.

Sleep-onset association type. Even as infants, children begin to associate certain conditions with sleep, and will need these conditions to be present in order to fall asleep. Positive sleep associations are conditions that the child can provide him/herself such as thumb sucking. On the other hand, negative sleep associations are conditions that require parental intervention such as a nighttime feeding or rocking. Children with sleep-onset association behavioral insomnia of childhood have negative sleep-onset associations. They are thereby unable to soothe themselves to sleep, whether for the initiation of sleep or after a nighttime arousal. Parents will describe the child as having difficulty falling asleep unless a particular condition is present. If the condition is present, sleep is easily initiated and the child has sleep of normal duration and quality.

Limit-setting type. Children with limit-setting behavioral insomnia of childhood have not had consistent limits set regarding their bedtime. Onset of this sleep disorder usually begins in the toddler years as the child gains individual mobility and language with which the child can test his/her limits. Manifestations of this disorder include difficulty initiating sleep at the appropriate time by stalling or refusing to go to bed. Children will stall by asking to complete an activity "just one more time" before going to bed or with "curtain calls" (i.e., requests made after the lights are out, such as another kiss or hug). The child tends to exhibit behaviors or make requests for things that they know the parent will respond to.

Primary prevention of this sleep disorder can be accomplished with sleep-based anticipatory guidance such as placing the infant to sleep while drowsy but awake, eliminating night feedings after 6 months of age, introducing a transitional object, establishing a "short and sweet" positive bedtime routine, and consistent reinforcement of bedtime. Once the sleep disorder has been established, it can be treated with standard behavioral techniques including standard and graduated extinction strategies. Behavioral strategies begin with the enforcement of good sleep hygiene. This includes a bedtime routine of soothing activities and an age- and time-appropriate napping schedule. As with any type of behavioral modification, children respond best to positive reinforcement for appropriate behaviors. Children with intractable sleep-onset and night-waking difficulties unresponsive to simple interventions, especially those with underlying neuropsychiatric comorbidities or medical conditions, may benefit from referral to a sleep and/or mental health specialist.

Other disturbances that can present as insomnia

Nighttime fears

The development of a child's imagination may be accompanied by the development of nighttime fears. These fears are usually developmentally appropriate with pre-schoolers being frightened of imaginary creatures in the dark while older children may have a fear of being hurt by a burglar. Onset of these fears usually begins around 3 years of age and tends to disappear by age 6, although a resurgence of fears in school-aged girls may occur, particularly in those who have anxiety issues. Nighttime fears may be managed by parental reassurance of safety to the child; however, parents should be advised to limit their interventions at night so that the child does not begin using the complaint of a nighttime fear as a means of bedtime resistance. Avoiding multimedia with frightening connotations, and giving children an object that relays a sense of safety, can help. Children with recurrent disruptive nightmares should be referred to a mental health professional and evaluated for other conditions including anxiety disorders, post traumatic stress disorder (PTSD), and possibly child abuse.

Medications for insomnia in children

Pediatric insomnia has been defined as "repeated difficulty with sleep initiation, duration, consolidation, or quality that occurs despite age-appropriate time and opportunity for sleep and results in daytime functional impairment for the child and/or family". Children with attention-deficit/hyperactivity disorder (ADHD) and those with pervasive developmental disorders/autism spectrum disorder are special populations of children with an increased prevalence of problem insomnia who may benefit from pharmacotherapy. While there is a need for pharmacologic management of pediatric insomnia, the widespread use of hypnotic and psychotropic medications for sleep problems in children in the absence of safety and efficacy data indicates a knowledge gap about the best pharmacologic practices for management of pediatric insomnia. Before appropriate pharmacologic management guidelines can be developed, rigorous, large-scale clinical trials of pediatric insomnia treatment are vitally needed to provide information to the clinician on the safety and efficacy of prescription and over-the-counter agents for the management of pediatric insomnia.

Sleep-disordered breathing

Obstructive sleep apnea

Obstructive sleep apnea (OSA) is a common health problem, affecting 2% of children. It is characterized by repetitive episodes of upper airway obstruction during sleep, causing intermittent hypoxemia and hypercapnia, and sleep disruption. Habitual snoring, the most common symptom of OSA, is seen in 10% of children, but not all of these children have clinically significant OSA requiring treatment. OSA peaks in 2–8-year-olds, paralleling the rapid growth of the tonsils and adenoids in relation to the oropharynx. On the other hand, the degree of tonsillar and adenoidal hypertrophy does not have a predictable linear relationship with the severity of OSA. Risk factors include African-American descent, obesity, prematurity, large adenoids and tonsils, craniofacial abnormalities involving midface hypoplasia and micrognathia, nasal allergies, lower airway tract inflammation, neuromuscular disease causing decreased upper airway tone (e.g., cerebral palsy and muscular dystrophy), genetic or craniofacial syndromes associated with small airways (e.g., Down syndrome), neuromuscular problems associated with reduced upper airway tone and sickle cell disease. Unlike adults, there is no sex predilection in prepubertal children. In teenagers, OSA is also associated with obesity, similar to adults.

Clinical signs of OSA include snoring, difficulty breathing (tachypnea, paradoxical breathing, retractions, gasping, and choking), and witnessed apnea (respiratory efforts without airflow which terminate with a gasp or choke). Diaphoresis can be an indication of hypercapnia or hypoxia. Daytime symptoms can include mouth breathing and neurobehavioral problems with attention, behavior, learning, and mood. Daytime sleepiness is not as common in children as in adults because sleep architecture is generally well preserved. Severe OSA can cause impaired growth with failure to thrive in very young children, especially in the presence of craniofacial or other comorbidities. Very severe, untreated OSA can cause pulmonary hypertension, cor pulmonale, diastolic hypertension, and ventricular hypertrophy and dysfunction. Clinical evaluation of a child can be insufficient for diagnosing OSA because of low sensitivity and specificity for predicting OSA in children. Overnight polysomnography can help detect the presence and severity of suspected OSA.

Intranasal corticosteroid sprays can improve nasal obstruction and decrease adenoidal hypertrophy. Weight management should be a long-term goal for an obese child. However, adenotonsillectomy is generally considered the first-line treatment for childhood OSA, and results in "cure" or improvement in 75–100% of children. Continuous positive airway pressure (CPAP) is a second line of therapy for children who have previously undergone adenotonsillectomy or who are not surgical candidates. CPAP therapy requires an overnight sleep study to titrate and determine the optimal pressure. Application in children can be challenging, especially when the children have other medical or developmental comorbidities. CPAP cases should be referred to a specialist who has experience using this therapy in children. This specialist can evaluate and prepare the child and family prior to scheduling an overnight titration study. Tracheostomy should be considered in the most severe OSA cases unresponsive to adenotonsillectomy and CPAP when life-threatening complications such as pulmonary hypertension or heart failure are present. Children with craniofacial anomalies and OSA must be seen in a multidisciplinary craniofacial center with expertise in facial reconstruction.

Hypersomnias: excessive somnolence disorders

Narcolepsy

Narcolepsy is a hypersomnolence disorder characterized by constant sleepiness and a tendency to fall asleep at inappropriate times. Onset of narcolepsy typically occurs between 15 and 25 years of age with a prevalence rate of 2 per 1000. The four most common symptoms of narcolepsy are:

(1) excessive daytime sleepiness
(2) cataplexy (sudden loss of muscle tone triggered by a strong emotion, most commonly laughter)
(3) sleep paralysis (inability to move upon waking)
(4) hallucinations (vivid visual or auditory experiences that occur with sleep onset, during naps, or upon waking).

A fifth feature is fragmented sleep.

Children with narcolepsy are sleepy no matter how much sleep they get, and present with the reappearance of daytime napping and falling asleep on school days as well as on the weekends. The hypersomnolence is more prominent during monotonous activities, and naps are highly irresistible but refreshing. Children can experience declining academic performance and may be misdiagnosed with attention-deficit disorder. Cataplexy is a very specific symptom of narcolepsy, found in approximately 80% of those with narcolepsy, but it may not appear until years after the onset of hypersomnolence. The loss of tone may involve postural muscles, resulting in a fall to the ground or just a mild buckling of the knees, and typically lasts less than 2 minutes. It can be misdiagnosed as a conversion reaction. Other muscle groups may be involved – jaw, neck, eyelids, or tongue and speech. Hypnagogic hallucinations and sleep paralysis are less specific than cataplexy because they occasionally occur in the general population, especially with sleep deprivation.

Low levels of hypocretin 1 in the spinal fluid are highly sensitive and specific for narcolepsy with cataplexy, but testing is not readily available. Hypocretin is a neurotransmitter that is involved in CNS arousal mechanisms. Genetic influences are also present, as evidenced by the human leukocyte antigen DQB1*0602 allele in 85–93% of people who have narcolepsy with cataplexy. Presence of this allele is highly sensitive but not specific for narcolepsy with cataplexy, since 20% of the population carry this allele.

The diagnosis is clinical, but specialized testing in a sleep laboratory and consultation with a sleep medicine specialist are recommended. Multiple sleep latency testing (MSLT), which consists of five opportunities to try to fall asleep during the day, measures the propensity to fall asleep and how the individual enters sleep. A mean sleep latency of less than 8 minutes and two sleep-onset REM periods during multiple sleep latency testing are highly suggestive of the diagnosis. However, MSLT findings in prepubertal children can be more variable. An overnight polysomnogram (PSG) is performed the night before the MSLT to rule out other sleep disorders that may disrupt sleep and cause hypersomnolence. Secondary narcolepsy can be seen in children who have had CNS tumors, surgery, radiation, or trauma. The differential diagnosis includes other causes of hypersomnolence: idiopathic hypersomnia, hypersomnia due to other medical disorders, insufficient sleep, medication effects, malingering, and depression.

Prescription medications which promote wakefulness (methylphenidate, mixed amphetamine salts, and modafinil) are needed to control the sleepiness. "One size does not fit all," so effort is needed to identify the optimal medication class and dose for an individual child. Caffeine is ineffective. Long-acting preparations may be taken prior to the start of the school day. Severe cataplexy may require the administration of a REM-suppressant class of medication (for example, an alerting selective serotonin reuptake inhibitor or a tricyclic antidepressant). Sodium oxybate, a highly regulated formulation of gamma-hydroxybutyrate, an endogenous neurotransmitter and metabolite of gamma-aminobutyric acid, is a newer medication that reduces daytime cataplexy, consolidates fragmented sleep, and improves daytime sleepiness, but pediatric experience is limited. In addition to educating the child about his or her condition, family, friends, and teachers should be educated as well. Individuals with narcolepsy are often misperceived as being lazy and inattentive. They have been misdiagnosed with medical, psychiatric, and behavioral disorders from syncope to schizophrenia and conversion disorder. Healthy sleep habits and working with the school to provide scheduled naps of at least 30 minutes' duration can help decrease somnolence, improve reaction times, and minimize the amount of stimulant medication that a child needs. Particularly in adolescents, counseling regarding careers (avoidance of shift work and monotonous or repetitive work) and determination of fitness for driving must be addressed.

Circadian rhythm disorders

Multiple physiologic processes of our bodies, including our sleep/wake cycle, follow circadian rhythms with a periodicity of roughly 24 hours. Sleep disorders may arise when a person's circadian rhythm and thus sleep/wake cycle falls out of synch with environmental cues.

Delayed sleep phase type

In delayed sleep phase type (DSPT), a person's sleep/wake cycle is shifted forward in time, making him or her feel sleepy later at night and arise later in the day compared to conventional norms. Attempts to sleep at a conventionally normal time result in complaints of insomnia, and efforts to wake up at an appropriate time may feel nearly impossible. On the other hand, attempts to fall asleep or arise at one's own preferred times are effortless. DSPT most commonly occurs in teenagers and young adults. It is estimated to affect 10% of teens. After puberty, adolescents experience a phase delay in their circadian rhythm that makes them feel sleepy 2–3 hours later than usual. The combination of this physiologic delay with multiple academic and social pressures enforcing an irregular sleep schedule places them at risk of developing DSPT. Other predisposing factors include having an evening chronotype, and a positive family history. Presenting complaints are frequently insomnia and/or excessive daytime sleepiness. The differential diagnosis includes normal sleep patterns, school avoidance, familial/social dysfunction, and primary and secondary insomnias. Diagnosis requires that other causes for the sleep problem are ruled out, that the history is consistent with a shift in the person's sleep and wake times later than what they would conventionally like to do, that this sleep delay is consistently documented in a 1–2-week sleep diary or by actigraphy, and that if these individuals are allowed to sleep and awaken on their own accord, they have no difficulty doing so.

Management of DSPT requires motivation and cooperation. It begins with educating both the adolescent and the parent(s) about the normal physiologic phase delay in sleep that occurs after puberty. Good sleep hygiene should be enforced and should include consistent sleep/wake times throughout the entire week including weekends. Activities that may delay falling asleep at night should be eliminated or minimized. Examples include late-day napping, drinking caffeinated beverages, exercising at night, and the use of multimedia devices close to bedtime. Minimizing bright light at night but maximizing it in the morning may help. The goal of these behavioral modifications is to shift the teen's sleep/wake schedule back to a time that is conventionally appropriate. Other specific therapies for DSPT include bright-light therapy, chronotherapy (delaying the teen's bedtime in two- or three-hour increments every night until his/her body clock has shifted around the clock), then strict maintenance of the new schedule once a more appropriate schedule has been achieved, and oral melatonin as a "phase shifter": all have potential therapeutic roles. A motivated teen, a supportive family, and a physician who has either adolescent or sleep medicine expertise can usually manage this problem. However, referral to a mental health specialist may be needed when other factors such as oppositional defiant disorder, mood disorder, or possible substance abuse may be present.

Parasomnias

NREM parasomnias
Sleep terrors, confusional arousals, and sleepwalking are all disorders of arousal that arise from NREM sleep, with considerable clinical overlap. NREM parasomnias are more common in children than in adults because children spend more time in the deeper stages of NREM sleep known as slow-wave sleep. These disorders usually occur within 1–2 hours after sleep onset, coincide with the transition from the first period of slow-wave sleep, and usually occur only once a night. If they do recur, their periodicity matches ultradian sleep cycles. Other common features include difficult arousal, amnesia for the event, and a range of automatic behavior and autonomic arousals. Any conditions that lead to sleep fragmentation or deprivation or that increase slow-wave sleep (e.g., increased body temperature) can predispose a child to parasomnias. Studies have also linked parasomnias with sleep-disordered breathing. Because sleep-disordered breathing, e.g., upper airway resistance syndrome, may occur unnoticed by the parents, a formal evaluation is appropriate. Genetics are important, with 60% of those affected reporting a first-degree relative who has parasomnias. In children, insufficient sleep is an important trigger; correcting sleep debt alone by increasing total sleep time may be a sufficient intervention.

Sleepwalking is common between the ages of 3 and 13 years, occurring in up to 17% of children, with most episodes resolving after age 10 years. Sleepwalking consists of complex movements that are normally made in the awake state. Children have been found crawling in bed, sitting up, and standing or sleeping in a different part of the house or even outside of the house. Complicated pathways may be achieved if the route is familiar to them. The child appears to be awake, but is not very responsive to his or her surroundings. Others may be agitated during an episode. Usually, episodes last 5–15 minutes. The morbidity associated with sleepwalking is typically a result of injury in this unresponsive state.

Confusional arousals primarily affect infants and toddlers, and tend to resolve by age 5 years. They include movements, usually with vocalization, including uncontrollable crying in infants. Episodes last 5–15 minutes and begin with some movement, moaning, or utterances that progress into thrashing, yelling, and inconsolable crying. The child may appear to be awake, but is unresponsive to his or her environment, including parents. Efforts to comfort the child are met with resistance, and exacerbate the episode by increasing agitation and prolonging it. Episodes typically end with the child spontaneously settling into sleep.

Sleep terrors are less common, affecting 3% of children, but are more extreme and disturbing for parents. A loud scream may initiate the event. The child will appear tremulous and diaphoretic, with an expression of extreme terror on his or her face. The child may flee from the bed and yell incoherently. The child appears alert, but is not responsive to those around him or her. Attempts at waking or comforting the child are met with increased agitation. After a few minutes, the episode suddenly stops and the child falls abruptly back to sleep, typically without recall of the event in the morning. Again, these are usually brief, lasting 5–15 minutes. If any recollection of the event is present, it is usually fragmented. Onset is usually between 2 and 4 years of age, with a peak at 5–7 years and spontaneous resolution usually by adolescence. The differential diagnosis for the NREM parasomnias includes nightmares, seizures, nocturnal panic attacks, cluster headaches, and PTSD.

Evaluation of parasomnias requires special emphasis on a detailed description of the nocturnal episodes, including the following: timing, presence of stereotypic movements, odd postures or rhythmic behaviors, response to intervention, recall of the event, daytime occurrences, and enuresis. Overnight polysomnography becomes part of the evaluation when (1) there are concerns about an underlying sleep disorder like OSA, (2) atypical features (i.e., repetitive, stereotypic behaviors, odd posturing, and timing associated with transition to sleep) are suggestive of a seizure disorder, or (3) the episode has resulted in a serious injury. When nocturnal seizures are suspected, the evaluation should include a baseline clinical EEG and consultation with a neurologist.

The management of NREM parasomnias includes parent education as to the benign nature of these phenomena and the importance of adequate sleep. Most parasomnias resolve spontaneously in adolescence. Modifiable triggers such as hot baths and late-night exercise should be avoided, and comorbid sleep disorders that fragment sleep such as OSA should be treated in children who are prone to problem parasomnias. Certain medications such as stimulants, antihistamines, neuroleptics, and sedative-hypnotics are also associated with inducing sleep terrors. Parents should avoid intervening with the episode since their actions can exacerbate the incident, but they should protect the child from injury. For children who have nightly, predictable episodes, up to one month of scheduled awakenings 15–30 minutes before a sleep terror normally occurs may abort the episodes. This technique has had variable success. Children who sleepwalk need to have a safe sleep environment that minimizes opportunities for injury or unsafe exit from the house. Pharmacotherapy is available; however, caution is advised in using medications for what is typically a self-limited problem. Extreme cases with disruption to the family or the child's sleep, cases that risk injury to the child or others, and cases that do not resolve in adolescence should be referred to a sleep specialist. If other comorbid sleep, medical, or psychiatric disorders are ruled out, these children may benefit from medications that suppress slow-wave sleep. Clonazepam is the most widely used medication in the treatment of these disorders, but good controlled studies are lacking.

Other parasomnias

Nightmares

Nightmares are frightening, REM-related phenomena that primarily manifest in the last half or third of the night. In contrast to NREM parasomnias, nightmares usually result in the child fully awakening. Once awake, the child is oriented and responsive to the environment. The child's behavior is typified by emotional arousal from being upset by the dream, rather than the fight-or-flight autonomic response that occurs in sleep terrors. The child remembers the dream and, depending on his or her developmental level, is able to tell the dream with a story-line sequence. The child can be comforted, but falling back to sleep tends to take some time. As with other parasomnias, stress, sleep deprivation, and anxiety can lead to nightmares. Other precipitating factors include traumatic events and medications that affect REM sleep, including amphetamines, sedative-hypnotics, dopamine agonists, beta-blockers, montelukast, erythromycin, and nonsteroidal anti-inflammatory medications. Withdrawal of a REM-suppressant medication such as clonidine can also trigger nightmares or vivid dreams as part of a "REM rebound" phenomenon.

Nightmares are diagnosed clinically and should be differentiated from sleep terrors, confusional arousals, an anxiety disorder, and PTSD. Management begins with parental reassurance and elimination of any drugs that may be triggering nightmares. Encourage good sleep hygiene and discourage frightening television shows, movies, and games prior to bedtime. Reading bedtime stories in which a child overcomes a fear may be useful. Children may be taught relaxation techniques to help them fall asleep. A child with severe, persistent nightmares may have PTSD and should be referred to a mental health specialist.

Sleep-related movement disorders

Restless legs syndrome

Restless legs syndrome (RLS) is a sensorimotor disorder that is very common in adults (prevalence estimate 10%), but increasingly recognized in children, with an estimated prevalence of 0.5–2%. RLS is diagnosed clinically based on the following four criteria:
- an urge to move the legs
- urge is initiated or exacerbated with rest

- moving the extremity results in symptom resolution
- symptom onset begins in the evening (although as the disease worsens, symptoms may begin earlier in the day).

For a child to be diagnosed with RLS, he or she must meet all four adult criteria and the child (as opposed to the parent) must be able to describe the sensation felt in the legs. Common descriptions from children are "oowies, boo-boos, tickle, bugs, spiders, ants, want to run, a lot of energy in my legs." A history of periodic limb movement disorder or a family history of RLS strengthens the diagnosis of RLS. It is possible that nocturnal symptoms previously attributed to "growing pains" may actually represent the onset of RLS in children. Causes of RLS include genetic predisposition, underactivity of dopamine, iron deficiency, and renal disease. Low iron levels have been found in the substantia nigra and CSF of adults with RLS. Of note, iron is necessary for dopaminergic function.

Referral to a specialist is recommended for evaluation and management. An iron profile should be done, because iron levels in the low or low-normal range can cause RLS even if there is no concomitant anemia. Since ferritin is an acute-phase reactant, it should not be checked when the child is acutely ill. A PSG may be done to rule out other sleep disorders. Management of RLS begins with good sleep hygiene, which may result in symptom resolution. A serum ferritin level below 35 µg/L should be treated with the same age-appropriate dose of iron that is given for iron-deficiency anemia. Advice should be given to take vitamin C, which helps the body absorb the iron. Conversely, food, tea, and calcium can decrease iron absorption. Once serum ferritin levels lie in the 35–50 µg/L range, oral iron therapy can be stopped and replaced with a multivitamin that contains iron. Dopaminergic agents are the mainstay of therapy in adults, but are not well studied in children and should be used with caution. Other medications used to treat RLS include clonidine, short-acting benzodiazepines, and gabapentin. These medications should also be used with caution and with consideration of their side-effect profiles.

Sleep-related rhythmic movement disorder

Sleep-related rhythmic movement disorder (RMD) is characterized by stereotyped movements of any part of the body at a frequency of 0.5–2 Hz (or 30–120 times a minute). These episodes include body rocking and head banging. Movements usually occur during transitions between sleep and wakefulness and last roughly 15 minutes. As many as two-thirds of healthy normal infants, more commonly male, have RMD. A majority outgrow it by age 5 years. RMD has been associated with mental retardation, ADHD, obsessive–compulsive disorder, and autism. Proposed causes include sensory deprivation, abuse, and self-soothing from vestibular stimulation. The differential diagnosis for RMD includes hypnagogic foot tremor, stereotypic movement disorder, akathisia, RLS, autoerotic behavior, epilepsy, tic disorder, autism, and pervasive developmental disorder. Neurodevelopmental, psychiatric, and social pathology should be ruled out. Parents of neurodevelopmentally normal children can be reassured that RMD is a normal and common phenomenon that the child will outgrow. Most children do not have brain injury from head banging, but for some children the movements can be violent. These children may benefit from a helmet or bed padding. Treatment methods include kinesthetic stimulation (i.e., rocking before bedtime), hypnosis, behavioral modifications, benzodiazepines, antihistamines, and tricyclic antidepressants, but success with these treatment modalities has been inconsistent. Children with neurodevelopmental, psychiatric, or social pathology should be referred to the appropriate subspecialist.

Summary

Pediatric sleep problems are common, underdiagnosed, and treatable. Because of the impact of sleep on children's physical, psychological, academic, and overall functioning, the impact of increased recognition, evaluation, and management of pediatric sleep disorders will likely have a significant positive impact on the general health and wellbeing of children. Since children referred for sleep disorders frequently have other comorbid medical, neuropsychiatric, or behavioral comorbidities, a multi-disciplinary approach to clinical assessment and coordination of care at the specialty level is often needed.

REFERENCES

American Academy of Pediatrics. Clinical practice guideline: diagnosis and management of childhood obstructive sleep apnea syndrome. *Pediatrics* 2002; **109**: 704–12.

American Academy of Sleep Medicine. *The International Classification of Sleep Disorders: Diagnostic and Coding Manual*, 2nd edn (ICSD-2). Westchester, IL: American Academy of Sleep Medicine, 2005.

Dauvilliers Y, Baumann CR, Carlander B, *et al.* CSF hypocretin-1 levels in narcolepsy, Kleine–Levin syndrome, and other hypersomnias and neurological conditions. *J Neurol Neurosurg Psychiatry* 2003; **74**: 1667–73.

Hoban TF. Rhythmic movement disorder in children. *CNS Spectr* 2003; **8**: 135–8.

Iglowstein I, Jenni OG, Molinari L, *et al.* Sleep duration from infancy to adolescence: reference values and generational trends. *Pediatrics* 2003; **111**: 302–7.

Johnson EO, Roth T, Schultz L, *et al.* Epidemiology of DSM-IV insomnia in adolescence: lifetime prevalence, chronicity, and an emergent gender difference. *Pediatrics* 2006; **117**: e247–56.

Kotagal S, Pianosi P. Sleep disorders in children and adolescents. *BMJ* 2006; **332**: 828–32.

Laberge L, Tremblay RE, Vitaro F, *et al.* Development of parasomnias from childhood to early adolescence. *Pediatrics* 2000; **106**: 67–74.

Mindell JA, Owens JA. *A Clinical Guide to Pediatric Sleep: Diagnosis and Management of Sleep Problems*. Philadelphia, PA: Lippincott Williams & Wilkins, 2003.

Mindell JA, Kuhn B, Lewin DS, *et al.* Behavioral treatment of bedtime problems and night wakings in infants and young children. *Sleep* 2006; **29**: 1263–76.

Mindell JA, Emslie G, Blumer J, *et al.* Pharmacologic management of insomnia in children and adolescents: consensus statement. *Pediatrics* 2006; **117**: e1223–32.

Moore M, Allison D, Rosen CL. A review of pediatric nonrespiratory sleep disorders. *Chest* 2006; **130**: 1252–62.

National Sleep Foundation. *Adolescent Sleep Needs and Patterns: Research Report and Resource Guide*. Washington, DC: National Sleep Foundation, 2000. www.sleepfoundation.org.

National Sleep Foundation. *Sleep in America Polls.* Washington, DC: National Sleep Foundation, 2004–07. www.sleepfoundation.org.

Owens JA, Rosen CL, Mindell JA. Medication use in the treatment of pediatric insomnia: results of a survey of community-based pediatricians. *Pediatrics* 2003; **111**: e628–35.

Owens J, Dalzell V. Use of the "BEARS" sleep screening tool in a pediatric residents' continuity clinic: a pilot study. *Sleep Med* 2005; **6**: 63–9.

Owens J, Mindell J. *Take Charge of Your Child's Sleep.* New York, NY: Marlow, 2005.

Picchietti D, Allen R, Walters A, *et al.* Restless legs syndrome: prevalence and impact in children and adolescents: the PEDS REST study. *Sleep* 2006; **29** (abstract supplement): A70.

Schechter MS. Technical report: diagnosis and management of childhood obstructive sleep apnea syndrome. *Pediatrics* 2002; **109**: e69.

Sheldon SH, Ferber R, Kryger MH, Dahl RE, *eds. Principles and Practice of Pediatric Sleep Medicine.* Philadelphia, PA: Saunders, 2005.

Wills L, Garcia J. Parasomnias: epidemiology and management. *CNS Drugs* 2002; **16**: 803–10.

13　Sleep and geriatrics

Marcel Hungs

Aging and its impact on sleep

While physiological sleep needs and patterns change throughout life, sleep disorders are not part of the normal aging process. As more is learned about the relationship of sleep to quality of life and conditions such as memory impairment and cardiovascular problems, it is the responsibility of healthcare providers to address sleep and its disturbances in the care of older individuals. The description of "older" is arbitrary, but it is clear that as persons age, the sleep problems they experience are different from those experienced by the younger adult population. One widely accepted paradigm defines older people to be 65 years or over. Estimates project that by 2050, 85 million Americans will be over 65. Many European countries project that at least 10% of their population will be aged 80 years or over by 2050.

The analysis of age-related changes in sleep requires the accumulation of data on a healthy population over 65 years of age. However, increased age raises the risk of cardiovascular, metabolic, cognitive, psychiatric, musculoskeletal, renal, hepatic, and hematological conditions. Therefore, it might be difficult to study a group of "healthy" individuals over 65 years of age, as it is largely the advances in medical knowledge, and the diagnostic and treatment techniques of medical conditions, that allow these individuals to grow old. The subjective experience and the physiology of sleep, as well as its electrophysiological correlates, change with age.

Subjective sleep perception in the elderly

The daily circadian rhythm and homeostatic balance of sleep and alertness are the main factors controlling the physiological need for sleep. Sleep-related symptoms are reported more frequently with increasing age. Approximately 50% of people 50 years and older suffer from lack of adequate sleep, and 46% of people 50 years and older sleep less than 7 hours each night. Eight percent find sleep never to be restful for them. Subjective sleep quality is reduced with increasing age. Sleep initiation tends to be more difficult as people age. Although most seniors actually get approximately the same amount of total sleep time they did as a younger person, a reduced amount of *night* sleep is observed in the healthy non-complaining older adults. Elderly individuals notice frequent nocturnal awakenings and spend more time

Sleep Medicine, ed. Harold R. Smith, Cynthia L. Comella, and Birgit Högl. Published by Cambridge University Press. © Cambridge University Press 2008.

in bed awake. Changes in circadian rhythm result in many older people both going to bed and waking up earlier. Frequency and duration of daytime naps can lead to a reversal of the sleep/wake cycle. Screening tools, such as the Epworth Sleepiness Scale, assess daytime sleepiness. The practitioner should be aware that screening tools might not accurately reflect the presence of sleepiness in the elderly, as items on the scales may not properly reflect daytime activities of an older person. A more objective assessment of daytime sleepiness is the multiple sleep latency test, a test managed in a sleep laboratory, which measures the propensity of a subject to fall asleep during four to five 20-minute periods throughout the day.

Physiological changes affecting sleep in the elderly

While the impact of physiological aging on the sleep process is not yet well understood, aging can impact all aspects of body function. Structural decline in the elderly, including reduced brain mass and numbers of neurons, might lead to functional brain loss. Such a structural decline has special significance in the hypothalamic suprachiasmatic nucleus, resulting in impaired melatonin response and altered circadian rhythm. Age-related decline in cerebral blood flow predisposes the brain to compromised blood supply during sleep. A decrease in slow-wave sleep leads to a reduction in growth hormone levels. As ovarian function declines and blood estradiol levels drop, menopausal and postmenopausal women may experience insomnia and nonrestorative night sleep.

Electrophysiological features in the elderly

Most electroencephalographic recordings in the elderly are similar to recordings of younger individuals, with 10 Hz average alpha rhythm. Some studies observe a mild to moderate slowing of the alpha rhythm with diffuse or focal slowing, reduced alpha blockade and photostimulation. Prominent focal slowing should raise the suspicion of a focal pathology in the brain.

Normal sleep architecture includes non-rapid eye movement (NREM) with light sleep (stages 1 and 2) and deep sleep (stages 3 and 4, also called delta/slow-wave sleep) as well as REM sleep. Stages 3 and 4 are generally observed during the first half of the sleep period and considered to be restorative sleep. REM sleep occurs more during the second half of the night, though characteristically occurring every 90 minutes throughout the night. Sleep architecture changes with increasing age.

Distinguishing polysomnographic (PSG) features seen with increasing age include:

- reduction in total sleep time
- decreased sleep efficiency
- increased percentage of stage 1 and 2 sleep
- decreased percentage of stage 3 and 4 sleep
- reduced amplitude of the delta waves
- reduced sleep spindles in amplitude, frequency, and amount
- reduced REM density (number of eye movements per minute of sleep) and total REM sleep time
- increased sleep fragmentation due to increased microarousals.

Primary sleep disorders affecting sleep in the elderly

Insomnia

Clinical presentation

Insomnia is a subjective report of insufficient or nonrestorative sleep despite adequate opportunity to sleep. Insomnia may affect up to 50% of the elderly, and perhaps more of those in institutional settings. Lower income, lower education, and being a widow/widower increase the risk for insomnia. Typical symptoms of sleep impairment in the elderly are difficulty falling asleep and maintaining sleep, early morning awakening, unrefreshing night sleep, and excessive daytime sleepiness. "Sundowning" is discussed in the dementia section of this chapter.

Insomnia is divided into transient (lasting for no more than a few nights), acute (lasting up to four weeks), and chronic (four or more weeks). Precipitating factors for eliciting transient and acute insomnia are medical or psychiatric conditions, medication effects, and stressful life events such as loss of a lifetime partner or family member. Pathophysiologically, insomnia in the elderly is often similar to insomnia in younger individuals, characterized by hyperarousal or somatized tension and anxiety. Predisposing factors for insomnia are anxiety, depression, increased focus on sleep onset with worry and stress about sleep, as well as a decreased homeostatic sleep drive. Once the insomnia persists without improvement, perpetuating factors complicating the insomnia include counterproductive behaviors, poor sleep hygiene, and psychological conditioning. The impact of chronic insomnia in the elderly is dramatic, and includes impaired daytime functioning and reduced quality of life. Seniors with insomnia have a higher healthcare utilization and higher mortality, and frequently require psychiatric care.

Diagnosis

The diagnosis of insomnia is made on clinical grounds. It is useful to determine whether the insomnia is transient, acute, or chronic to guide the evaluation and treatment approach. Transient or acute insomnia usually occurs in people with no history of sleep disturbances, and it is often related to an identifiable cause. Chronic insomnia is often seen in those with underlying medical conditions including psychiatric disorders, pain, arthritis, reflux disease, or dyspnea. Poor sleep hygiene and maladaptive sleep habits serve as perpetuating factors. As bedtime approaches, individuals become more tense, anxious, and worried about health, work, and personal problems. Insomnia may cause physical and mental fatigue, anxiety, and irritability. Once the symptoms persist, persons might develop psychophysiological insomnia, experiencing a heightened arousal level at bedtime and a "racing mind."

The assessment of insomnia should focus on the sleep history, onset, duration, pattern, and severity of symptoms. The 24-hour sleep/wakefulness patterns can be assessed by using a sleep diary for 1–2 weeks, along with an interview of the bed partner. After careful review of potential causes of insomnia (Table 13.1), a comprehensive physical examination should be performed. Laboratory investigations are

Table 13.1. *Common causes of chronic insomnia in the elderly.*

(1) Primary sleep disorders
    (a) Circadian rhythm disorders: advanced and delayed sleep phase type
    (b) Sleep-disordered breathing: sleep apnea (obstructive, central, or mixed)
    (c) Nocturnal movements: restless legs syndrome, periodic limb movement disorder, REM sleep behavior disorder
(2) Poor sleep hygiene: daytime nap, too early bedtime, use of bed for other activities (e.g., reading, paying bills, watching television), heavy or late meals, lack of exercise, sedentary lifestyle
(3) Medical conditions
    (a) Pain: arthritis, musculoskeletal pain, neuropathy
    (b) Cardiovascular: heart failure, nocturnal dyspnea, angina
    (c) Pulmonary: chronic obstructive pulmonary disease, allergic rhinitis
    (d) Gastrointestinal: gastroesophageal reflux disease, peptic ulcer disease, constipation, diarrhea
    (e) Urinary: nocturia, urinary retention, bladder incontinence
    (f) Central nervous system: stroke, Parkinson's disease, dementia, seizures
    (g) Psychiatric: anxiety, depression, psychosis, delirium
    (h) Endocrine: menopause, thyroid dysfunction, diabetes mellitus
(4) Environmental: noise, light and other disturbances, extreme bedroom temperatures, uncomfortable bedding, lack of exposure to sunlight
(5) Medications: central nervous system stimulants, antidepressants, antiepileptic medications, decongestants, bronchodilators, diuretics, antihypertensives, anticholinergics

chosen based on the potential causes of the insomnia and might include in part thyroid, electrolyte, hepatic, and renal values.

Treatment

The treatment plan in an elderly person suffering from insomnia will focus on a discussion of the individual's expectations. One focus in the treatment is improvement of sleep hygiene measures. Based on the individual situation, recommendations to improve sleep hygiene may include:

(1) avoid and minimize use of caffeine, cigarettes, stimulants, and alcohol
(2) if appropriate, increase activity level in the afternoon or early evening by walking or exercising
(3) follow the circadian rhythm, increasing exposure to natural light and bright light during the day and avoiding bright light in the evening
(4) avoid daytime napping
(5) maintain a comfortable temperature in the bedroom
(6) minimize light and noise exposure at night
(7) eat a light snack if hungry but avoid heavy meals at bedtime
(8) limit liquids in the evening.

The healthcare provider should address a primary sleep disorder and initiate a work-up including polysomnography if individuals experience excessive daytime sleepiness or if the bed partner witnesses snoring, apnea, frequent awakening, or unusual movements at night.

In the senior population the improvement of general medical disorders affecting sleep onset and sleep maintenance (Table 13.1) can be very useful. Improvement of nocturia, nocturnal dyspnea, or pain may positively impact nocturnal awakenings and insomnia.

Over the long term, *nonpharmacologic measures* are frequently more successful in improving insomnia than pharmacological treatments. Behavior therapy aims to change maladaptive sleep habits, reduce autonomic arousal, and alter dysfunctional beliefs and attitudes that can perpetuate insomnia. Interventions include relaxation therapy, sleep restriction, stimulus control, and cognitive therapies. If the individual has a disturbed circadian pattern, exposure to bright-light therapy is an effective way to establish a healthy sleep/wake cycle. Benefits are seen after 60–120 minutes of artificial light treatment with an appropriate intensity of 6000–8000 lux (see circadian disorder section of this chapter for further details).

Pharmacologic intervention: non-prescription sleeping aids are widely used by individuals to improve sleep onset and sleep maintenance. Diphenhydramine and doxylamine, often in combination with products such as acetaminophen, are "sleep aids" available without a prescription. Although they might be effective in a small number of persons, these medications are known for next-day sedation, fall risk at night, cognitive impairment, as well as dry mouth, all side effects to be avoided in the elderly. Alcohol is widely used as a hypnotic, but it is a poor choice. Among other negative impacts on health, alcohol causes initial CNS depression followed by rebound excitation, which disrupts sleep. Melatonin supplementation is known to improve sleep, but adequate controlled trials are lacking, and the purity, hypnotic dose, and adverse effects have not been established. Valerian root may have a mild hypnotic effect on sleep.

The use of sleep-enhancing prescription medications is a well-established treatment in persons with insomnia. Pharmacological goals of the treatment include improved sleep initiation, sleep maintenance without hangover effects, and improved next-day functioning. When treating the elderly population, additional points should be considered. Medications with shorter half-lives are preferred to minimize daytime side effects such as sedation. One should use only the lowest effective dose, intermittently (2–4 times weekly) with a short-term prescription (not more than 3–4 weeks). The medication should be gradually weaned off to avoid rebound insomnia. Many medications used for insomnia are used off-label (Table 13.2).

Often, the treatment of insomnia in the elderly poses a challenge. One should consider an initial combined treatment of pharmacologic and behavior therapy, with the goal of weaning the pharmacological treatment while continuing long-term cognitive behavioral therapy.

Table 13.2. *Commonly used prescription medications to treat insomnia in the elderly.*

Type of medication	Example	Dosing in the elderly	Considerations for each category
Sedating antidepressants	Trazodone	50–150 mg taken before bedtime	Oversedation, alpha-adrenergic blockade, including orthostatic hypotension, priapism, atrial and ventricular arrhythmias
Tricyclic antidepressants	Amitriptyline Doxepin Mirtazapine	10–25 mg 10–25 mg 7.5–15 mg taken before bedtime	Daytime sedation, anticholinergic effects, alpha-adrenergic blockade, cardiac conduction prolongations
Benzodiazepine	Triazolam[a] Oxazepam[b] Estazolam[b] Lorazepam[b] Temazepam[b] Clonazepam[c] Diazepam[c] Flurazepam[c]	0.125 mg 10–15 mg 0.5–1 mg 0.25–1 mg 7.5–15 mg 0.25 mg 2.5–5 mg 7.5 mg taken before bedtime	Daytime sedation, ataxia with fall risk, psychomotor slowing, cognitive effects, anterograde amnesia, respiratory depression, tolerance and withdrawal, rebound insomnia, potential for abuse and dependence
Non-benzodiazepine GABA-A receptor agonist	Zaleplon Zolpidem Zolpidem ext. release Eszopiclone	5 mg 5 mg 6.25 mg 1–2 mg taken before bedtime	Daytime sedation, ataxia with fall risk, psychomotor slowing, anterograde amnesia, rebound insomnia
Melatonin receptor agonist	Ramelteon	8 mg taken before bedtime	Somnolence, dizziness, nausea, fatigue, headache.

Note:
Duration effect:
[a]short
[b]intermediate
[c]long

Sleep-disordered breathing

Clinical presentation

Sleep-disordered breathing (SDB) describes a group of disorders characterized by abnormalities of respiratory patterns or the quantity of ventilation during sleep. Obstructive sleep apnea (OSA) is characterized by the repetitive collapse or partial collapse of the pharyngeal airway during sleep and the need to arouse to resume ventilation. These episodes of obstruction are frequently associated with recurrent oxygen desaturation triggering arousals from sleep. The recurrent hypoxemia contributes to the observed sleep fragmentation, leading to daytime somnolence and diminished cognitive performance. Central sleep apnea describes abnormalities of the respiratory pattern associated with a temporary cessation of the respiratory effort, often associated with heart failure and CNS conditions.

SDB is common in older adults, with up to 20% of people aged 60 and older having an apnea/hypopnea index (AHI) of 15 or more per hour of sleep. Elderly men and women often lack the traditional symptoms and signs of SDB such as snoring, high BMI, and large neck circumference. OSA prevalence increases with age, independent of the observed rise in BMI with age. The AHI nearly doubles every 10 years. While snoring is a common symptom in the general population, with high sensitivity for the diagnosis of OSA, low prevalence of snoring in older adults makes it a less useful screening tool. The frequency of *symptomatic* sleep apnea declines in the older population. It is unclear whether this decline is due to underreporting of symptoms in elderly persons or because sleep apnea has fewer observable symptoms and consequences in older individuals.

Diagnosis

Symptoms of SDB in the elderly may include:
- excessive daytime sleepiness
- snoring
- choking or gasping for air during sleep
- witnessed apnea
- night sweats
- morning confusion
- cognitive impairment
- impotence
- frequent nocturnal awakening
- nocturia
- unrefreshing night sleep
- dry mouth
- headache on awakening
- worsening of underlying comorbidities.

Tools such as the Berlin Questionnaire can be used to screen for sleep apnea. The Berlin Questionnaire assesses risk factors for sleep apnea, namely snoring behavior, waketime sleepiness or fatigue, and the presence of obesity or hypertension; it is a useful instrument in identifying persons with sleep apnea.

The physical exam might show:

- drowsiness or sleepiness
- obesity
- increased neck circumference (> 43 cm [17 inches] for men, > 38 cm [15 inches] for women)
- crowding of the oropharynx
- low-lying soft palate
- large uvula
- prominent tonsils
- micrognathia
- retrognathia
- macroglossia

The gold standard for diagnosing SDB is polysomnography. Frequently used terms in the description of SDB are:

- *Apnea:* cessation of airflow for at least 10 seconds
- *Hypopnea:* decrease in airflow or effort of at least 30% associated with a drop in oxygen saturation of 4%
- *Obstructive event:* occurs in the presence of continued respiratory effort
- *Central event:* associated with absence of respiratory effort
- *Apnea/hypopnea index (AHI):* the number of apneas and hypopneas per hour of sleep.

An AHI of 5 events per hour is normal, 6–15 is considered mild OSA, 16–30 is considered moderate OSA, and an AHI of over 30 events per hour is considered severe.

Treatment

Treatment of OSA in the general adult population makes an impact not only on excessive daytime sleepiness, but also on the overall health of the individual. Among others, cognitive deficits, arterial and pulmonary hypertension, cardiac function, and arrhythmias improve with the elimination of the disrupted night sleep, intermittent hypoxemia, and increased sympathetic activity of obstructive sleep apnea. In contrast, it is not yet precisely known how elderly individuals per se benefit from SDB treatment. The decision to treat is guided by the clinical presentation and comorbidities. Even though only limited evidence exists to justify treatment of the highly prevalent asymptomatic OSA with AHI > 15 in the elderly, OSA treatment should, in theory, benefit this group of persons. Conservative treatment approaches include normalizing an increased BMI, avoidance of the supine sleeping position (by placing a foam wedge or tennis ball in the back of the sleepwear), elevation of the upper body at 30 degrees, avoidance of sedative medications, especially muscle-relaxing agents, and avoidance of alcohol too close to bedtime. There is no effective pharmacologic therapy for OSA.

Gold standard for the treatment of OSA is continuous positive airway pressure (CPAP) delivered by way of a nasal mask. CPAP delivers a continuous flow of air, splinting the airway open and preventing the recurrent collapse of the upper airway, which occurs during apneas and hypopneas. This treatment is effective in eliminating obstructive respiratory events, maintaining normal oxygen saturation, and decreasing sleep fragmentation. Compliance can be increased by using a heated humidifier with the CPAP device and choosing the optimal CPAP mask for the individual.

Improvement of underlying cardiac failure is a critical component in the treatment of central sleep apnea (CSA) and Cheyne–Stokes breathing. Bilevel positive airway pressure is used to assist in treatment of severe OSA, CSA, and Cheyne–Stokes breathing by providing two different pressures: a higher pressure during inhalation and a lower pressure during exhalation. Devices using technology that automatically titrates positive airway pressure, as needed, to maintain airway patency are increasingly used in the treatment of sleep apnea.

Surgical approaches such as septoplasty, tonsillectomy/adenoidectomy, uvulopalatopharyngoplasty and laser-assisted uvuloplasty for the treatment of OSA are available but should be used with caution in the elderly population. The increased surgical risk for an older adult with underlying comorbidities needs to be weighed against the benefits of the procedure and other treatment options. Tracheotomy is very rarely necessary.

Periodic limb movement disorder and restless legs syndrome
Clinical presentation
Periodic limb movements are a common finding in up to 60% of healthy elderly individuals. Periodic limb movement disorder (PLMD) is defined as periodic episodes of repetitive and highly stereotyped limb movements during sleep. Movements may be associated with arousals and contribute to sleep fragmentation and difficulty maintaining sleep or may be asymptomatic and found incidentally on polysomnography. The individual is not able to describe the limb movements, since the events occur during sleep, but the associated sleep fragmentation can cause impairment of daytime function, including excessive sleepiness. The bed partner or family members are the best sources for obtaining a description of the limb movements.

A related condition is restless legs syndrome (RLS), a neurological movement disorder characterized by an irresistible urge to move the legs as a reaction to uncomfortable sensations that often occur in the evening or when at rest. The pathophysiology of RLS is not yet fully understood, with observations suggesting involvement of the dopaminergic and opioidergic systems, leading to the symptoms of RLS. There is a genetic component in RLS, with increased risk of RLS among first-degree relatives. Iron deficiency might be seen in RLS. Clinical indications for diagnosing RLS may include:

- urge to move legs and/or arms, accompanied or caused by uncomfortable/ unpleasant sensations
- temporary relief with movement, partial or total relief from discomfort by walking or stretching
- onset or worsening of symptoms at rest or inactivity, such as when lying or sitting
- worsening or onset of symptoms in the evening or at night
- sleep disturbances
- frequently a positive family history for RLS
- positive response to dopaminergic therapy.

Diagnosis

PLMD is diagnosed by correlation of clinical symptoms and polysomnography findings. The significance of PLMD on polysomnography is uncertain in elderly asymptomatic persons. PLMD may be associated with peripheral neuropathies, rheumatologic conditions, iron-deficiency anemia, and chronic renal failure. Caffeine and antidepressants (tricyclic and SSRI) are known to worsen PLMD and RLS. Individuals with insomnia, nonrestorative night sleep, sleep fragmentation, daytime sleepiness, and documented microarousals related to limb movements should be considered for treatment.

While people with PLMD may not have any sleep complaints, RLS sufferers may describe symptoms of discomfort when initiating sleep or at rest. RLS is diagnosed clinically on the basis of the key diagnostic elements, including unpleasant sensations in the lower extremities which improve when moving legs and return when the movement stops. RLS can be seen in iron-deficiency anemia, renal disease, rheumatoid arthritis, peripheral neuropathy, and excessive caffeine intake.

Treatment

Treatment recommendations for RLS include reducing caffeine and tobacco use and improving the homeostatic drive by increasing daytime alerting activities. Medications used for PLMD and RLS include dopamine agonists, benzodiazepines, opiates, GABA agonists, and antiepileptic drugs (Table 13.3). Ferritin level should be over 45 µg/L for optimal treatment benefit.

Circadian rhythm sleep disorders
Clinical presentation

Circadian rhythms are seen in physiological functions such as endogenous hormone secretions, core body temperature, and the sleep/wake cycle. Central control of the circadian sleep/wake rhythm is localized in the suprachiasmatic nucleus of the hypothalamus. The circadian rhythm is synchronized by an external zeitgeber signal (external light/dark rhythm) and internal rhythms (such as internal core body temperature and endogenous melatonin cycle). A two-process model explains the sleep/wake cycle: on one hand is the homeostatic drive, which increases with the duration of waking and is entrained by the need for sleep, and on the other hand the circadian rhythm, influenced by the light/dark cycle, allows for the switch of sleep and waking into different phases on a daily basis.

The sleep/wake circadian rhythm becomes less synchronized with increased age, leading to a weaker response to external cues. Consequences of the altered sleep/wake cycle advance or delay the sleep rhythm.

A common presentation in elderly persons with the *advanced sleep phase type* (ASPT) of circadian rhythm disorder is an advancing of their sleep time. They sleep early in the evening or late afternoon before traditional bedtimes and wake up in the early morning hours. The advancing of the sleep time is paralleled by a drop of the core body temperature earlier in the evening and rising eight hours later (for example at 03:00 or 04:00), leading to complaints of waking up in the middle of the

Table 13.3. *Treatment recommendations in periodic limb movement disorder (PLMD) and restless legs syndrome (RLS).*

Type of medication	Example	Dosing in the elderly	Side effects
Supplement	Ferrous gluconate	Taken 2–3 times a day with vitamin C Recommended for ferritin <45 μg/L	Constipation
Dopaminergic agonists	Pramipexole	Start at 0.125 mg c. 1–2 hours prior to bedtime with snack and titrate to effect (target 0.5 mg)	Nausea, constipation, orthostatic dysregulation, dizziness, somnolence, hallucinations, impulse control disorders
	Ropinirole	Start at 0.25 mg c. 1 hour prior to bedtime with snack and titrate to effect (target 1–2 mg)	
Dopaminergic agents	Levodopa-carbidopa or levodopa-benserazide	100/25 mg: ½–1 tab 30 min before bedtime; 200/50 mg: ½–1 tab; immediate and slow-release formulations may be combined; total daily levodopa dose not higher than 200 mg	Nausea, sleepiness, augmentation, and rebound of daytime symptoms, insomnia, gastrointestinal disturbances
Benzodiazepine	Clonazepam	0.25 mg at bedtime initially; carefully increase daily dose by 0.25 mg each week; not to exceed 2.0 mg per day	CNS and respiratory depression, confusion, depression, amnesia, paradoxical reactions including excitability, irritability, aggressive behavior, agitation, nervousness, tolerance, daytime drowsiness and confusion, unsteadiness, falls, aggravation of sleep apnea; withdrawal symptoms

Anticonvulsants	Gabapentin	100–300 mg at bedtime with maximum of 3600 mg/d divided tid	Daytime sleepiness, nausea, cognitive slowing
Antihypertensive medications	Clonidine	0.1 mg twice a day	Dry mouth, drowsiness, constipation, sedation, weakness, depression, hypotension
Opiates	Propoxyphene	50–100 mg at bedtime to a maximum of 300 mg per day	Nausea, vomiting, restlessness, constipation
	Codeine	15 mg at bedtime to a maximum of 120 mg per day	Addiction, tolerance
	Hydrocodone	5–10 mg at bedtime to a maximum of 10 mg 3 times a day	Respiratory depression, hepatotoxicity dependency, abuse, lightheadedness dizziness, sedation, nausea/vomiting constipation, drowsiness, psychomotor impairment
	Methadone	5–10 mg at bedtime; use lowest effective dose	Respiratory depression, hypotension, cardiac arrest, QT prolongation, torsades de pointes, arrhythmias, ventricular tachycardia, ventricular fibrillation, cardiomyopathy, seizures, pulmonary edema, substance abuse

night and being unable to return to sleep. Individuals might try to stay awake in the evening, but still wake up early in the morning, reducing their total sleep time and causing sleep deprivation.

Another circadian rhythm disturbance is the *delayed sleep phase type* (DSPT) in which a person experiences a delay in sleep time. The individual will not be tired at the usual, socially accepted bedtime; he or she initiates sleep several hours later and wakes up much later in the morning. If the person gets up earlier in the morning, total sleep time will be reduced and there is a risk of an accumulation of significant sleep deprivation.

Irregular sleep patterns are frequently observed in institutionalized individuals, requiring supervision by caregivers (see the dementia section of this chapter for details).

Diagnosis

Circadian rhythm disorder should be considered when there is a misalignment between the person's sleep pattern and the desired or socially accepted sleep and wake times. The diagnosis of delayed or advanced sleep phase type is based on a clinical history and a sleep diary. A PSG is not required for the diagnosis; however, if a PSG is performed at the preferred, shifted sleep times, the sleep architecture is normal for age. Wrist actigraphy monitoring documents the shifted sleep phases.

Treatment

The treatment of circadian rhythm disorder starts with addressing and improving sleep hygiene. If the history, sleep log, and optional actigraphy data support the diagnosis, a customized treatment plan should be discussed with the individual. For DSPT, bright light in the morning and melatonin and dim light in the evening are recommended (Fig. 13.1). Bright light (2500–10 000 lux) can be used for 2 hours in

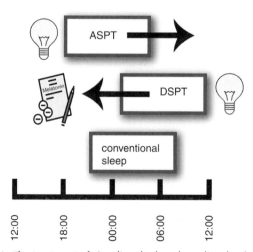

Fig. 13.1. The treatment of circadian rhythm sleep disorder: bright light in the evening for advanced sleep phase type (ASPT); melatonin in the evening and bright light in the morning for delayed sleep phase type (DSPT).

the morning upon awakening for 2 weeks along with restricted evening light to advance sleep onset and improve morning alertness. Compliance with bright-light therapy is often limited because of the need to awaken at an earlier time. Oral melatonin (0.3–5 mg at 22:00) or the melatonin receptor agonist ramelteon (8 mg at 22:00) will advance the sleep onset and help with resetting the circadian sleep delay to the desired sleep time in the evening.

The treatment of ASPT follows a similar mechanism, including bright-light exposure, timed light exposure in the evening, chronotherapy, and pharmacotherapy with hypnotics to maintain sleep during the early morning (Fig. 13.1). In chronotherapy for ASPT, sleep times are advanced by up to 3 hours every 2 days until the desired sleep schedule is achieved. Bright-light therapy for 2 hours in the evening, typically between 19:00 and 21:00, is often successful for changing sleep/wake times. Hypnotics are used with caution in the elderly.

Sleep in dementia

Clinical presentation

Sleep disturbances in persons with dementia include nocturnal sleep disruption, insomnia, and unpredictable nocturnal behavior with subsequent daytime sleepiness. Individuals with dementia may experience agitation, vocalizations, wandering, and combativeness at night. The agitation worsens frequently around sunset and lasts through the nocturnal hours, leading to the frequently used concept of *sundowning*. Nocturnal agitation, when present, usually requires expeditious pharmacologic, behavioral, and/or environmental intervention. Persons with dementia experience a sleep phase delay with higher levels of overall nocturnal activity. A vicious cycle may develop, with disrupted night sleep and daytime naps resulting in insomnia.

Dementia may lead to a decreased cell number in the suprachiasmatic nucleus and subsequent decreased melatonin responsiveness, with impairment of the circadian rhythm function and variations of the sleep/wake cycle. A decreased exposure to light during daytime, limited social interaction or stimulation, lack of physical activity, and disrupting caregiver schedule contribute to sleep disturbances in the demented individual. Institutionalized persons in particular are not exposed to sufficient light during the day, adding to the impaired function of the suprachiasmatic nucleus. Disruptive nighttime routines, such as bathing combined with bright-light exposure throughout the night in the nursing home or hospital, add to the interrupted sleep/wake cycle. Ophthalmological conditions such as macular degeneration or optic nerve degeneration add to the impaired effect of light and worsen the imbalance of the sleep/wake cycle in those suffering from dementia. The limited social interaction and reduced range of physical activity also lead to decreased wake-promoting stimulation and increased napping during the day.

Diagnosis

Evaluation for sleep disturbances in individuals with dementia includes a complete history and physical examination with a focus on drug interactions. Laboratory studies may include a complete blood count, chemistry, and thyroid function. The identification of treatable factors causing delirium and impaired sleep in an older person, even without the presence of dementia, includes uremia, diabetes, liver dysfunction, vitamin B_{12} and folate deficiencies, systemic infection, and anemia.

Defining the underlying cognitive decline is helpful in adapting the treatment for an individual. Polysomnographic features in persons with dementia include increased wakefulness after sleep onset, reduced nocturnal total sleep time, reduced sleep efficiency, and reduced REM sleep. Special attention should be given if REM sleep behavior disorder (RBD) is present, since this may be a precursor of synucleinopathy. RBD may herald the onset of neurodegenerative conditions such as Parkinson's disease or Lewy body dementia. In RBD, one experiences dream-enactment behavior and florid dream recall. Polysomnography can document complex movement, vocalization, and acting out during REM sleep, where normally no movements are seen. Surface electromyographic activity during sleep shows high levels of tonic and phasic muscle activity in REM sleep. Disrupted sleep patterns, nocturnal agitation, and daytime sleepiness usually require pharmacologic, behavioral, and environmental intervention.

Treatment

The first approach in treatment of sleep disturbances in dementia is the identification of comorbidities, causes for delirium such as infectious, metabolic, and toxic conditions, and polypharmacy. If a suspicion of specific sleep-related conditions such as OSA or RBD is raised, polysomnography should be considered.

Once comorbidities and underlying specific sleep disorders are addressed, pharmacologic and nonpharmacologic treatment options should be considered to improve the sleep of the demented elderly person.

(1) If the demented person with disrupted night sleep is not exposed to sufficient bright light in the morning and later afternoon, increasing this exposure improves nocturnal sleep and the sleep/wake cycle.

(2) Daytime physical activity and intellectual stimulation improve sleep onset and sleep maintenance, and reduce nighttime agitation.

(3) Caregivers of institutionalized persons can implement behavioral interventions such as daytime sleep restriction, physical activity, and phototherapy to improve nocturnal sleep patterns.

(4) Common medication choices in demented individuals with disrupted sleep include rapid-elimination and short-half-life benzodiazepine or GABA-A agonists (e.g., zolpidem, zaleplon, zopiclone). Although these medications may be of help, significant side effects in the fragile elderly and cognitively impaired population need to be considered. Ataxia, fall risk, confusion, amnesia, paradoxal reaction, and daytime drowsiness are frequently observed.

(5) Melatonin (3–10 mg) offers a potential treatment option for sleep-onset and sleep-maintenance insomnia, but has only limited clinical success.

(6) A melatonin-receptor agonist, ramelteon 8 mg, is significantly more potent than melatonin, has fewer general side effects than melatonin, and has less risk of

ataxia, amnesia, and other side effects, such as those seen in benzodiazepine or GABAergic drugs.

(7) Antipsychotic medications have often been used for sleep in individuals with agitated dementia. Newer, atypical antipsychotic medications, such as olanzapine (5–10 mg), quetiapine (25–100 mg), and risperidone (0.5–2.0 mg), may be considered for the management of the nocturnal agitation.

Conclusion

As sleep and its restorative function become more widely recognized for their impact on both medical conditions and quality of life in the elderly, the healthcare community has ever-increasing responsibility for translating the growing knowledge of sleep medicine into clinical practice in geriatric medicine. Addressing sleep-related concerns in elderly persons may provide the opportunity for improving not only their sleep, but also their overall morbidity and mortality.

FURTHER READING

Ancoli-Israel S. Sleep and aging: prevalence of disturbed sleep and treatment considerations in older adults. *J Clin Psychiatry* 2005; **66** (Suppl 9): 24–30.

Ancoli-Israel S, Ayalon L. Diagnosis and treatment of sleep disorders in older adults. *Am J Geriatr Psychiatry* 2006; **14**: 95–103.

Avidan AY. Sleep disorders in the older patient. *Prim Care* 2005; **32**: 563–86.

Bliwise DL. Sleep disorders in Alzheimer's disease and other dementias. *Clin Cornerstone* 2004; **6** (Suppl 1A): S16–28.

Bruce AS, Aloia MS. Sleep and cognition in older adults. *Sleep Med Clin* 2006; **1**: 207–20.

Conn DK, Madan R. Use of sleep-promoting medications in nursing home residents : risks versus benefits. *Drugs Aging* 2006; **23**: 271–87.

Grigg-Damberger MM. Sleep in aging and neurodegenerative diseases. *Suppl Clin Neurophysiol* 2004; **57**: 508–20.

Hungs M, Smith HR. Sleep disorders associated with medical disorders. In: Gilman S, ed. *MedLink Neurology*. San Diego, CA: MedLink Corporation. www.medlink.com. Accessed April 11, 2007.

Kamel NS, Gammack JK. Insomnia in the elderly: cause, approach, and treatment. *Am J Med* 2006; **119**: 463–9.

Naylor E, Zee PC. Circadian rhythm alterations with aging. *Sleep Med Clin* 2006; **1**: 187–96.

Schnelle JF, Alessi CA, Al-Samarrai NR, Fricker RD Jr, Ouslander JG. The nursing home at night: effects of an intervention on noise, light, and sleep. *J Am Geriatr Soc* 1999; **47**: 430–8.

Vitiello MV. Sleep in normal aging. *Sleep Med Clin* 2006; **1**: 171–6.

14 Forensic sleep medicine issues: violent parasomnias

Michel A. Cramer Bornemann, Mark W. Mahowald, and Carlos H. Schenck

Actus non facit reum nisi mens sit rea – the deed does not make a man guilty unless his mind is guilty

Edward Coke (1552–1634)

Introduction

Increasingly, parasomnias are invoked as an explanation for a wide variety of illegal and/or violent behaviors ostensibly arising from the sleep period, with the hope that if such behavior is deemed sleep-related, it may serve to exonerate the perpetrator. In such cases, sleep medicine practitioners are asked to render opinions regarding legal issues pertaining to violent or injurious behaviors purported to have arisen from sleep. Such acts, if having arisen from sleep without conscious awareness, would constitute an "automatism." Recent advances in the understanding of wake/sleep behaviors and consciousness have made it apparent that some complex behaviors, occasionally violent or injurious with forensic science implications, are exquisitely state-dependent, meaning that they arise exclusively, or predominantly, from the sleep period. They may therefore be without conscious awareness, and therefore possibly without culpability.

It is likely that violence arising from the sleep period is more frequent than previously assumed. One recent survey found that 2% of the adult population report violent behaviors arising from the sleep period.

Case example

AJT was a white male in early adulthood who was the son of a wealthy shoe manufacturer with a factory near Weymouth, Massachusetts. Despite being married with two young daughters, AJT was known to frequently engage in "debauchery" and had been known to squander his affluence in "revelries associated with his aberrant actions." Unbeknownst to his wife, AJT had long been involved in an affair with MAB, a young woman with a slight graceful figure and of "exquisite beauty." She had recently become estranged from her husband in Maine and had taken up residence in Boston. MAB had several wealthy suitors, and it had been reported that she did not object to

Sleep Medicine, ed. Harold R. Smith, Cynthia L. Comella, and Birgit Högl. Published by Cambridge University Press. © Cambridge University Press 2008.

providing female companionship or using sex to obtain material gifts and their perceptible status.

AJT's relationship with MAB apparently was quite volatile, but nonetheless MAB liked to quarrel with AJT because "they had such a good time making up." On at least one such occasion AJT lavished upon MAB an incredibly extravagant gown. The couple continued their tumultuous affair, and it was not uncommon for MAB's neighbor to be aware of their increasingly quarrelsome relationship. Late one night a neighbor heard a loud shriek coming from MAB's residence, followed by a displeasingly heavy thud. The neighbor then heard someone stumbling down the stairs to make their way out of the front door. The neighbor assumed that the individual leaving was AJT, as he had been seen visiting with MAB earlier that evening.

Moments thereafter MAB was found on the floor of her room with her jugular vein and trachea completely severed, her hair partially consumed by fire, and her face charred and blackened by flames. The walls in the room where the body was found were splattered with blood. A bloodstained razor and articles of men's clothing belonging to AJT were discovered near the foot of the bed. AJT quickly became the prime suspect, especially when an acquaintance of MAB relayed to authorities that at the time of MAB's death she was planning to elope with an old lover and move to western New York. MAB was noted to have said that "she was tired of the way she had been living, and was resolved that her future life should atone for her past follies."

AJT evaded arrest by fleeing north into Canada. From Montreal, he wrote to his family to inform them of his intent to abscond to Liverpool, England. Having been denied access to Europe, AJT was eventually located and apprehended by Louisiana authorities on an ocean vessel in the Gulf off of the coast of New Orleans. AJT was consequently returned to Massachusetts, where he was represented by a well-respected attorney. This case, which was brought to trial in 1846, has come to be known as the Albert Jackson Tirrell case. It is widely regarded as the first successful defense in the United States using sleepwalking that resulted in a full acquittal of the criminal charges related to a death. Further review of this case also underscores the many sociologic factors at play within the judicial process which ultimately render a decision. In contrast to today's cultural moral climate, it is interesting to note that Albert Tirrell was eventually found guilty of adultery and "lascivious cohabitation," for which he pleaded nolo contendere. Mr. Tirrell was sentenced to three years of hard labor at a state penitentiary. This case was used over 150 years later as precedent to acquit a Massachusetts college student accused of sexual assault in 2001.

State-dependent violence

Sleep is an active, rather than a passive, process, comprising two completely different states: non-rapid eye movement (NREM) sleep and rapid eye movement (REM) sleep. Therefore, our lives are spent in three entirely different states of being – wakefulness, REM sleep, and NREM sleep. Recent studies have indicated that bizarre behavioral syndromes can, and do, occur as a result of the incomplete declaration or rapid oscillation of these states. Although the automatic behaviors of some "mixed states" are relatively benign (e.g., shoplifting in narcolepsy), others may be associated with very violent or injurious behaviors.

Sleep-related disorders associated with violence

Violent sleep-related behaviors have been reviewed in the context of automatic behavior in general, with many well-documented cases resulting from a wide variety of disorders. Conditions associated with sleep-period-related violence fall into two major categories, as listed in Table 14.1: neurologic and psychiatric.

Neurologic conditions

Extrapolating from animal experimental data to the human condition, it has been shown that structural lesions at multiple levels of the nervous system may result in wakeful violence. The animal studies provide insights to violent sleep-related behaviors in disorders of arousal, REM sleep behavior disorder (RBD), and sleep-related seizures.

Disorders of arousal

The disorders of arousal comprise a spectrum ranging from confusional arousals (sleep drunkenness) to sleepwalking to sleep terrors. Although there is usually amnesia for the event, vivid dream-like mentation may occasionally be experienced and reported. The older prevailing concept that disorders of arousal, particularly if persisting into or beginning during adulthood, were indicative of underlying psychiatric disease has been firmly dispelled. Disorders of arousal, in any age group, are infrequently associated with psychopathology. Recent population surveys indicate that, in contrast to what was previously thought, the disorders of arousal are quite prevalent in the adult population, being reported by 3–4% of all adults, occurring weekly in 0.4%.

Table 14.1. *Conditions associated with automatic behavior arising from the sleep period.*

Primary sleep disorders (neurologic conditions)
Disorders of arousal (confusional arousals, sleepwalking, sleep terrors)
REM sleep behavior disorder
Nocturnal seizures
Compelling hypnagogic hallucinations
Somniloquy (sleeptalking)
Catathrenia
Psychiatric conditions
Dissociative states (may arise exclusively from sleep)
Posttraumatic stress disorder
Malingering
Munchausen's syndrome by proxy

Febrile illness, alcohol, prior sleep deprivation, and emotional stress may serve as primers to disorders of arousal in susceptible individuals. Sleep deprivation is well known to result in confusion, disorientation, and hallucinatory phenomena. Medications such as sedative-hypnotics, neuroleptics, minor tranquilizers, stimulants, and antihistamines, often in combination with each other or with alcohol, may also play a role. Many of the reported forensic cases of sleepwalking-related violence involved alcohol consumption in an individual prone to experience spontaneous disorders of arousal. It may be difficult to determine the relative role of sleepwalking versus frank intoxication in such cases. The role of alcohol and recreational drugs in legal cases is discussed below.

Pathophysiology of disorders of arousal

The pathophysiology of disorders of arousal is incompletely understood. However, studies of central pattern generators (in animals), state dissociation (in humans and animals), and sleep inertia (in humans) provide insight.

Central pattern generators/locomotor centers

The fact that violent or injurious behaviors may arise in the absence of conscious wakefulness raises the crucial question of how such complex behaviors can occur. The widely held concept that the brainstem and other more "primitive" neural structures primarily participate in elemental/vegetative rather than behavioral activities is inaccurate. There is clear evidence that highly complex emotional and motor behaviors may originate from these more "primitive" structures – without involvement of more rostral neural structures.

There are striking behavioral similarities between documented sleepwalking-related violence in humans and "sham rage" in animals and the "hypothalamic savage" syndrome in humans (the induction of rage and aggressive behavior by stimulation or lesions of the hypothalamic region). Although it has been assumed that the "sham rage" animal preparations are "awake", there is some suggestion that similar preparations are behaviorally awake, and yet (partially) physiologically asleep, with apparent "hallucinatory" behavior possibly representing REM sleep dreaming occurring during wakefulness, dissociated from other REM state markers. The neural bases of aggression and rage in the cat also support an anatomic basis for some forms of violent behavior. In humans, during arousals which can result in confusion or aggression there may be clear electroencephalographic evidence of rapid oscillations between wakefulness and sleep. It is likely that such behaviors occurring in states other than wakefulness are the expression of motor/affective activity generated by lower structures – unmonitored and unmodified by more rostral regions.

These animal studies provide insights to sleep-related violent behaviors in humans: structural lesions at multiple levels of the nervous system have been implicated in wakeful violence. A common thread linking two parasomnias, the REM sleep behavior disorder (RBD) discussed below and disorders of arousal, is the appearance of motor activity dissociated from waking consciousness. In RBD the motor behavior closely correlates with dream imagery, and in disorders of arousal it often occurs in the absence of (remembered) mentation. This dissociation of behavior from consciousness may be explained by the presence of locomotor centers, from the mesencephalon to the medulla, which are capable of generating complex behaviors without cortical input. These areas project to the central pattern generator of the spinal cord, which itself is able to produce complex stepping movements in the absence of supraspinal influence. This accounts for the fact that decorticate experimental and barnyard animals are capable of performing very complex, integrated motor acts.

Keeping in mind that not only is sleep a very active process, but that the generators or effectors of many components of both REM and NREM sleep reside in the brainstem and other "lower" centers, it is not surprising that, during sleep, prominent motoric and affective behaviors do occur. Central pattern generators are in close proximity to a number of the brainstem sleep generators. One explanation for the similar clinical behaviors observed in different parasomnias has been offered by Tassinari. His concept is that parasomnia behaviors are similar because parasomnia behaviors are generated by central pattern generators – released via different mechanisms in different parasomnias.

State dissociation

There is compelling evidence that there is extensive reorganization of the central nervous system activity as it moves across states of being. Factors involved in state generation are complex, and include a wide variety of neurotransmitters, neuromodulators, neurohormones, and a vast array of "sleep factors" which act upon the multiple neural networks. These facts lead to the conclusion that sleep is a fundamental property of numerous neuronal groups, rather than a phenomenon that requires the whole brain. Therefore, state determination is the result of a dynamic interaction among many variables, including circadian, neural network, neurotransmitter, and myriad sleep-promoting substances. Some identical neuronal groups are extremely active in more than one state, with differing state-dependent effects – i.e., many REM sleep phenomena are similar to the alerting response seen in wakefulness. Some brainstem regions effect motor suppression in REM sleep but motor facilitation in wakefulness.

The recurrent recruitment of state-determining parameters is amazingly consistent. However, there are multiple experimental examples of state component dissociation (simultaneous admixtures of clinical and neurophysiologic elements of the three states of being – wakefulness, NREM sleep, and REM sleep). These fall into three categories, as reviewed by Mahowald and Schenck (1999):

Lesion/stimulation – Hypothalamic, thalamic, and brainstem manipulation/stimulation induces state dissociation. Recent studies in molecular biology may add a fascinating new dimension to such dissociation. For example, 6-hydroxydopamine (6-OHDA) lesions of the locus ceruleus inhibit the expected immediate early gene (*c-Fos*) expression (normally expected during wakefulness) in the cortex and hippocampus without changing the EEG. Therefore, following such lesions, the cortex may be at least partially functionally asleep, without a sleep EEG pattern.

Pharmacologic – Manipulation of the cholinergic/glutamate neurotransmitter systems results in a variety of state dissociations.

Sleep deprivation – REM sleep deprivation in cats results in the appearance of PGO (ponto-geniculo-occipital) spikes during NREM sleep.

In addition to these experimental dissociations, there is evidence in animals for the natural occurrence of clinically wakeful behavior during physiologic sleep. Two examples which dispel the concept of "all or none" state declaration are (1) the concurrence of swimming or flight during sleep in birds and (2) the phenomenon of unihemispheric sleep in some aquatic mammals (bottle-nosed dolphin, common porpoise, and northern fur seal) guaranteeing continued respiration while "sleeping." Another naturally occurring dissociated state is seen during the arousal from torpor in hibernating ground squirrels, when there is what Krilowicz and colleagues have described as an "uncoupling between thalamic, EMG, and cortical REM correlates."

Both experimentally induced and naturally occurring state dissociations in animals serve to predict spontaneously occurring "experiments in nature" and drug-induced state dissociation in humans, which undoubtedly exist on a broad spectrum of expression. Such state dissociations are the consequence of timing or switching errors in the normal process of the dynamic reorganization of the CNS as it moves from one state (or mode) to another. Elements of one state persist, or are recruited, erroneously into another state, often with fascinating and dramatic consequences. The concept of state dissociation in humans helps to explain such phenomena as waking hallucinations, narcolepsy, RBD, lucid dreaming, out-of-body experiences, alien abductions, near-death experiences, repressed/recovered memories of childhood sexual abuse, and disorders of arousal.

Sleep inertia

Sleep inertia (also termed "sleep drunkenness") likely also plays a role in sleep-related complex behaviors. Sleep inertia refers to a period of impaired performance and reduced vigilance following awakening from the regular sleep episode or from a nap. This impairment may be severe, last from minutes to hours, and be accompanied by polygraphically recorded microsleep episodes. Recent studies have clearly proven that sleep inertia is a potent phenomenon, resulting in impaired performance and vigilance, averaging 1 hour, and requiring up to 2–4 hours to dissipate, in normal, non-sleep-deprived individuals, and is worse following sleep deprivation, one of the known priming factors in sleepwalking. Impaired performance during the transition from sleep to wake has important implications for rapid decision making upon forced awakenings (such as a middle-of-the-night telephone call) and for performance following scheduled naps in the workplace. There appears to be great inter-individual variability in the extent and duration of sleep inertia – both following spontaneous awakening after the major sleep period and following naps. Sleep inertia may be thought of as the "confusional arousal" potential in all of us, and it may be that disorders of arousal represent an extreme form of sleep inertia.

Other, very important factors beyond the scope of this chapter include (1) the known effect of genetics on violence, and (2) the well-demonstrated effects of environmental and social factors upon the structure and function of the nervous system. The plasticity of the nervous system in response to environmental influences is greater than previously thought. Psychobiological and sociocultural factors are undoubtedly operant in both wakeful and sleep-related violence.

Treatment of the disorders of arousal include both pharmacologic (benzodiazepine and tricyclic antidepressant) and behavioral (hypnosis) approaches.

Importantly, there are associations between obstructive sleep apnea and confusional arousals. Patients suffering from obstructive sleep apnea may experience frequent arousals, which may serve to precipitate arousal-induced precipitous motor activity. Therefore, the observed clinical behavior – a confusional arousal – may actually be due to another underlying primary sleep disorder: obstructive sleep apnea. This is another example of why overnight PSG studies with extensive physiologic monitoring are mandatory in the clinical evaluation of problematic motor parasomnias.

Disorders of arousal and human violence

The behaviors associated with disorders of arousal are not necessarily benign: they may be violent, and result in considerable injury to the individual or to others, or in damage to the environment. The proposition that sleep disorders may be a legitimate defense in cases of violence arising from the sleep period has understandably been met with great skepticism. Such behaviors are not new. Criminal acts without conscious awareness occurring during sleep drunkenness (formerly termed "somnolentia") were described over a century ago. Sleepwalking resulting in injury to self or others has been termed Elpenor's syndrome, after an incident in Homer's *Odyssey* (Book 10). A youth named Elpenor became intoxicated and fell asleep on the roof of a house. He was suddenly awakened by noise of others preparing to leave the island of Aeoli, and ran off the rooftop rather than taking the staircase, sustaining a fatal cervical fracture.

Specific sleep-related incidents have included:

(1) somnambulistic homicide, attempted homicide, filicide
(2) murders and other crimes with sleep drunkenness, including sleep apnea and narcolepsy
(3) suicide, or fear of committing suicide
(4) sleep terrors/sleepwalking with potential violence or injury
(5) inappropriate sexual behaviors during the sleep state.

Violent sleep-related behaviors have resulted in symptoms of posttraumatic stress in a spouse.

In addition to the one described at the beginning of this chapter, some very dramatic cases have been tried using the confusional arousal or sleepwalking defense. In the Parks case in Canada, the defendant drove 23 km, killed his mother-in-law, and attempted to kill his father-in-law. Somnambulism was the legal defense, and he was acquitted. In the Butler, PA, case, a confusional arousal attributed to underlying obstructive sleep apnea was offered as a criminal defense for a man who fatally shot his wife during his usual sleeping hours. He was found guilty. In the Falater case, a man stabbed his wife 44 times and drowned her in their swimming pool while a neighbor watched and their two children were sleeping in their house. His claim of sleepwalking was not endorsed by the jury, who convicted him.

Accidental death resulting from self-injury incurred during sleepwalking may be erroneously attributed to suicide – a situation termed "parasomnia pseudosuicide." Proper designation of cause of death is of the utmost importance, given the religious, cultural, moral, and insurance implications of suicide.

REM sleep behavior disorder

REM sleep behavior disorder (RBD) represents an experiment of nature, predicted in 1965 by animal experiments and subsequently identified in humans. One of the defining features of REM sleep is atonia – active paralysis of all somatic musculature (sparing the diaphragm, to permit respiration). In RBD, REM sleep atonia is absent, which permits the "acting out" of dreams, often with dramatic and violent or injurious behaviors. The oneiric (dream) behavior demonstrated by cats with bilateral perilocus ceruleus lesions and by humans with spontaneously occurring RBD clearly arises from and continues to occur *during* REM sleep. These oneiric behaviors displayed by people with RBD are often misdiagnosed as manifestations of a seizure or psychiatric disorder. RBD is seen most often in men over 50 years of age and is often associated with underlying neurologic disorders, most notably Parkinson's disease and dementia with Lewy body disease. The violent and injurious nature of RBD behaviors has been extensively reviewed by Schenck and Mahowald (2005). Treatment with clonazepam is highly effective.

Other sleep disorders such as disorders of arousal, underlying sleep apnea, and nocturnal seizures may perfectly simulate RBD.

Nocturnal seizures

The association between seizures and violence has long been debated. Infrequently, seizures may result in violent, murderous, or injurious behaviors. Of particular note is the frantic, elaborate, and complex nocturnal motor activity that may result from seizures originating in the orbital, mesial, or prefrontal region. "Episodic nocturnal wanderings," a condition clinically indistinguishable from other forms of sleep-related motor activity such as complex sleepwalking, but which is responsive to anti-epileptic medication, has also been described, and appears to be one form of nocturnal frontal lobe epilepsy. Aggression and violence may be seen preictally, ictally, and postictally. Postictal wanderings may result in confused or violent behaviors. Some postictal violence is induced or perpetuated by well-intended bystanders trying to "calm" a person following a seizure.

Other sleep disorders such as obstructive sleep apnea or RBD may masquerade as nocturnal seizures.

Compelling hypnagogic hallucinations

Conversely, recurrent sexually oriented hypnagogic hallucinations experienced by individuals with narcolepsy may be so vivid and convincing to the victim that they may serve as false accusations.

Sleeptalking

Sleeptalking has also been addressed by the legal system. It is interesting to speculate whether utterances made during sleep could be admissible in court.

Psychiatric conditions

Psychogenic dissociative states

Psychogenic dissociative disorders may arise exclusively or predominantly from the sleep period. Most, if not all, persons with nocturnal dissociative disorders were victims of repeated childhood physical and/or sexual abuse.

Posttraumatic stress disorder

Dissociative states and injury related to "nightmare" behaviors have been reported in association with posttraumatic stress disorder (PTSD). The "limbic psychotic trigger reaction" in which motiveless unplanned homicidal acts occur is speculated to represent partial limbic seizures that are "kindled" by highly individualized and specific trigger stimuli, reviving past repetitive stress.

Malingering

Malingering must also be considered in cases of apparent sleep-related violence. Our center has seen a young adult male who developed progressively violent behaviors apparently arising from sleep directed exclusively at his wife. This behavior included beating her and chasing her with a hammer. Following exhaustive neurologic, psychiatric, and polysomnographic evaluation, it was determined that this behavior represented malingering. It was suspected that he was attempting to have the sleep center "legitimize" his behaviors, should his wife be murdered during one of these episodes.

Munchausen syndrome by proxy

In this syndrome, a child is reported to have apparently medically serious symptoms, which in fact are induced by an adult, usually a caregiver, often a parent. The use of surreptitious video monitoring in sleep disorder centers during sleep (with the parent present) has documented the true etiology for some cases of reported sleep apnea and other unusual nocturnal spells.

Our center has evaluated one case in which it was suspected that a wife was attributing self-inflicted injuries to her husband's "violent sleepwalking." This subsequently led to his being jailed for domestic abuse, undergoing a divorce, and subsequently being sued by his ex-wife for "posttraumatic stress" symptoms.

The role of alcohol or drugs in sleep-related violent behavior

Some forensic sleepwalking cases involve large amounts of alcohol, medications, or recreational drugs, and these agents have been implicated in inducing sleepwalking. There is very little, if any, scientific evidence that these agents actually cause sleepwalking. Certainly in the setting of large amounts of alcohol or drugs, the behaviors are better attributed to the drug, rather than to sleepwalking.

Medicolegal evaluation

Automatisms and the law

The concept of automatic behavior (automatism) as it pertains to legal culpability varies by jurisdiction. The medical and legal concepts of automatism are very different. The medical concept is relatively straightforward (complex behavior in the absence of conscious awareness or volitional intent), while the judicial concept is quite different. Legally, in most common-law jurisdictions, there are two forms of automatism, "sane" and "insane." The "sane" automatism results from an external or extrinsic factor, the "insane" from an internal or endogenous cause. This choice results in two very different consequences for the accused: commitment to a mental hospital for an indefinite period of time if "insane," or acquittal without any mandated medical consultation or follow-up if "sane." For example, a criminal act resulting from altered behavior due to hypoglycemia induced by injection of too much insulin would be a "sane" automatism, whereas the same act, if due to hypoglycemia caused by an insulinoma, would be an "insane" automatism. By this unscientific paradigm, criminal behavior associated with epilepsy is, by definition, an "insane" automatism. The current common-law legal system unfortunately must consider a sleep-related violence case strictly in terms of choosing between "insane" or "non-insane" automatism, without any stipulated deterrent concerning a recurrence of sleepwalking with criminal charges that was induced by a recurrence of the high-risk behavior. If sleepwalking is deemed an "insane" automatism, then a significant percentage of the general population is legally insane. Clearly, dialogue between the medical and legal professions regarding this important area would be helpful to both professions, and to those arrested during automatisms.

One reasonable approach in dealing with the above-mentioned automatisms from a legal standpoint would be to add a category of acquittal which allowed for innocence based on lack of guilt consequent to set diagnoses – specific illnesses which could be categorized by a group of subspecialty clinicians in consultation with the legal profession.

Another suggestion has been a two-stage trial, which would first establish who committed the act, and then deal separately with the issue of culpability. The first part would be held before a jury, the second in front of a judge with medical advisors present.

One fortunate, and unexplained, fact is that nocturnal sleep-related violence is hardly ever a recurrent phenomenon. Rarely, recurrence is reported, and possibly should be termed a "non-insane automatism." Thorough evaluation and effective treatment are mandatory before the patient can be regarded as no longer a menace to society. In some cases, clear precipitating events can be identified, and must be avoided to be exonerated from legal culpability. These concepts have led us to propose two new forensic categories: (1) "parasomnia with continuing danger as a non-insane automatism" and (2) "(intermittent) state-dependent continuing danger."

The role of the sleep medicine specialist

Recent interest in the forensic aspects of parasomnias provides sleep medicine professionals with an opportunity to educate and assist the legal profession in cases of sleep-related violence. One infrequently used tactic to improve scientific testimony is to use a court-appointed "impartial expert." When approached to testify, volunteering to serve as a court-appointed expert, rather than one appointed by either the prosecution or defense, may encourage this practice. Other proposed measures include the development of a specific section in scientific journals dedicated to expert witness testimony extracted from public documents, with request for opinions and consensus statements from appropriate specialists, or the development of a library of circulating expert testimony which could be used to discredit irresponsible professional witnesses. Good science is not determined by the credentials of the expert witness, but rather, by scientific consensus.

To address the problem of junk science in the courtroom, many professional societies are calling for, and some have developed, guidelines for expert witness qualifications and testimony. The American Sleep Disorders Association and the American Academy of Neurology have adopted their own guidelines, which include:
(A) Expert witness qualifications
  (1) Must have a current, valid, unrestricted license.
  (2) Must be a Diplomat of the American Board of Sleep Medicine.
  (3) Must be familiar with the clinical practice of sleep medicine and should have been actively involved in clinical practice at the time of the event.
(B) Guidelines for expert testimony
  (1) Must be impartial: ultimate test for accuracy and impartiality is a willingness to prepare testimony that could be presented unchanged for use by either the plaintiff or the defendant.
  (2) Fees should relate to time and effort, not contingent upon the outcome of the claim. Fees should not exceed 20% of the practitioner's annual income.
  (3) Practitioner should be willing to submit such testimony for peer review.
  (4) To establish consistency, the expert witness should make records from his/her previous expert witness testimony available to the attorneys and expert witnesses of both parties.
  (5) The expert witness must not become a partisan or advocate in the legal proceeding.

Familiarizing oneself with these guidelines may be helpful in a given case, as the expert witness from each side should be held to the same standards.

Clinical and laboratory evaluation of violence in the context of sleep and wakefulness

A history of complex, violent, or potentially injurious motor behavior arising from the sleep period should suggest the possibility of one of the conditions mentioned in this chapter. Two questions accompany each case of reportedly sleep-related violence: (1) Is it possible for behavior this complex to have arisen in a mixed state of wakefulness and sleep without conscious awareness or responsibility for the act?

(2) Is that what happened at the time of the incident? The answer to the first is often "yes." The second can never be determined with surety, as "the thief has fled in the night."

To assist in the determination of the putative role of an underlying sleep disorder in a specific violent act, we have proposed guidelines:

(1) There should be reason (by history or formal sleep laboratory evaluation) to suspect a bona fide sleep disorder. Similar episodes, with benign or morbid outcome, should have occurred previously. (It must be remembered that disorders of arousal may *begin* in adulthood.)

(2) The duration of the action is usually brief (minutes).

(3) The behavior is usually abrupt, immediate, impulsive, and senseless – without apparent motivation. Although ostensibly purposeful, it is completely inappropriate to the total situation, out of (waking) character for the individual, and without evidence of premeditation.

(4) The victim is someone who merely happened to be present, and who may have been the stimulus for the arousal.

(5) Immediately following return of consciousness, there is perplexity or horror, without attempt to escape, conceal, or cover up the action. There is evidence of lack of awareness on the part of the individual during the event.

(6) There is usually some degree of amnesia for the event. However, this amnesia need not be complete.

(7) In the case of sleep terrors/sleepwalking or sleep drunkenness, the act may:
  (a) occur upon awakening (rarely immediately upon falling asleep), usually at least one hour after sleep onset
  (b) occur upon attempts to awaken the subject
  (c) have been potentiated by sedative/hypnotic administration or prior sleep deprivation.

Guidelines have also been proposed for dealing with those cases in which alcohol purportedly played a role.

A recent review has clearly established that polysomnography performed after the fact is of absolutely no value in determining whether the accused was sleepwalking at the time of the criminal behavior. Even frank sleepwalking during a formal sleep study would only indicate that the individual was a sleepwalker – not that sleepwalking was involved at the time of the crime.

Summary and future directions

It is abundantly clear that violence may occur during any one of the three states of being. That which occurs during REM or NREM sleep may have occurred without conscious awareness, and is due to one of a number of completely different disorders. Violent behaviors during sleep may result in events which have forensic science implications. The apparent suicide (e.g., leap to death from a second-storey window), assault or murder (e.g., molestation, strangulation, stabbing, shooting) may be the unintentional, non-culpable but catastrophic result of disorders of arousal, sleep-related seizures, RBD, or psychogenic dissociative states.

More research, both basic science and clinical, is urgently needed to further identify and elaborate upon the components of both waking and sleep-related violence, with particular emphasis upon neurobiologic, neuroplastic, genetic, and socioenvironmental factors. The study of violence and aggression will be greatly enhanced by close cooperation among sleep medicine clinicians, basic science sleep researchers, and social scientists.

FURTHER READING

Achermann P, Werth E, Dijk DJ, Borbely AA. Time course of sleep inertia after nighttime and daytime sleep episodes. *Arch Ital Biol* 1995; **134**: 109–19.

Beran RG. Automatisms: the current legal position related to clinical practice and medicolegal interpretation. *Clin Exp Neurol* 1992; **29**: 81–91.

Berntson GG, Micco DJ. Organization of brainstem behavioral systems. *Brain Res Bull* 1976; **1**: 471–83.

Bisson JI. Automatism and post-traumatic stress disorder. *Br J Psychiatry* 1993; **163**: 830–2.

Blake PY, Pincus JH, Buckner C. Neurologic abnormalities in murderers. *Neurology* 1995; **45**: 1641–7.

Bonkalo A. Impulsive acts and confusional states during incomplete arousal from sleep: criminological and forensic implications. *Psychiatr Q* 1974; **48**: 400–9.

Borum R, Appelbaum KL. Epilepsy, aggression, and criminal responsibility. *Psychiatr Serv* 1996; **47**: 762–3.

Bowker RM, Morrison AR. The startle reflex and PGO spikes. *Brain Res* 1976; **102**: 185–90.

Broughton RJ, Shimizu T. Sleep-related violence: a medical and forensic challenge. *Sleep* 1995; **18**: 727–30.

Charney DS, Kales A, Soldatos CR, Nelson JC. Somnambulistic-like episodes secondary to combined lithium-neuroleptic treatment. *Br J Psychiatry* 1979; **135**: 418–24.

Chase MH. The motor functions of the reticular formation are multifaceted and state-determined. In: Hobson JA, Brazier MAB, eds. *The Reticular Formation Revisited*. New York, NY: Raven Press, 1980: 449–72.

Cirelli C, Pompeiano M, Tononi G. Neuronal gene expression in the waking state: a role for the locus coeruleus. *Science* 1996; **274**: 1211–15.

Cohen DA. *Pillars of Salt, Monuments of Grace: New England Crime Literature and the Origins of American Popular Culture, 1674–1860*. Amherst, MA: University of Massachusetts Press, 2006.

D'Cruz OF, Vaughn BV. Nocturnal seizures mimic REM behavior disorder. *Am J Electroneurodiagnostic Technol* 1997; **37**: 258–64.

Dinges DF. Are you awake? Cognitive performance and reverie during the hypnopompic state. In: Bootzin RR, Kihlstrom JF, Schacter DL, eds. *Sleep and Cognition*. Washington, DC: American Psychological Association, 1990: 159–75.

Elliott FA. Neuroanatomy and neurology of aggression. *Psychiatr Ann* 1987; **17**: 385–8.

Elliott FA. Violence: the neurologic contribution. An overview. *Arch Neurol* 1992; **49**: 595–603.

Fenwick P. Automatism, medicine, and the law. *Psychol Med Monogr Suppl* 1990; **17**: 1–27.

Fenwick P. Sleep and sexual offending. *Med Sci Law* 1996; **36**: 122–34.

Fenwick P. Epilepsy, automatism, and the English law. *Med Law* 1997; **16**: 349–58.

Ferrara M, Curcio G, Fratello F, *et al.* The electroencephalographic substratum of the awakening. *Behav Brain Res* 2006; **167**: 237–44.

Fisher C, Kahn E, Edwards A, Davis DM, Fine J. A psychophysiological study of nightmares and night terrors. III. Mental content and recall of stage 4 night terrors. *J Nerv Ment Dis* 1974; **158**: 174–88.

Fleming J. Dissociative episodes presenting as somnambulism. *Sleep Res* 1987; **16**: 263.

Glenn LL. Brainstem and spinal control of lower limb motoneurons with special reference to phasic events and startle reflexes. In: McGinty DJ, Drucker-Colin R, Morrison A, Parmeggiani PL, eds. *Brain Mechanisms of Sleep*. New York, NY: Raven Press, 1985: 81–95.

Golden CJ, Jackson ML, Peterson-Rohne A, Gontkovsky ST. Neuropsychological correlates of violence and aggression: a review of the clinical literature. *Aggress Violent Behav* 1996; **1**: 3–25.

Greene AF, Lynch TF, Decker B, Coles CJ. A psychobiological theoretical characterization of interpersonal violence offenders. *Aggress Violent Behav* 1997; **2**: 273–84.

Guilleminault C, Silvestri R. Disorders of arousal and epilepsy during sleep. In: Sterman MB, Shouse MN, Passouant PP, eds. *Sleep and Epilepsy*. New York, NY: Academic Press, 1982: 513–31.

Guilleminault C, Moscovitch A, Leger D. Forensic sleep medicine: nocturnal wandering and violence. *Sleep* 1995; **18**: 740–8.

Hammond WA. *Sleep and Its Derangements*, Philadelphia, PA: Lippincott, 1869.

Hartmann E, Greenwald D, Brune P. Night-terrors-sleep walking: personality characteristics. *Sleep Res* 1982; **11**: 121.

Hays P. False but sincere accusations of sexual assault made by narcoleptic patients. *Med Leg J* 1992; **60**: 265–71.

Hendricks JC, Morrison AR, Mann GL. Different behaviors during paradoxical sleep without atonia depend upon lesion site. *Brain Res* 1982; **239**: 81–105.

Hindler CG. Epilepsy and violence. *Br J Psychiatry* 1989; **155**: 246–9.

Hobson JA. Sleep is of the brain, by the brain, and for the brain. *Nature* 2005; **437**: 1254–6.

Jewett ME, Wyatt JK, Ritz-de Cecco A, *et al.* Time course of sleep inertia dissipation in human performance and alertness. *J Sleep Res* 1999; **8**: 1–8.

Krilowicz BL, Glotzbach SF, Heller HC. Neuronal activity during sleep and completed bouts of hibernation. *Am J Physiol* 1988; **255**: R1008–19.

Mahowald MW, Schenck CH. Dissociated states of wakefulness and sleep. *Neurology* 1992; **42**: 44–52.

Mahowald MW, Schenck CH. Complex motor behavior arising during the sleep period: forensic science implications. *Sleep* 1995; **18**: 724–7.

Mahowald MW, Schenck CH. Dissociated states of wakefulness and sleep. In: Lydic R, Baghdoyan HA, eds. *Handbook of Behavioral State Control: Cellular and Molecular Mechanisms*. Boca Raton, FL: CRC Press, 1999: 143–58.

Mahowald MW, Schenck CH. Parasomnias: sleepwalking and the law. *Sleep Med Rev* 2000; **4**: 321–39.

Mahowald MW, Schenck CH. Evolving concepts of human state dissociation. *Arch Ital Biol* 2001; **139**: 269–300.

Mahowald MW, Schenck CH. Insights from studying human sleep disorders. *Nature* 2005; **437**: 1279–85.

Mahowald MW, Schenck CH. Non-rapid eye movement sleep parasomnias. *Neurol Clin* 2005; **23**: 1077–106.

Mahowald MW, Schenck CH. Violent parasomnias: forensic medicine issues. In: Kryger MH, Roth T, Dement WC, eds. *Principles and Practice of Sleep Medicine*, 4th edn. Philadelphia, PA: Elsevier/Saunders, 2005: 960–8.

Mahowald MW, Bundlie SR, Hurwitz TD, Schenck CH. Sleep violence–forensic science implications: polygraphic and video documentation. *J Forensic Sci* 1990; **35**: 413–32.

Mahowald MW, Schenck CH, Rosen GR, Hurwitz TD. The role of a sleep disorders center in evaluating sleep violence. *Arch Neurol* 1992; **49**: 604–7.

Mahowald MW, Woods SR, Schenck CH. Sleeping dreams, waking hallucinations, and the central nervous system. *Dreaming* 1998; **8**: 89–102.

Mahowald MW, Schenck CH, Goldner M, Bachelder V, Cramer-Bornemann M. Parasomnia pseudo-suicide. *J Forensic Sci* 2003; **48**: 1158–62.

McNally RJ, Clancy SA. Sleep paralysis in adults reporting repressed, recovered, or continuous memories of childhood sexual abuse. *J Anxiety Disord* 2005; **19**: 595–602.

McNally RJ, Clancy SA. Sleep paralysis, sexual abuse, and space alien abduction. *Transcult Psychiatry* 2005; **42**: 113–22.

Mogenson GJ. Limbic-motor integration. *Prog Psychobiol Physiol Psychol* 1986; **12**: 117–70.

Morrison A. Paradoxical sleep and alert wakefulness: variations on a theme. In: Chase MH, Weitzman ED, eds. *Sleep Disorders: Basic and Clinical Research*. New York, NY: SP Medical and Scientific, 1983: 95–122.

Nelson KR, Lee SA, Schmitt FA. Does the arousal system contribute to near death experience? *Neurology* 2006; **66**: 1003–9.

Ohayon MM, Caulet M, Priest RG. Violent behavior during sleep. *J Clin Psychiatry* 1997; **58**: 369–76.

Pontius AA. Homicide linked to moderate repetitive stresses kindling limbic seizures in 14 cases of limbic psychotic trigger reaction. *Aggress Violent Behav* 1997; **2**: 125–41.

Pressman MR. Factors that predispose, prime, and precipitate NREM parasomnias in adults: clinical and forensic implications. *Sleep Med Rev* 2007; **11**: 5–30.

Pressman MR, Mahowald MW, Schenck CH, Cramer Bornemann MA. Alcohol-induced sleepwalking or confusional arousal as a defense to criminal behavior: a review of scientific evidence, methods and forensic considerations. *J Sleep Res* 2007; **16**: 198–212.

Raschka LB. Sleep and violence. *Can J Psychiatry* 1984; **29**: 132–4.

Roth B, Nevsimalova S, Rechtschaffen A. Hypersomnia with "sleep drunkenness". *Arch Gen Psychiatry* 1972; **26**: 456–62.

Roth B, Nevsimalova S, Sagova V, Paroubkova D, Horakova A. Neurological, psychological and polygraphic findings in sleep drunkenness. *Arch Suisses Neurol Neurochir Psychiatr* 1981; **129**: 209–22.

Schenck CH, Mahowald MW. REM sleep behavior disorder: clinical, developmental, and neuroscience perspectives 16 years after its formal identification in *Sleep*. *Sleep* 2002; **25**: 120–30.

Schenck CH, Mahowald MW. Rapid eye movement sleep parasomnias. *Neurol Clin* 2005; **23**: 1107–26.

Schenck CH, Bundlie SR, Ettinger MG, Mahowald MW. Chronic behavioral disorders of human REM sleep: a new category of parasomnia. *Sleep* 1986; **9**: 293–308.

Schenck CH, Hurwitz TD, Bundlie SR, Mahowald MW. Sleep-related injury in 100 adult patients: a polysomnographic and clinical report. *Am J Psychiatry* 1989; **146**: 1166–73.

Schenck CS, Milner DM, Hurwitz TD, Bundlie SR, Mahowald MW. Dissociative disorders presenting as somnambulism: polysomnographic, video, and clinical documentation (8 cases). *Dissociation* 1989; **4**: 194–204.

Shik ML, Orlovsky GN. Neurophysiology of locomotor automatism. *Physiol Rev* 1976; **56**: 465–501.

Tassinari CA, Rubboli G, Gardella E, *et al.* Central pattern generators for a common semiology in fronto-limbic seizures and in parasomnias: a neuroethologic approach. *Neurol Sci* 2005; **26**: s225–32.

Thomas TN. Sleepwalking disorder and *mens rea*: a review and case report. *J Forensic Sci* 1997; **42**: 17–24.

Tinuper P, Provini F, Bisulli F, Lugaresi E. Hyperkinetic manifestations in nocturnal frontal lobe epilepsy: semiological features and physiopathological hypotheses. *Neurol Sci* 2005; **26**: s210–14.

Valzelli L. *Psychobiology of Aggression and Violence*. New York, NY: Raven Press, 1981.

Weiger WA, Bear DM. An approach to the neurology of aggression. *J Psychiatr Res* 1988; **22**: 85–98.

Wills N, Chase MH. Brain stem control of masseteric reflex activity during sleep and wakefulness: mesencephalon and pons. *Exp Neurol* 1979; **64**: 98–117.

Index